OXFORD MEDICAL PUBLICATIONS

Emergencies in
Supportive and
Palliative Care

**Published and forthcoming titles in
the Emergencies in . . . series:**

Emergencies in Anaesthesia, Third Edition
Edited by Keith Allman, Andrew McIndoe, and Iain H. Wilson

Emergencies in Clinical Medicine, Second Edition
Edited by Piers Page, Asif Shah, Greg Skinner, Alan Weir, and Natasha Eagles

Emergencies in Critical Care, Second Edition
Edited by Martin Beed, Richard Sherman, and Ravi Mahajan

Emergencies in Gastroenterology and Hepatology
Marcus Harbord and Daniel Marks

Emergencies in Obstetrics and Gynaecology, Second Edition
Edited by Stergios K. Doumouchtsis and S. Arulkumaran

Emergencies in Paediatrics and Neonatology, Second Edition
Edited by Stuart Crisp and Jo Rainbow

Emergencies in Supportive and Palliative Care, Second Edition
David Currow, Katherine Clark, and Paul Kleinig

Emergencies in Sports Medicine
Edited by Julian Redhead and Jonathan Gordon

Head, Neck, and Dental Emergencies, Second Edition
Edited by Mike Perry

Emergencies in Supportive and Palliative Care

SECOND EDITION

David Currow

Deputy Vice-Chancellor (Research and Sustainable Futures),
University of Wollongong, Wollongong, Australia; Matthew
Flinders Distinguished Professor, Flinders University, Adelaide,
Australia

Katherine Clark

Senior Staff Specialist, Royal North Shore Hospital, Sydney,
Australia; Area Director of Palliative Services, Northern Sydney
Local Health District; Conjoint Professor, University of Sydney;
Senior Clinical Advisor, Palliative Care, Ministry of Health, New
South Wales, Sydney, Australia

Paul Kleinig

Senior Staff Specialist, Southern Adelaide Palliative Services;
General Physician, Southern Adelaide Local Health Network;
Clinical Lecturer, Flinders University, Adelaide, Australia

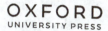

OXFORD
UNIVERSITY PRESS

OXFORD
UNIVERSITY PRESS

Great Clarendon Street, Oxford, OX2 6DP,
United Kingdom

Oxford University Press is a department of the University of Oxford.
It furthers the University's objective of excellence in research, scholarship,
and education by publishing worldwide. Oxford is a registered trade mark of
Oxford University Press in the UK and in certain other countries

Published in the United States of America by Oxford University Press
198 Madison Avenue, New York, NY 10016, United States of America

British Library Cataloguing in Publication Data
Data available

Library of Congress Control Number: 2023952604

ISBN 978–0–19–289833–3

DOI: 10.1093/med/9780192898333.001.0001

Printed in the UK by
Ashford Colour Press Ltd, Gosport, Hampshire

'... give us strength:
strength to hang on,
strength to let go.'

Michael Leunig
The Common Prayer Collection
Penguin 1990

'Quick! I'm not dead yet ...'

Anon

Preface

Supportive and palliative care is a rich and challenging area of clinical practice. Clinicians need to have a clear understanding of the life-limiting illness, the comorbid illnesses that impact so greatly on the population we serve, and the knowledge of both disease-modifying and symptomatic measures that ultimately optimize comfort and function.

Comprehensive assessment will help each person with a life-limiting illness increase the likelihood that they can achieve their priorities at a time of life that can be challenging for everyone involved. We hope that this book will provide a simple but thorough framework for quality, day-to-day clinical care dealing with unexpected changes in the clinical condition of people with life-limiting illnesses.

An emergency is subjective. Emergencies are so often dictated by their life-threatening nature and the potential for improved outcomes. In clinical practice, we tend to think of emergencies as life-and-death situations. As clinicians, until we know whether it is a life-and-death situation, any unexpected change is an emergency to the person with the life-limiting illness, their family, and health professionals until we have more information.

In patient-centred supportive and palliative care, emergencies also need to be defined by the potential distress that a particular clinical issue raises for that person and their family, together with the symptoms that herald this unexpected change. With the background of a life-limiting illness, many people quite reasonably interpret unexpected change as the harbinger of imminent death.

Therefore, the unexpected onset of new symptoms in someone with a life-limiting illness is a very challenging part of clinical practice:
• How aggressively should this person be investigated?
• What disease-modifying and symptomatic treatments are reasonable options?

Good supportive and palliative care relies on the full range of clinical skills in order to deliver outcomes appropriate to *this* person with *their* life-limiting illness. Through careful history, physical examination, and the judicious use of investigations, clinicians can negotiate treatment choices best tailored to this person's needs. For many people with a life-limiting illness, the best symptom control remains treatment of the underlying pathology causing the change in the person's clinical condition.

This book is for clinicians in emergency departments, acute care hospitals, inpatient palliative care units including hospices, residential aged care facilities, and when people are still in their own homes. It addresses the immediate clinical challenges while more definitive measures are being put in place.

Knowing the tempo of this person's life-limiting illness will allow health professionals to give appropriate advice. Guiding this decision-making process is an understanding of where this person is on their disease trajectory.

This book uses three categories which consider how this person's needs are changing as their disease progresses:

- In the *terminal stages* of their life-limiting illness with poor level of function.
- *Deteriorating*, and needing increasing support.
- *Stable* with a good level of function.

These three categories broadly reflect the natural history of the disease with no intervening complications. The first generally equates to an expected prognosis of days or hours, the second to weeks, and the third to at least months or years (or in the case of many people receiving supportive care, a prognosis otherwise not limited by the disease at this time).

An acute deterioration in someone who is otherwise stable may become a terminal event if it is not treated. Clinically, this unexpected deterioration needs to be distinguished from the terminal stage of an advanced illness where the life-limiting illness is now expected to lead rapidly to death. Such distinctions do not override individual choice where, despite a good level of function, fully informed people may choose a less aggressive option.

Assessment includes a comprehensive overview of:

- where this person is on the disease trajectory of their life-limiting illness (rate of weight loss, presence of fatigue or anorexia, and the rate of functional decline)
- the natural history of this life-limiting illness and the comorbid illnesses that this person has
- how this person sees their future emotionally and existentially.

Knowing how this person's disease is manifesting itself systemically provides insight into future expected decline. It is the *unexpected* changes in condition that this book addresses.

How to get the most out of this book

Section 1 is designed to help clinicians **make the diagnosis** of the cause of an unexpected change. It is presented as a series of symptoms which may present without warning, and where there may be potentially reversible causes that need to be excluded before the symptom should be labelled 'refractory' or 'intractable'. Looking for treatable problems that mimic the untreatable in people with life-limiting illnesses forms the basis of differential diagnosis in supportive and palliative care. The interventions considered need to be appropriate to the severity of the symptom, the stage of disease, and the likelihood of improving that symptom through the clinical path proposed. In palliative and supportive care, a symptom can only be considered refractory when:

- easily reversible causes have been excluded, or
- by agreement; a fully informed person with a life-limiting illness chooses not to define further any underlying pathology even if it is potentially reversible.

Section 2 focuses on **detailed evaluation and treatment options** tailored to the needs of people with life-limiting illnesses. It looks at the underlying reversible clinical pathology that can cause symptoms and the treatment options, ranging from attempting full reversal of the new pathology through to symptom support. This range of options will need to be discussed with people who have a life-limiting illness to inform their decision-making, particularly if they are relatively well.

Symptom control includes an adequate assessment for **all people** with a new symptom. Optimizing level of comfort and level of function is pivotal for **all people**, irrespective of their stage of disease.

For **some people** with a good or reasonable level of function and prognosis, discussions are needed to determine whether the more intensive investigations and interventions should be contemplated. This is not always a simple decision and will require input from a number of health professionals in advising the person and their family about the potential benefits and burdens of the proposed intervention.

This book provides guidance for all members of the multidisciplinary team—allied health practitioners, nurses, and doctors—in assessing this person in the context of a sudden or unexpected change in their clinical condition while facing a life-limiting illness.

David Currow,
Katherine Clark,
and Paul Kleinig

Acknowledgements

Thanks go to all the people who helped to bring together the first edition of this book. It is exciting to have the opportunity to revise and update this for the next generation of clinicians in supportive and palliative care.

Debbie Marriott is the consummate professional—focused, calm, and meticulous. Her work on the manuscript (and everything else that continues at the same time) is simply remarkable.

Kit provides the most wonderful support (even for the hare-brained ideas), while working tirelessly herself to make the world a better place.

How could one man always be so present? After so many years, Paul continues to keep the coffee flowing and computers working with an equanimity that continues to defy belief.

This book is the result.

Contents

Key to the book *xiii*
Emergency symbols *xv*
High-grade emergencies *xvii*
Abbreviations *xix*

Section 1 Frequently encountered symptoms

1 Frequently encountered symptoms | 3

Section 2 Specific clinical presentations

2 Clinical pharmacology | 59
3 Dermatological problems | 83
4 Cardiovascular problems | 99
5 Respiratory problems | 125
6 Gastrointestinal disorders | 147
7 Haematological disorders | 183
8 Renal and metabolic disorders | 207
9 Endocrine problems | 225
10 Neurology | 239
11 Mental health | 263
12 Orthopaedic disorders | 273
13 Genitourological disorders | 281

Appendices

1 Australia-modified Karnofsky Performance Scale (AKPS) | 301
2 The LANSS pain scale: Leeds Assessment
of Neuropathic Symptoms and Signs | 302
3 Glasgow Coma Score | 304

Index *305*

Contents

... to the book xiii
Emergency symbols xv
High-grade emergencies xvi
Abbreviations xix

Section 1 Frequently encountered symptoms
1 Frequently encountered symptoms

Section 2 Specific clinical presentations
2 Clinical pharmacology
3 Dermatological problems
4 Cardiovascular problems
5 Respiratory problems
6 Gastrointestinal disorders
7 Haematological disorders
8 Renal and metabolic disorders
9 Endocrine problems
10 Neurology
11 Mental health
12 Orthopaedic disorders
13 Genitourinary disorders

Appendices
1 Australia modified Karnofsky Performance Scale (AKP)
2 The LANSS pain scale: Leeds Assessment of Neuropathic Symptoms and Signs
3 Glasgow Coma Score

Index 303

Key to the book

Section 1 Frequently encountered symptoms

Symptoms

- Symptoms: e.g. shortness of breath and fever.
- Time frame for onset: acute, subacute, longer term.
- Possible causes: e.g. community-acquired pneumonia—go to relevant part of Section 2.

Reversibility

- Factors which are likely to have a reversible component and may require prompt intervention. The best symptom control remains, where possible, to treat the underlying cause of the symptom.
- Factors unlikely to have an easily reversible component will need symptomatic treatment.

Symptomatic treatment for this clinical presentation

- Non-pharmacological interventions.
- Pharmacological interventions.

Section 2 Specific clinical presentations

Having made the clinical diagnosis from the presenting symptom, obtain more detailed information from the chapters in this section.

Assessment

- Key history to help in the differential diagnosis and define potentially reversible causes.
- Key physical examination.

Investigations and treatment

Potential investigations, how they will help clinical decision-making, and treatment options including symptom control by prognosis/current global functional status *before* this acute change. Prognosis is estimated as the following:

- Hours or days *or* needing a great deal of support and spending most of their time in bed (symptom control is the focus here).
- Weeks to months *or* starting to need support, with limited energy, spending more time at home. This should be read in addition to the section where people's prognosis is estimated as hours to days.
- Months to years *or* still playing golf. This section adds to the sections 'Hours to days' and 'Weeks to months' for people with a better prognosis.

Books for additional information

Oxford Textbook of Medicine (6th edition)
J. Firth, C. Conlon, and T. Cox (Eds.)
Oxford University Press, 2020

Oxford Textbook of Palliative Medicine (6th edition)
N.I. Cherny, M.T. Fallon, S. Kaasa, R.K. Portenoy, M. Fallon, and D.C. Currow (Eds.)
Oxford University Press, 2021

Oxford Handbook of Palliative Care (3rd edition)
M. Watson, S. Ward, N. Vallath, J. Wells, and R. Campbell (Eds.)
Oxford University Press, 2019

Oxford Handbook of Oncology (4th edition)
J. Cassidy, D. Bissett, R.A.J. Spence OBE, M. Payne, and G. Morris-Stiff (Eds.)
Oxford University Press, 2015

Emergency symbols

☀: A true life-threatening emergency. Memorizing these conditions may help. Call immediately for help. Try to remain calm and quickly assess ABC. Once the problem has been dealt with remember to reassess—other problems may have been forgotten or missed in the heat of the moment.

☀: These people need to be assessed very quickly, because they can rapidly deteriorate. Consider senior help/advice as you assess the person.

① These conditions require careful assessment and correction but are unlikely to become life-threatening emergencies.

⑦ These sections cover management guidelines or advice on clinical dilemmas. The timing of clinical intervention is under the control of you, their caring clinician.

High-grade emergencies

Topic	Emergency	Page
Drug-related	Malignant hyperthermia	70
Dermatology	Severe cutaneous adverse reactions (SCARS)	84
	Hypersensitivity reactions	87
Cardiovascular	Acute cardiac decompensation	100
	Cardiac tamponade	104
	Thoracic aortic dissection	110
	Bleeding abdominal aortic aneurysm	112
	Cutaneous arterial bleed	114
	Acute limb ischaemia	116
	Venous thromboembolic disease	119
Respiratory	Pneumothorax	133
	Mediastinitis	136
	Large-airway obstruction	138
	Haemoptysis	140
Gastrointestinal	Upper gastrointestinal bleeding	158
	Lower gastrointestinal bleeding	161
	Perforated gut	156
	Acute hepatocellular failure	177
Haematology	Neutropenic sepsis	184
	Thrombocytopenia	191
	Disseminated intravascular coagulation	196

Topic	Emergency	Page
Renal and metabolic	Acute kidney injury	208
	Hyperkalaemia	212
	Hyponatraemia	219
Endocrine	Hypoglycaemia	226
	Hyperglycaemia	228
	Hypoadrenal crisis	232
	Thyroid storm	235
Neurology	Acute stroke	240
	Spinal cord compromise	242
	Delirium: acute confusional states	246
	Seizures	249
	Meningitis	252
	Intracranial bleed	256
	Raised intracranial pressure	259
Mental health	Suicide assessment	264
Orthopaedic	Fat embolism syndrome	278
Genitourological	Acute renal artery occlusion	290

Abbreviations

5-HT$_3$	5-hydroxytryptamine type 3	Hb	haemoglobin
ACE	angiotensin-converting enzyme	HUS	haemolytic uraemic syndrome
ACTH	adrenocorticotropic hormone	ICD	implantable cardioverter defibrillator
AGEP	acute generalized exanthematous pustulosis	IDC	indwelling (urinary) catheter
AMI	acute myocardial infarction	IM	intramuscular
AML	acute myeloid leukaemia	INR	international normalized ratio
APTT	activated partial thromboplastin time	ITP	immune thrombocytopenic purpura
BSL	blood sugar level	IV	intravenous
CAP	community-acquired pneumonia	JVP	jugular venous pressure
		LDH	lactate dehydrogenase
CNS	central nervous system	LFT	liver function test
COPD	chronic obstructive pulmonary disease	LMWH	low molecular weight heparin
COVID-19	coronavirus disease 2019	MAOI	monoamine oxidase inhibitor
COX	cyclooxygenase	MRI	magnetic resonance imaging
CrCl	creatinine clearance	MRSA	methicillin-resistant *Staphylococcus aureus*
CRP	C-reactive protein	NaCl	sodium chloride
CSF	cerebrospinal fluid	NG	nasogastric
CT	computed tomography	NSAID	non-steroidal anti-inflammatory drug
CTPA	computed tomography pulmonary angiogram	PCA	patient-controlled analgesia
CVA	cerebrovascular accident	PPI	proton pump inhibitor
CXR	chest X-ray	PT	prothrombin time
CYP	cytochrome P450	RDW	red cell distribution width
DIC	disseminated intravascular coagulation	SC	subcutaneous
		SCAR	severe cutaneous adverse reaction
DRESS	drug reaction with eosinophilia and systemic symptoms	SIADH	syndrome of inappropriate antidiuretic hormone secretion
DVT	deep vein thrombosis	SJS	Stevens–Johnson syndrome
ECG	electrocardiogram	SL	sublingual
ERCP	endoscopic retrograde cholangiopancreatography	SLE	systemic lupus erythematosus
		SNRI	serotonin and noradrenaline reuptake inhibitor
ESR	erythrocyte sedimentation rate	SSRI	selective serotonin reuptake inhibitor
EUC	electrolytes, urea, and creatinine	SVC	superior vena cava
FBC	full blood count	T$_3$	tri-iodothyronine
FFP	fresh frozen plasma	T$_4$	thyroxine
GFR	glomerular filtration rate	TB	tuberculosis
GI	gastrointestinal	TEN	toxic epidermal necrolysis
GIT	gastrointestinal tract		
HAP	hospital-acquired pneumonia		

TFT	thyroid function test	VAP	ventilator-associated pneumonia
TOF	tracheo-oesophageal fistula	VP	ventriculoperitoneal
TTP	thrombotic thrombocytopenic purpura	WCC	white cell count
		WHO	World Health Organization

Section 1

Frequently encountered symptoms

Frequently encountered symptoms

The 'WHY' framework 4
Global assessment of the person with palliative or supportive
    care needs 6
Chest pain 7
Abdominal pain 11
Pelvic pain 14
Low back pain 18
Neuropathic pain 20
Headache 21
Pain in the setting of previous substance misuse 24
Breathlessness 26
Acute confusional state (delirium) 29
Decreased level of consciousness 32
Agitation 35
Constipation 37
Diarrhoea 39
Nausea (and vomiting) 41
Unheralded vomiting 44
Fever 46
Care in the last hours of life 50
Catastrophic terminal events 53
Implantable defibrillators 54
Making a request for organ donation 55

The 'WHY' framework

Clinical decision-making in palliative care—fundamental questions that underlie good palliative practice for health professionals.

Does this person have a life-limiting illness?

Every health professional involved in the care of a person should satisfy themselves that this person has a progressive, life-limiting illness. Admission to a palliative care service without a life-limiting illness has occurred, at times with disastrous consequences. There have also been examples where, in the presence of a life-limiting illness, a new intercurrent problem has been wrongly attributed to the life-limiting illness.

The supportive care needs of people who are seriously unwell with a potential life-limiting illness are also considered in this book.

The question 'Why?' arises when someone's clinical course does not reflect the known course of the illness. Therefore, knowing the natural history of the illness is the foundation on which the answer to this question is built. Is today's new symptom:
- an expected manifestation of the disease?
- an unexpected manifestation of the disease?
- an exacerbation of an intercurrent problem?
- a new intercurrent problem?

When there is deterioration, the following question will need to be asked:

> **'Is this person unwell today because of overall progression in (maximally) treated disease or because of the effects of an acute problem with an easily reversible cause?'**

Another way to approach the assessment is to ask:

> **'Is this an expected or an unexpected deterioration?'**

For most people with cancer and end-stage organ failure, death is a result of shutdown of the whole body, not simply where the cancer is growing or which organ is failing. Uncontrolled cancer or end-stage organ failure are systemic diseases where many changes are 'expected', leading to a gradual and predictable global decline. Unexpected changes need to be carefully evaluated (including the possibility that the problem is iatrogenic).

Screening questions that need to be included if you are to have an overview of all that is going on for this person include:

> **Why has a change in condition occurred?**
> **What is the time frame for the change?** (Acute changes often have a potentially reversible cause.)
> **What else has changed in or around the same time period?**

Throughout the course of an illness, these questions need to be asked explicitly with every change that is encountered.

Can we do something about the problem?

'Yes' does not mean that we should start to treat. We need to consider:
- this presenting problem
- the underlying life-limiting illness and its current systemic manifestations (fatigue, weight loss, anorexia)

- whether the problem is likely to be reversible or not
- the person's wishes under these circumstances.

(Therefore, we also need to assess the person's testamentary capacity. If the person is unable to give guidance because of their illness, ask the next of kin/guardian/significant person/medical power of attorney what *this person* (not their next of kin) would want or not want to be done in these circumstances.)

Although this level of questioning may seem excessive, most people at the end of life want to be included in decision-making about their care and ensure that simple things to improve their level of function and comfort are discussed.

Where possible, the best treatment of any symptom is still to treat the cause of the problem.

What can we reasonably do to maintain or improve comfort or function for this person?

Global assessment of the person with palliative or supportive care needs

Five key considerations

The life-limiting illness

- Each life-limiting illness has its own natural history. Being aware of how it affects someone, where it manifests itself, and how it limits life are crucial. What is the median, 1-year, and 5-year survival with this person's known extent of disease?

Intercurrent illnesses

- What are the intercurrent illnesses that are actively contributing to the symptoms this person is experiencing?
- Can the treatment of any active intercurrent problems improve this person's prognosis, level of function, or level of comfort?
- What are the intercurrent illnesses that are inactive and not limiting prognosis, function, or comfort?

Response to disease- or prognosis-modifying therapies

- How has the person responded to therapy for their life-limiting illness in the past?
- How is the person responding to current therapies?
- Can the course of the illness be modified (with therapies that are acceptable and reasonable given the person's overall level of function and prognosis)?
- Will such interventions predictably improve prognosis, or help maintain or improve function or comfort?

Change in functional status over time

- Is global functioning stable or changing over months, weeks, days, or hours? (This is a key index for the future course of the life-limiting illness if nothing else can be modified.)
- How quickly are systemic indices including level of function, energy levels, appetite, and weight changing? (See Appendix 1.)

The person's perception of their future

- Always listen carefully to the goals, dreams, and fears of the person with a life-limiting illness—they have a great deal of insight. What does this person most need in order to live life fully at this time?

Further reading

Watson M et al. (eds) (2019). Ethical issues and the person in the patient (Chapter 1). In: *Oxford Handbook of Palliative Care*, 3rd ed. Oxford: Oxford University Press. Available at: https://doi.org/10.1093/med/9780198745655.003.0001

Chest pain

Onset of symptom

Acute onset (<24 h) of chest pain
- **Retrosternal and heavy**, associated with shortness of breath, radiation of pain to the jaw, neck, or either hand, and an impending sense of doom is typical of myocardial ischaemic pain (p.8). Identical pain may be experienced with oesophagitis or oesophageal spasm (p.9).
- **Sharp and central**, worsens with respiration, relieved by sitting forward, fevers, increasing breathlessness, and a pericardial rub are typical of pericarditis (p.106).
- **Radiating to the back, with a sudden onset and a retrosternal component**, very distressing and associated with nausea and breathlessness is typical of aortic dissection (p.110) and is usually associated with a history of long-standing hypertension.
- **Worse with respiration, sharp, and well localized** is typical of pleural pain. This may be associated with acute breathlessness, fever, and cough. Differential diagnoses include pulmonary embolism (p.119), pleurisy secondary to infection (p.126), pneumothorax (p.133), costochondritis, rib fracture, or local trauma.
- **Arising from the scapula and radiating anteriorly to the chest**, associated with fever, sweats, and tachycardia is suggestive of mediastinitis (p.136). These people may be very unwell. The association of recent oesophageal surgery or stenting raises this possibility.
- **Associated with abdominal pain** may indicate pancreatitis (p.174), oesophageal disorders (spasm, oesophagitis, ulceration, reflux, mucositis (p.150)), or biliary disorders (gallstones, malignant obstruction, sepsis (p.172)).
- **Associated with anxiety:** normal physical examination may indicate an emotional cause of chest pain. This is not uncommon, although physical causes must first be carefully excluded.

Subacute onset (1–3 days) of chest pain
- **Difficult to localize** but described as a deep aching discomfort in people with cancer may be due to malignant pericardial invasion.
- **More gradual onset of pleuritic pain** may represent malignant invasion of the pleura, rib fractures or infiltration, chest wall invasion, or zoster infection.
- **Dermatomal in distribution** may occur because of intercostal nerve damage (malignant infiltration, post-thoracotomy, or post-pleurodesis), or may be due to a radiculopathy (acute herpes zoster, malignant thoracic cord disease). (See Appendix 2.)

Insidious onset (days to weeks) of chest pain
Chronic chest pain may develop from local trauma (including instrumentation) or because of neuropathy. Promptly diagnose and treat in people with a good prognosis.

Can you modify anything contributing to the symptom?

The pain of an **acute coronary syndrome**, regardless of the person's estimated prognosis, may be modified by the administration of oxygen, sub-lingual (SL) or topical nitrates (if a person's blood pressure is sufficient), and morphine (intravenous (IV) or subcutaneous (SC) 2.5–5 mg as re-quired in people who are opioid naïve), with the aim of limiting ischaemia. If the prognosis of the individual prior to the onset of this problem is con-sidered greater than weeks, antiplatelet treatment (aspirin 100 mg daily) and antithrombin treatment (low-molecular-weight heparin (LMWH)) should be initiated. For people with a longer prognosis, promptly consider reperfusion therapy (thrombolysis, stenting).

The pain of **pericarditis**, regardless of prognosis, may be modified by non-steroidal anti-inflammatory drugs (NSAIDs) (p.106).

An **aortic dissection** may propagate and lead to aortic rupture if asso-ciated hypertension is not managed. The aim in all but the terminal stages of an illness is to prevent this complication. The initial antihypertensive agent must be a beta-blocker. Failure to treat initially with a beta-blocker may provoke catecholamine release and exacerbation of hypertension (p.110).

All people with a **pulmonary embolus** (p.119) require oxygen to maintain oxygen saturation >92%. This may improve chest pain and reduce breathlessness from hypoxaemia, increased pulmonary artery pressures, and increased pulmonary vascular resistance. In people with a longer prog-nosis, mortality is lessened by treatment and, unless there are contraindica-tions, anticoagulation should be initiated.

Acute onset of unilateral chest pain and absence of air entry associ-ated with shortness of breath may indicate a **pneumothorax** (p.133). **Consider whether the pneumothorax is under tension**.

Acute mediastinitis (p.136) occurs most commonly as the result of a ruptured trachea or oesophagus, or a serious infection (pleura, lung, sternum, or descending from the neck or oropharynx). If the rupture is not limited to the mediastinum or is between the visceral pleura and the medi-astinum, surgical advice should be sought if a person's prognosis otherwise warrants it.

Pericardial effusions (p.104) in people with a prognosis of greater than weeks are best palliated with pericardiocentesis. If this is a recurrent problem, consider a surgical pericardial window.

Chest infections causing pleuritic chest pain will usually respond to antibiotics. These may be offered regardless of prognosis (p.126).

The pain of **herpes zoster** may precede the rash. When the rash oc-curs, it is vesicular and later crusts. Promptly commencing antiviral medi-cations may not prevent post-herpetic neuralgia (oral famciclovir 250 mg three times daily in people who are not immunocompromised and 500 mg three times daily in those who are immunocompromised for 7 days, or aciclovir 800 mg five times daily for 7 days, both requiring dose reduction in people with impaired renal function) but duration or intensity of pain may be lessened. Concomitant administration of corticosteroids with anti-viral treatment may improve acute herpetic pain and healing of vesicles, without preventing post-herpetic neuralgia. (Corticosteroids must not be prescribed in the acute phase without antivirals.)

The onset of chest and back pain secondary to a threatened **cord compression** (p.242) is a vitally important diagnosis to consider. The first sign of a cord compression is often back pain, usually in the absence of a neurological deficit. Dexamethasone (16 mg in 24 h) may limit cord damage, regardless of prognosis. Early imaging in someone who is otherwise mobile is urgently required.

Malignant bone disease requires combinations of interventions, including opioid analgesia, paracetamol, anti-inflammatory agents (dexamethasone, NSAIDs, cyclooxygenase (COX)-II inhibitors), bisphosphonates, and, if symptoms are not settling or with a pathological fracture, radiotherapy.

Chest pain arising from **oesophageal spasm** may respond to calcium channel blockers or nitrates. Additionally, **oesophagitis** secondary to any cause should prompt prescription of proton pump inhibitors, metoclopramide 10 mg three or four times daily, and sucralfate 1 g four times daily. Opioid analgesia may still be required. A similar approach may be taken in pain occurring secondary to peptic ulcer disease.

Post-thoracotomy pain is difficult to predict and to modify. Failure to improve using a systematic approach with stepwise addition of analgesia prompts consideration of interventional pain relief such as an intercostal block. (See Appendix 2.)

What underlying factors cannot be improved?

People with a large or **saddle pulmonary embolus**, who present with shock, have a grave prognosis. The groups at risk include people with cancer, immobile people, and elderly people. This is the group who are least likely to tolerate aggressive interventions with thrombolysis, which carries its own risks of morbidity and mortality.

People with **descending necrotic mediastinitis** have a poor prognosis due to severe sepsis.

Symptomatic treatment

Non-pharmacological intervention

People with ischaemic chest pain may require a combined approach to management that includes rest and oxygen.

People with rib fractures or malignant bone disease may benefit from review by a physiotherapist to teach them how to support the affected region while still performing breathing exercises to avoid secondary chest infections.

People with bone metastases causing pain or cord compromise should promptly receive a radiotherapy consultation.

Pharmacological intervention

All people with chest pain require adequate analgesia for the severity of the pain they are experiencing. Individuals with strong pain require opioids. The most widely recommended initial opioid, except when a true history of allergy exists, remains morphine. True contraindications to morphine are rare and must be excluded on history. When initiating opioids, low doses administered 'around the clock', always with breakthrough or rescue analgesia available, should be used. An appropriate dose to start with is 2.5–5.0 mg of oral morphine given every 4 h with a smaller dose used for breakthrough analgesia as necessary. Modifications to this depend upon the individual's past exposure to opioids, their frailty, and their renal function.

People with ischaemic chest pain may benefit from a nitrate (SL, oral, or transdermal), a calcium channel blocker, and opioids. Starting doses depend upon current blood pressure.

People with pleuritic pain may be treated with an opioid in severe cases and an anti-inflammatory agent, either steroidal or non-steroidal.

People with chest pain secondary to malignant disease require the prescription of opioids and appropriate adjuvant analgesia. In malignant bone disease, this includes regular paracetamol (1 g three times daily). Other useful adjuvant agents include NSAIDs and bisphosphonates (IV pamidronate 60–90 mg or IV zoledronic acid 4 mg).

Neuropathic pain also requires the use of adjuvant agents. Recommended agents include tricyclic antidepressants (amitriptyline, doxepin) or anti-convulsants (carbamazepine, sodium valproate, clonazepam, gabapentin, pregabalin).

Further reading

Chang VT (2021). Management issues in visceral pain (Chapter 7.16). In: *Oxford Textbook of Palliative Medicine*, 6th ed. Oxford: Oxford University Press. Available at: https://doi.org/10.1093/med/9780198821328.003.0049

Abdominal pain

Onset of symptom

Acute onset (<24 h) of abdominal pain

- **Guarding**, worse with palpation or coughing, suggests inflammation. Fever, confusion, nausea, and vomiting suggest infection. Infections include peritonitis (primary, secondary), cholecystitis or cholangitis (p.172), pancreatitis (p.174), appendicitis, lower lobe pneumonia (p.126), or myocardial ischaemia (p.8). A rigid abdomen suggests a ruptured viscus.
- **Left lower quadrant pain** associated with loose bowel actions and a low-grade fever suggests diverticulitis. Bright rectal blood loss can be caused by mucositis (p.150), colitis (p.153), diverticulitis, colon cancer, polyp, or angiodysplasia. Torrential gut bleeding may cause shock. Generalized lower abdominal pain and loose bowel actions suggests colitis or enteritis (p.153).
- **Pain with few physical findings** is typical of gut ischaemia secondary to obstruction of the mesenteric vessels (p.156). Later changes include gastrointestinal (GI) bleeding, abdominal distension, and a rigid tender abdomen with guarding. These people may be shocked.
- **Cramping, associated with altered bowel habits** (constipation progressing to obstipation, nausea, and vomiting) may be due to gastrointestinal tract (GIT) obstruction (p.163). This pain may initially be intermittent but become more severe and constant with progressive obstruction. Obstructive pain may develop secondary to constipation, functional obstruction, adhesions, tumours, strangulated hernia, volvulus, or gallstone ileus. Distal large bowel obstruction is less frequently associated with vomiting.
- **Sudden-onset upper quadrant pain** may represent splenic or renal infarction, usually associated with fever, nausea, and vomiting. It is seen in people with haematological disorders (sickle cell anaemia, lymphoma, or leukaemia), embolic disorders (cardiac arrhythmias, septic emboli, antiphospholipid disorders), vascular disorders (aortic dissection, vasculitis), or splenic torsion.
- **Severe right upper quadrant pain** may represent a subcapsular hepatic bleed (sometimes relieved by sitting forward).

Subacute onset (1–3 days) of abdominal pain

- **In the upper abdomen and associated with back pain, nausea, vomiting, and fever**, may be due to acute pancreatitis (p.174). The presence of hypotension, tachycardia, and associated sepsis indicates severity. Any periumbilical or flank bruising reflect haemorrhagic pancreatitis.
- **Epigastric pain** may indicate peptic ulcer disease (*Helicobacter pylori*, NSAIDs, corticosteroids, delayed gastric emptying, smoking) or gastritis.
- **Localized right upper quadrant**, associated with jaundice and encephalopathy, may indicate acute liver failure, most often with history of hepatic cirrhosis or occur *de novo* (p.177).

Insidious onset (days to weeks) of abdominal pain

- **Acute worsening in the right upper quadrant** radiating around to the back or across the epigastrium in a person with a liver malignancy (either primary or metastatic) may represent capsule stretch or a bleed into a metastasis. This pain may be severe and worsen with respiration. The liver will be tender to palpation.
- **Epigastric pain radiating through to the back** and a past history of pancreatitis may indicate a pancreatic cyst, pancreatic necrosis, chronic pancreatitis, or pain from cancer of the pancreas.
- **Epigastric pain** in individuals with known dyspepsia may represent development of an ulcer, ulcer perforation, or an underlying malignancy.
- **Poor localization of pain that occurs 30–60 min after meals** may be due to mesenteric angina, due to vascular disease or compression of more than two branches of the mesenteric artery.

Can you modify anything contributing to the symptom?

Peritonitis may be primary (spontaneous bacterial peritonitis) or secondary (peritoneal dialysis, ruptured viscus including appendicitis). Spontaneous bacterial peritonitis is suggested in people with cirrhosis and decompensated liver disease. A diagnostic tap for white cell count (WCC) (polymorphs), lactate dehydrogenase (LDH), glucose, and protein should be performed.

Secondary peritonitis due to perforation or transmural ischaemia has a very high mortality rate untreated. Well people require surgical intervention and broad-spectrum antibiotics.

Epigastric pain radiating to the right upper quadrant and right shoulder tip is characteristic of **cholecystitis** (p.172) treated with hydration, analgesia, and antibiotics. In critically unwell people, percutaneous drainage of the gall bladder may provide analgesia and reduce mortality.

The most important complication of impacted gallstones is **acute pancreatitis**. Consider endoscopic retrograde cholangiopancreatography (ERCP) to relieve the obstruction. Complications include a pseudocyst, abscess, or chronic pancreatitis.

In right lower quadrant pain, consider **appendicitis**.

There are multiple causes of **colitis** (infectious, ischaemic, ulcerative, granulomatosis) (p.153). The most likely cause will be identified on history. The most common cause is *Clostridium difficile* toxin. If diarrhoea persists, cholestyramine 4 g may reduce symptoms.

Mucositis occurring secondary to radiotherapy or chemotherapy may improve with supportive hydration and, in cases that persist, regular octreotide.

Simple **diverticulitis** requires adequate hydration and antibiotics. A perforated diverticulum may lead to peritonitis or an abscess. A surgical review may be indicated.

In the case of **peptic ulcer disease**, symptoms may be improved by decreasing acid secretion (ranitidine 300 mg daily or omeprazole 20 mg daily), and reducing contact of acid with the ulcer to promote healing (sucralfate 1 g four times daily). Treat *H. pylori* if present.

Acute liver failure (p.177) requires discontinuation of hepatotoxic medications. Treat reversible causes (paracetamol overdose), maintain blood glucose with a 5% dextrose infusion, and restrict protein intake and protein absorption (lactulose 20 mL two to three times daily).

What underlying factors cannot be improved?

Catastrophic intra-abdominal events carry a very poor prognosis and are unlikely to be reversible in people with advanced life-limiting illnesses. These include gut necrosis secondary to **mesenteric infarction** or **ruptured aortic aneurysm**. Although the symptoms of a bowel obstruction can be palliated, a multilevel obstruction can rarely be reversed surgically and heralds a poor prognosis.

Further reading

Chang VT (2021). Management issues in visceral pain (Chapter 7.16). In: *Oxford Textbook of Palliative Medicine*, 6th ed. Oxford: Oxford University Press. Available at: https://doi.org/10.1093/med/9780198821328.003.0049

Pelvic pain

Onset of symptom

Pelvic disease can cause several different types of pain (visceral, neuro-pathic, musculoskeletal).

Acute onset (<24 h) of pelvic pain

- **Abrupt onset, severe, associated with guarding, worse with palpation and coughing** may represent an inflammatory cause of pain, such as peritonitis (primary, secondary) (p.156).
- **In women** the differential diagnosis of acute onset of pain which is difficult to localize, and which may be associated with nausea and vomiting includes a ruptured ovarian cyst or uterus, ovarian torsion, or pelvic inflammatory disease. This diagnosis is often missed and must be considered in women with pelvic pain and fevers. Consider fallopian tube disorders (torsion, salpingitis) or haemorrhage into an ovarian cyst.
- **In men or women, better localized pain** leads to consideration of appendicitis, with pain originating in the right lower quadrant; diverticulitis with pain localized to left lower quadrant; pain in the midline or either iliac fossa with incarcerated inguinal or abdominal hernias; or generalized discomfort from colitis (p.153). Colorectal cancer, polyp, or angiodysplasia (p.161) can present with bright rectal blood loss.
- **Abrupt onset and associated with flank pain** raises the possibility of pyelonephritis (p.282), renal infarct (p.290), or renal colic (p.286). The association with flank to loin pain suggests the passage of stones, blood clot, or tissue along the ureter. All may occur with fever, haematuria, and nausea and vomiting.
- **Distressing midline suprapubic pain associated with a palpable mass** may be due to acute urinary retention (p.288). A history of dysuria, difficulty voiding, frequency, haematuria, and fever should be sought. Similar pain occurring more laterally, also associated with a palpable mass, may be due to ovarian cysts, ovarian malignancy, or a pelvic abscess.
- **In men, acute onset of scrotal pain** may include torsion of the testis (in young men), trauma, and acute epididymitis. An uncommon but very severe problem in debilitated or immunocompromised people is necrotizing fasciitis. Acute onset of scrotal pain may be referred pain from the prostate, prostatic urethra, bladder neck, or seminal vesicles.
- **In men, acute onset of penile pain may also be due to local problems or referred pain** including phimosis (with urinary retention), ischaemic priapism complicating sickle cell anaemia (p.205), vasculitis, or polycythaemia. Exclude spinal cord compression. Referred pain may be due to ureteric colic, renal pathology, or spinal cord compromise (p.242).

Subacute onset (1–3 days) of pelvic pain

- **Dull, aching, poorly localized at rest, but more defined with movement, may represent bony invasion**. Prostate cancer metastasizes commonly to bones along with cancers of the breast, lung, kidney, thyroid, and GIT. Any cancer in the pelvis may cause pain through local pressure.

- **Dull, aching, and associated with a dragging sensation when standing may be due to visceral pelvic pain**. Infiltration of the uterus (cancer, adenomas, endometriosis, and stretching of the broad ligament) tends to lead to pain that is felt in the midline of the hypogastrium. Cervical pain (cancer, infections) is usually perceived in the lower back, sacrum, and hypogastrium. Ovarian pain tends to be the most poorly localized due to interconnection of ovarian nerves with other pelvic nerves. It is usually perceived towards the edge of the pelvis.

- Prostatic pain tends to be experienced in the perineum, scrotum, and penis. Prostate discomfort may result from malignant infiltration or prostatitis. Men with **prostatitis** present with perineal pain and may have urinary retention that has been preceded by dysuria and fevers. People with pelvic cancers often have a mixture of nociceptive, neuropathic, and somatic pains.

Acute-on-chronic onset (days to weeks) of pelvic pain

- **Chronic pelvic pain with acute exacerbations in women is a clinical challenge**. Aetiologies include gynaecological, urological, GIT, and musculoskeletal causes. An acute exacerbation of pelvic pain is most commonly due to endometriosis, pelvic inflammatory disease, adhesions, or irritable bowel syndrome.

- **Chronic pelvic pain in men with acute exacerbations may be due to chronic prostatitis**.

Men present with chronic perineal pain associated with low back pain and dysuria. This may be due to chronic infection, inflammation of the prostate, or chronic pelvic pain syndrome.

Can you modify anything contributing to the symptom?

Women with a **ruptured ovarian cyst** or **ovarian torsion** require pelvic ultrasound to confirm the diagnosis. Most pain from a ruptured cyst will settle with rest and analgesia.

Torsion of an ovary or other adnexal structure requires laparoscopy to ascertain if the structure can be saved or requires surgical resection.

Generalized abdominal pain that localizes to the right lower quadrant is typical of **appendicitis**. Escalating pain that suddenly lessens may reflect a ruptured appendix. This is predominantly a clinical diagnosis and requires antibiotics and an urgent surgical consultation.

Ischaemic colitis (p.153) occurs because of impaired blood supply to the gut wall. The best intervention is surgical resection of the affected area if the person is well enough. People with colitis secondary to **inflammatory bowel disease** require immunosuppressive therapy to be recommenced.

Mucositis (p.150) occurring secondary to radiotherapy or chemo-therapy may improve with hydration and gut rest.

Diverticulitis can cause pelvic pain that is often acute, but people will most often give a history of that pain over time.

People with **pyelonephritis** (p.282) will appear unwell with fever, rigor, and renal angle tenderness, often associated with dysuria and haematuria. If the person fails to settle, consider complications including papillary necrosis, renal calculi, or a fungal infection.

Acute disruption to the arterial blood supply to the kidney may result in a **renal infarct** associated with pain, fever, and haematuria. The most important steps are rapid diagnosis and initiation of anticoagulation (p.290).

Papillary necrosis and subsequent rupture and sloughing off of debris occurs secondary to a variety of disorders including urinary tract infections (especially fungal) and medications (NSAIDs, COX-II inhibitors, paracetamol). This is most likely to complicate urinary tract infections in people with diabetes and those with sickle cell anaemia. It is important to stop medications that may be contributing, and ensure adequate hydration and appropriate antibiotics.

Renal calculi may cause extremely severe pain. These people require hydration and adequate analgesia. Renal function must be checked and blood collected for blood and urine cultures. Appropriate antibiotics should be initiated (p.282).

Acute urinary retention requires urinary catheterization (p.288). Initially, a urethral catheter should be considered. Consult a urologist if catheterization is difficult. Heavily blood-stained urine should prompt bladder irrigation through a three-way catheter. Send a specimen of sterile urine for culture. Once catheterized, exclude a spinal cord or cauda equina lesion (p.242).

Acute scrotal pain in young men is a surgical emergency as it may herald torsion of the testis.

Epididymitis is almost certainly due to infection, and urine cultures must be collected and broad-spectrum antibiotics commenced immediately for 2 weeks (80 mg trimethoprim/400 mg sulfamethoxazole twice daily or ciprofloxacin 500 mg twice daily).

Necrotizing fasciitis is diagnosed by the appearance of the perineum which has early erythema followed by desquamation with underlying dark necrotic areas. These people require fluid resuscitation, antibiotics, and surgical debridement.

Phimosis may cause urinary retention. Consult a surgeon as the priority.

Ischaemic priapism is a medical emergency. If this is due to sickle cell anaemia, commence hydration, analgesia, and oxygen. Other causes require an urgent urology consultation.

Painful **bony metastases in the pelvis** may respond to combinations of analgesics (opioids, NSAIDs, paracetamol, bisphosphonates). Plain X-rays and bone can exclude a fracture. Consult radiotherapy.

Malignant visceral pain responds well to opioid analgesia. With pelvic metastases, there is often a neuropathic component that will require the addition of analgesia. For all people with cancer pain, consider modifying symptoms with radiotherapy, chemotherapy, or hormone therapy.

Prostate pain may be due to acute prostatitis, acute-on-chronic prostatitis, or prostate cancer. The pain of acute prostatitis should settle with antibiotics. More chronic pain should prompt a search for prostate cancer. Chronic prostatitis is more difficult to relieve.

What underlying factors cannot be improved?

Pre-existing long-term pelvic pain may not be modifiable in the face of a life-limiting illness.

Symptomatic treatment

Non-pharmacological intervention

In some cases, people with pelvic pain may have a long history of pain that worsens with their deteriorating condition. These people require comprehensive support that addresses their psychological, social, and emotional concerns.

Pharmacological intervention

Prescribe medications according to the severity and type of pain. This needs to be approached in a systematic manner with appropriate use of adjuvant analgesia. It is likely that people with advanced cancer will require opioid analgesia as part of their analgesic regimen.

Further reading

Chang VT (2021). Management issues in visceral pain (Chapter 7.16). In: *Oxford Textbook of Palliative Medicine*, 6th ed. Oxford: Oxford University Press. Available at: https://doi.org/10.1093/med/9780198821328.003.0049

Low back pain

Onset of symptom

Chronic low back pain is a major cause of long-term comorbidity in the community. It will often worsen at the end of life. The palliative dictum that pain can be relieved is often challenged in people who have had significant long-term back pain.

Acute onset (<24 h) of low back pain and ...

- **A history of osteoporosis or metastatic bone disease:** vertebral crush fractures can occur at any time without obvious trauma. In addition to the pain of the fracture, there may be significant neuropathic pain with entrapment of the nerve at the level of the fracture.
- **A history of glucocorticoid use:** consider accelerated osteoporosis with crush fracture.
- **Known metastatic malignancy in the central nervous system (CNS) that may directly affect the cord:** other sites of disease may become clinically apparent with cauda equina involvement (radicular pain involving the buttocks, decreased saddle sensation, and impaired sphincter control) or the lower cord (epidural, subdural, or intrathecal disease).
- **Fever (neutropenia, vascular access lines, or epidural or intrathecal lines):** consider epidural abscess or meningitis, and urgent initiation of systemic antibiotics and removal of the catheter line (depending upon the life expectancy).
- **Coagulopathy or thrombocytopenia:** exclude a local epidural bleed.
- **Sudden loss of mobility:** exclude a cord compression from direct tumour effects, vertebral collapse impinging on the cord, or local bleeding compromising the cord.
- **Atrial fibrillation and neurological deficits:** exclude anterior spinal artery occlusion.

Subacute onset (1–3 days) of low back pain

- **Bed-bound:** people may often experience increasing low back pain when they are bed-bound (without neurological deficit) at the end of life. Repositioning and alternating pressure mattresses may help.
- **Pressure areas:** extreme pain is often experienced as skin breaks down over the sacrum. Always inspect for compromised skin.
- **Metastatic bone disease (or a malignancy such as prostate, non-small cell lung, or breast cancer that has a propensity for bone metastases):** back pain is a common presentation of bone disease. (New back pain also precedes most episodes of cord compression, often by weeks.)

Insidious onset (days to weeks) of lower back pain

- **Cachexia:** people will often have worsening of long-term back pain as muscle bulk is lost (including paravertebral muscles). Although potentially pain free for many years, people with previous significant back pain may find that it worsens significantly as they decondition.

- **Spondyloarthropathy:** decreasing mobility at the end of life may worsen long-term back pain.

Can you modify anything contributing to the symptom?

Sepsis (epidural or intrathecal) requires urgent intervention (especially if iatrogenic) (p.243).

Cord compression requires urgent introduction of dexamethasone while the cause of the compression is defined (p.242). For most people with metastatic bone disease, radiotherapy (or chemotherapy in people with chemosensitive tumours) will be of benefit.

Careful management (including pressure-alternating mattresses) for anyone who is bed-bound, will help avoid pressure damage to skin. Programmes to maintain mobility (even in bed) are important so that people can shift their weight in bed.

Check for urinary retention/incontinence.

What underlying factors cannot be improved?

People with **deconditioning and cachexia** at the end of life will derive limited benefit from mobility interventions.

Long-term back pain will not suddenly be treatable just because the person has a life-limiting illness. Other clinicians will also have tried analgesics including medications for neuropathic pain over a much longer period of time.

Symptomatic treatment

Non-pharmacological intervention

For people who are mobile, maintaining mobility with tailored physical therapy is important. For those who can manage it, gentle strengthening exercises will be important both currently and in future care.

Pharmacological intervention

Data support the use of opioids, NSAIDs, and muscle relaxants such as diazepam 2.5–5 mg three times daily orally (when there is muscle spasm) when there is an acute exacerbation of low back pain.

Further reading

Caraceni A et al. (2021). Neurological problems in advanced cancer (Chapter 14.8). In: *Oxford Textbook of Palliative Medicine*, 6th ed. Oxford: Oxford University Press. Available at: https://doi.org/10.1093/med/9780198821328.003.0083

Neuropathic pain

Neuropathic pain is defined as pain which is caused by damage or inflammation to the somatosensory system, either in the central or peripheral nervous systems. Features supporting the diagnosis of neuropathic pain include the presence of paradoxical sensory perceptions such as burning, coldness, or tingling; the presence of abnormalities of sensation in the same region—either hypo- or hypersensitivity; or a pain experience that is random, episodic, or shooting in nature.

Patients may use vivid descriptive terminology, attempting to convey the nature of the pain.

Visceral neuropathic pain can lack typical neuropathic features. For example, coeliac plexus pain due to invasion by pancreatic adenocarcinoma typically presents as deep upper abdominal pain radiating to the back.

Onset of symptom

Acute or subacute onset (hours to days) of neuropathic pain and …

- **Subacute spinal pain:** spinal cord or cauda equina compression. This may be the first presentation of cord compromise. Ideally any cord lesion is diagnosed before muscle weakness.
- **Bony metastatic disease:** pathological fracture with acute neural compression.
- **Atrial fibrillation:** consider spinal cord infarct.
- **Lateralizing neurological deficit:** stroke.
- **Coagulopathy or thrombocytopenia:** consider bleeding: a retroperitoneal bleed leading to abdominal pain and associated unilateral neuropathic lower limb pain; epidural bleed leading to spinal pain and radicular trunk or arm pain and/or bilateral neuropathic lower limb pain.
- **Fever:** consider CNS infection.
- **With ascending symptomatology:** Guillain–Barré syndrome.

Chronic onset of neuropathic pain and …

- **Symmetrical peripheral (glove and stocking) pain:** peripheral neuropathy. Common causes are diabetes, alcohol, amyloidosis, hypothyroidism, chemotherapy (particularly oxaliplatin), nutritional deficiency, carcinoma-associated peripheral neuropathy, and chronic inflammatory polyneuropathy.
- **Single or adjacent radicular distribution:** focal neuropathy. Often due to direct invasion by tumour—common nerves involved are the brachial plexus, intercostal nerves, pelvic nerves, trigeminal nerve, sciatic nerve, and femoral nerve. Post-herpetic neuralgia, trigeminal neuralgia, diabetic mononeuropathy, radiation neuritis, and vascular compression due to aneurysm need to be considered.
- **Polyradicular or multiple peripheral nerves involved:** multifocal neuropathy. In the presence of metastatic cancer, particularly known central nervous disease, leptomeningeal carcinomatosis is most likely. Consider mononeuritis multiplex due to vasculitis.

Further reading

Ventzel L, Finnerup NB (2021). Management issues in neuropathic pain (Chapter 7.15). In: *Oxford Textbook of Palliative Medicine*, 6th ed. Oxford: Oxford University Press. Available at: https://doi.org/10.1093/med/9780198821328.003.0048

Headache

Onset of symptom

Most people experience headaches. The best way to categorize headaches is to classify them as either primary, secondary, or cranial neuralgias based on characteristics of the headache or headaches over the previous 12 months (Table 1.1).

There are many types of headaches. This section focuses on the most frequent pathologies.

Table 1.1 Categorization of headaches

Headache classification	Definition	Examples
Primary	Headaches for which no cause can be found	Migraine Cluster Tension-type
Secondary	The result of another condition causing traction on or inflammation of pain-sensitive structures The diagnosis is based on the problem beginning with or worsening as the result of an underlying pathological condition. If the underlying condition is resolved, the headaches disappear	Injury or trauma Hypertensive emergencies Idiopathic intracranial hypertension Carotid or vertebrobasilar dissection Space-occupying lesions (tumours, abscesses, cysts) Acute hydrocephalus Dural sinus thrombosis Intracranial haemorrhage Giant cell (temporal) arteritis Cerebrovascular accident or stroke Meningitis or encephalitis Carbon monoxide poisoning Toxin exposure or withdrawal Disorders of the neck, ears, oral cavity, sinuses, or eyes (including acute angle-closure) Medications including overuse
Cranial neuralgia	Idiopathic, infiltration, or compression	Trigeminal, occipital, or glossopharyngeal neuralgia

Acute onset (<24 h) of severe headache

- Sharp, maximal at onset, and often described as the worst headache ever experienced is typical of a thunderclap headache. While there may be no underlying pathology, urgently assess—this may be a **subarachnoid haemorrhage**. Other pathologies of this presentation include venous sinus thrombosis, hypertensive encephalopathy, pituitary apoplexy, or reversible cerebral vasospasm.

- A unilateral headache associated with tenderness to palpation over the temple, claudication of the jaw while chewing, and painless, monocular visual loss is typical of **temporal arteritis**.
- Headache, neck stiffness, fever, confusion, photophobia, seizures associated with nausea and vomiting with recent history of travel, skin lesions, poor vaccination record, or immune compromise require meningitis or encephalitis to be excluded.
- A new onset of headache and stroke-like symptoms in a younger person associated with neck pain, diplopia, unsteady gait, or dizziness should prompt consideration of carotid or vertebral artery dissection especially if there is a recent history of trauma to the neck or head.
- Acute angle glaucoma presents in older people with recent onset of unilateral or bilateral eye pain associated with acute headache, photophobia, and visual changes.
- Ischaemic or haemorrhagic strokes present with focal neurological deficits reflective of the area of the brain affected. The person often has new onset of headache, and nausea and vomiting.
- A new headache complicating a history of coagulopathy or viscosity disorders along with blurred vision, a visual field deficit, and nausea and vomiting suggest a dual vein thrombosis.
- Hypertensive emergencies most commonly occur due to non-compliance with medications. The symptoms reflect the end-organ affected and may include headache, dizziness, altered mental status, shortness of breath, chest pain, decreased urine output, vomiting, or changes in vision.

Subacute onset (1–3 days) of headaches
- New daily persistent headache for which no underlying pathology can be identified. Persistent daily headache is characterized by the fact that within 24 h of onset it may become constant and unresponsive to management.
- Space-occupying intracranial lesion including cerebral abscess, parasitic infections, and primary or metastatic tumours may present with headache, nausea, and vomiting, along with focal neurological signs or seizures.

Longer-term headaches
Chronic headaches can be diagnosed when a person experiences 15 or more headaches per month for at least 3 consecutive months.
The most common types of chronic headaches include the following:
- Chronic migraines may be associated with an aura. Other features may commonly include unilateral, throbbing headache that may be associated with photophobia, nausea, or vomiting.
- Chronic tension headaches are described as persistent, non-pulsatile, and associated with temporal tenderness.
- Medication overuse headache occurs when medications used to address the symptoms of headaches paradoxically worsen the headaches. Analgesic withdrawal often worsens them.
- Painful idiopathic cranial neuropathies. Trigeminal neuralgia is distinguished from other presentations of trigeminal distribution of pain. The main difference in this secondary group is that a cause of pain can be identified and this is accompanied by evidence of axonal damage.

This may be the result of herpes zoster infection, demyelination disorders such as multiple sclerosis, or a mass lesion.

Can you modify anything contributing to the symptom?

Headaches are a ubiquitous problem in the general population. At the same time, it may be the presenting symptom of a myriad of diseases. As such, an informed, systematic approach to assessment is required. The situation is even more challenging when people present with a new headache in the context of a long-standing primary headache disorder.

'Red flag' factors include age >50 years; new onset of fevers or other systemic illness; a change in the character of a long-standing headache; thunderclap headache; underlying illnesses; new neurological signs; and headaches that are worse with position changes or activities that increase intra-abdominal pressure.

Further reading

Cherny NI (2021). Acute cancer pain syndromes (Chapter 7.3). In: *Oxford Textbook of Palliative Medicine*, 6th ed. Oxford: Oxford University Press. Available at: https://doi.org/10.1093/med/9780198821328.003.0036

Pain in the setting of previous substance misuse

Onset of symptom

People with a history of substance misuse may develop a life-limiting illness. Managing symptoms of pain or anxiety requires the same level of careful assessment and therapy.

Distinguish between someone who is still using substances illicitly and those who may have had a history at some time earlier in life.

Carefully assess for the cause of pain in the same systematic way as one would for anyone else.

Acute onset (<24 h)

- **Fever and substance misuse:** consider recent IV drug use and the possibility of sepsis including infective endocarditis (p.108), osteomyelitis, or cerebral abscess.
- **Fever, tachycardia,** or **hypertension:** exclude drug withdrawal as a cause for diaphoretic signs.
- **Confusion and a history of alcohol use:** ensure that this person is not developing Wernicke's encephalopathy. Administer thiamine (up to 500 mg IV three times daily) to people with a history of excessive alcohol use and any suggestion of cognitive decompensation.

Can you modify anything contributing to the symptom?

Careful evaluation of current users of illicit drugs is crucial to their ongoing care. Acute withdrawal needs to recognized early and treated actively, depending on the substance(s) used.

What underlying factors cannot be improved?

In the setting of a life-limiting illness, it is unlikely that drug misuse patterns will change.

Symptomatic treatment

Non-pharmacological intervention

A supportive environment is important. Although it may seem obvious, a non-judgemental approach to the person and their support network is needed by **all** staff who come into contact with them. This can be difficult in an inpatient setting when, for example, substance misuse is continuing.

Pharmacological intervention

Medications for symptom control should be chosen as they would be for any other person. The doses of opioids in people with opioid-responsive pain who have recently used illicit opioids may need to be higher and dose intervals even reduced to obtain the same therapeutic benefit.

NSAIDs and paracetamol should be used as adjuvants for opioid-responsive pain. For pain with a neuropathic component, tricyclic antidepressants, membrane stabilizers, and steroids have roles.

For people who have used benzodiazepines for non-therapeutic indications, tolerance is likely to be a significant problem and their use (except in alcohol withdrawal) will have limited benefit.

Further reading

Pergolizzi JV et al. (2021). Opioid therapy: managing risks of abuse, addiction, and diversion (Chapter 7.7). In: *Oxford Textbook of Palliative Medicine*, 6th ed. Oxford: Oxford University Press. Available at: https://doi.org/10.1093/med/9780198821328.003.0040

Breathlessness

Onset of symptom

Breathlessness is one of the few symptoms which generally worsens as death approaches in a life-limiting illness.

Acute onset (<24 h) of breathlessness and …

- **Fever: community-acquired pneumonia** (p.126), **empyema** (p.131), **mediastinitis** (p.136) (which most often presents with a history of thoracic instrumentation), or a history of **valvular heart disease** with septic/inflammatory damage to the valve (p.108).
- **Asymmetrical signs on chest examination:** a **pneumothorax** (p.133) may be spontaneous but more frequently follows recent fine-needle biopsy of a chest mass.
- **Normal examination: acute pulmonary thromboembolism** (p.119), or **acute pancreatitis** (p.174) which can cause significant desaturation and can occur with malignant obstruction of the common bile duct.
- **History of chest pain: acute myocardial infarction** (AMI) (including those with no chest symptoms) can present with **cardiac decompensation** (p.100). Other causes of chest pain and breathlessness include **dissecting thoracic aneurysm** (p.110) and **pericarditis** (p.106).
- **Acute bleeding:** is likely to be obvious except in people on anticoagulation who have **GIT** (p.158) or **retroperitoneal bleeding**.
- **Following a fall or fracture:** consider **fat embolus syndrome**. Examine for a rash and increasing confusion (p.278).

Subacute onset (1–3 days) of breathlessness

- **With fever: atypical pneumonias** (p.126) often have a prodrome of a few days with influenza-like symptoms and low-grade fever. A productive cough and low-grade fever suggest **bronchitis**.
- **Relatively normal examination: lymphangitis carcinomatosis** (p.144) can present with a subtle, subacute onset but, once established, breathlessness often worsens quickly. Exacerbations of underlying **chronic obstructive pulmonary disease (COPD)** will often have an onset spread over days.
- **Asymmetrical signs on chest examination:** people with progressive **tracheal obstruction** (p.138) notice increasing shortness of breath and often a fixed wheeze as the lumen diameter diminishes. Obstruction of the more distal airways may also occur. Consider this in people presenting with breathlessness and a wheeze.
- **Fluid overload** can develop with either **cardiac decompensation** due to silent ischaemia/infarction (p.100) or end-stage renal failure. This may also be iatrogenic, particularly in frail people with a life-limiting illness.
- **Signs of anaemia:** rapid loss of haemoglobin (Hb) may occur with either **bleeding** or **haemolysis**. This is usually associated with fatigue, headache, impaired concentration, and chest tightness.

- **Unexplained hypotension, increasing fatigue, and cough** may be due to **cardiac tamponade** (p.104). This is most likely to occur in people with end-stage renal failure or a local effect of cancer.

Insidious onset (days to weeks) of breathlessness

- **Pleural effusions** (p.129) and **pericardial effusions** often have an insidious onset with progressive breathlessness that worsens from occurring on significant exertion to occurring at rest.
- **A cancer associated with lymphangitis carcinomatosis** (p.144): more often in a person with primary breast cancer.
- **Worsening cachexia:** in all end-stage illness breathlessness will worsen as death approaches.
- **Increasing ascites** reduces diaphragmatic excursion (p.166).
- **A history of bleomycin use:** often has an insidious onset.
- **A history of cardiomyopathy:** often has a gradual onset.
- **A history of chronic airways disease:** check for sputum production, fever, and wheezing. Consider an infective exacerbation. These people may have been smokers. If this is associated with weight loss and increasing fatigue, consider the development of primary lung cancers.

Can you modify anything contributing to the symptom?

Thromboembolism is treatable with the aim of reducing the incidence of fatal pulmonary emboli (p.119).

Community-acquired pneumonia in the presence of no other significant lung pathology and a functioning immune system can be treated (p.126).

People with **lymphangitis carcinomatosis** should be treated symptomatically (p.144).

For an **acute myocardial infarction**, further myocardial damage can be minimized (p.8). (Use of thrombolytics is limited to people with no recent GIT bleeding and no intracerebral pathology.)

Non-loculated **pleural effusions** can be treated with pleural drainage and ideally with pleurodesis (p.129).

Fluid overload can be improved in most people except in end-stage disease and hypoalbuminaemia (p.100).

Pericardial effusions can be drained, affording significant relief (p.104).

Increasing abdominal girth due to **ascites** can be quickly relieved by peritoneal tap. The addition of diuretics may also be effective (p.166).

People who present with worsening **heart failure** may improve by ensuring that anaemia is reversed and any associated infections are treated. Ensure that management of heart failure has been maximized (p.100).

People with **anaemia** may be transfused. Consider the burden of this intervention in very late-stage illness. Consider the role of iron, vitamin B_{12}, or folate replacement.

An **infective exacerbation of airways disease** warrants antibiotics, corticosteroids, and possibly bronchodilators.

What underlying factors cannot be improved?

Cachexia without an ability to reverse the underlying catabolic state will progress. Late **drug toxicity** is irreversible and often progresses. Although **loculated pleural effusions** can be treated with videoscopically assisted thoracentesis, the procedure is limited to people who have a good functional status.

Symptomatic treatment

Non-pharmacological intervention

There are good data to support energy conservation (in conjunction with an occupational therapist) and relaxation/visualization techniques to minimize breathlessness.

Avoid unnecessary exercise.

People's sense of impending doom is often overwhelming as breathlessness tends to worsen as the disease progresses. Addressing these understandable fears is central to supporting people at the end of life.

Pharmacological intervention

Regular low-dose oral morphine (10 mg per 24 h or 10 mg parenterally every 24 h) in opioid-naïve people with long-term breathlessness will help reduce breathlessness in many people. An increase of 30–50% per dose may be necessary in people already on opioids to help with their breathlessness.

A regular dose of an anxiolytic such as a long-acting benzodiazepine (clonazepam 0.5 mg twice daily or lorazepam 0.5–1.0 mg SL twice daily) may have a role late in disease or in someone with new onset of breathlessness while the cause of the symptom is being diagnosed.

Oxygen may be of benefit in people who are hypoxaemic. Flowing air may be of significant benefit in people with normal oxygen tension.

Any person with a wheeze should have a trial of a bronchodilator (salbutamol 2.5–5.0 mg nebulized four times daily, ipratropium bromide 250–500 micrograms nebulized four times daily, 0.9% NaCl 5 mL nebulized as required).

A person with late-stage disease and stridor or lymphangitis may have a trial of oral dexamethasone 4–8 mg in the mornings.

With noisy terminal respiratory secretions, hyoscine butylbromide 20 mg SC every 4 h may be of limited symptomatic benefit.

Further reading

Dwight J (2020). Chest pain, breathlessness, and fatigue (Chapter 16.2.1). In: *Oxford Textbook of Medicine*, 6th ed. Oxford: Oxford University Press. Available at: https://doi.org/10.1093/med/9780198746690.003.0340

Johnson MJ, Currow DC (2021). Breathlessness and other respiratory symptoms in palliative care (Chapter 41). In: *Oxford Textbook of Palliative Medicine*, 6th ed. Oxford: Oxford University Press. Available at: https://doi.org/10.1093/med/9780198821328.003.0058

Acute confusional state (delirium)

Onset of symptom

Delirium is characterized by a fluctuating mental state. Even late in disease, people value clear cognition (p.246).

Acute onset (<24 h) of confusion and ...

- **Recent new medications** can add to the existing anticholinergic load from long-term medications and cause an acute delirium (p.68).
- **Recently commenced corticosteroids** may precipitate an agitated delirium.
- **Asterixis:** metabolic factors including severe uraemia (p.208) or hepatic decompensation (p.177) especially with upper GIT bleeding may precipitate a delirium.
- **Hypoxaemia** can cause acute confusion. (Be concerned about the introduction of oxygen for breathlessness in a person with a history of carbon dioxide retention; this can cause respiratory depression in a small number of susceptible people with central hypoventilation states.)
- **Sepsis:** acute sepsis can include community-acquired pneumonia (p.126), biliary tract sepsis (p.172), meningitis (p.252), or a urinary tract infection (p.284) especially in the elderly.
- **Atrial fibrillation** or **mechanical heart valve:** consider a transient ischaemic event or stroke (p.240).
- **Recent change in physical place of care** may cause delirium in a person with an underlying dementia.
- Known past history of cerebral metastases, or past history of a cerebrovascular accident (CVA) should prompt consideration of **seizures** (p.249).

Subacute onset (1–3 days) of confusion

- **Recent medication withdrawal** (including benzodiazepines, glucocorticoids, tobacco, alcohol, or selective serotonin reuptake inhibitors (SSRIs)).
- **Febrile** or **hypotensive:** sepsis often causes a subtle onset of confusion. Sources include a urinary tract infection, atypical pneumonia, or cellulitis.
- **Continued use of antihypertensives** late into the course of a life-limiting illness can cause cerebral hypoperfusion as people start to become hypotensive.
- **Ascites:** consider spontaneous bacterial peritonitis.
- **Dehydration** may contribute significantly with increased insensible losses (air conditioning, hot weather), decreased oral intake, or high output states (ileostomies, fistulae (p.180)).
- **Metabolic derangements:** the onset masks a much longer time course over which **hypercalcaemia** (p.215) or **hyponatraemia** (p.219) develop. (Exclude diuretics as a cause for hyponatraemia.)
- **Hypoglycaemia** is rarely seen unless the person is taking hypoglycaemic agents (p.226), in which case review carefully as appetite or oral intake decreases.
- **Cerebral metastases** may directly contribute to confusion depending where the lesions are (this includes meningeal disease). CNS disease

of any aetiology may cause **hyponatraemia** with the syndrome of inappropriate antidiuretic hormone secretion (SIADH) (p.220).
- Recent radiological investigations using contrast may precipitate **hyperthyroidism** in some people (p.236).
- **In the terminal phase of a life-limiting illness** acute confusional states are frequently encountered towards death. If the deterioration is expected, treat symptomatically. If it is unexpected and appears to precipitate the terminal phase, consider differential diagnoses.

Insidious onset (days to weeks) of confusion
- A clear differential diagnosis needs to be drawn from **dementia**. Many people with subtle cognitive changes may be found to have short-term memory problems for the first time as the catabolic insult of an advanced, life-limiting illness unmasks a previously unrecognized dementia.
- **Untreated depression and anxiety** may present with features of delirium (p.266, p.270).
- **Progressive cachexia** may contribute to a susceptibility to delirium independent of identifiable nutritional deficiencies.
- **A history of alcohol misuse:** always have a low threshold for the introduction of thiamine until the cause for confusion becomes established.

Can you modify anything contributing to the symptom?
There is often a lag of days between reducing or reversing precipitating causes of delirium and seeing cognition improve.

All medications need to be reviewed. The newest medications (often opioids) may be adding to an anticholinergic load precipitating an acute confusional state (p.68). It may be possible to reduce long-term medications in order to reduce the anticholinergic load while continuing opioids, if needed.

Sepsis can be treated and this may be one of the most important aspects of reducing acute confusion. Recurrent sepsis or sepsis in the setting of severe immunocompromise or prolonged neutropenia may become untreatable.

Hepatic decompensation is often amenable to treatment; stop any GIT bleeding, use lactulose or neomycin to decrease gut transit time, and minimize protein intake (p.177).

Dehydration can be treated with the judicious use of parenteral hydration. In the terminal phases of a life-limiting illness, hydration needs are not great and small amounts of fluid are all that is necessary; larger volumes are likely to cause peripheral or pulmonary oedema and increased upper GIT secretions.

Hypercalcaemia may respond to bisphosphonates (p.215). Where **hyponatraemia** is secondary to SIADH, fluid restriction may be of benefit (although most people at the end of life already have low fluid intakes).

Resetting **glycaemic control** (8–14 mmol/L) is likely to reverse problems associated with hypoglycaemia (p.226) and protect from further symptomatic episodes.

Newly diagnosed **cerebral metastases** may benefit from oral dexa-methasone (4–16 mg daily).

Treat **hypoxaemia** with oxygen. Consider the person's past history of airways disease. In people who are well enough, collect arterial blood gases to guide oxygen flow rates.

Seizures may cause delirium in the postictal phase or in the presence of status epilepticus. Attempts to arrest seizure activity should be made with prompt administration of benzodiazepines and antiseizure medications (p.249).

What underlying factors cannot be improved?

Without an ability to reverse the underlying systemic illness, **cachexia** cannot be reversed. Often, despite attempts, reversing metabolic factors late in illness does not improve cognition.

Despite therapeutic advances, **dementia** is not yet amenable to treat-ment late in the course of a life-limiting illness.

Symptomatic treatment

Non-pharmacological intervention

Disorientation is frightening to people; the sensations of hallucinations are real and often overwhelming. A quiet, familiar environment with prompts that orientate a person to time and place helps. Family and staff sensitivity to acute confusion is crucial.

If this is occurring at the end of life, consider whether or not constipation, acute urinary retention, or pain due to uncomfortable positioning may be contributing.

Pharmacological intervention

Acute confusional states need to be treated actively.

Low-dose antipsychotics have a very limited role with no evidence to support that they help to treat the delirium or reduce its duration.

If someone is agitated or a risk to themselves or others, consider the role of sedation with a regular benzodiazepine. This may include diazepam 2–5 mg once to three times daily or lorazepam 0.5–1.0 mg SL once to four times daily in doses sufficient to ensure that the amnesic effects of benzodiazep-ines are not worsening the confusion.

Further reading

Agar M et al. (2021). Delirium (Chapter 13.4). In: *Oxford Textbook of Palliative Medicine*, 6th ed. Oxford: Oxford University Press. Available at: https://doi.org/10.1093/med/9780198821 328.003.0074

Sheehan B (2020). Delirium (Chapter 26.5.1). In: *Oxford Textbook of Medicine*, 6th ed. Oxford: Oxford University Press. Available at: https://doi.org/10.1093/med/9780198746690.003.0627

Decreased level of consciousness

Onset of symptom

Acute onset (<24 h) of decreased level of consciousness and ...

- **A history of falls, anticoagulation, or coagulopathy:** subarachnoid bleed is an urgent diagnosis of exclusion (p.256).
- **A CNS tumour:** consider raised intracranial pressure (p.259) (with hydrocephalus, intracranial bleed, or coning), or seizures (p.249).
- **New medications:** consider medications with sedating effects including opioids, benzodiazepines, tricyclic antidepressants, or anticonvulsants (e.g. phenytoin has non-linear pharmacokinetics) (p.61).
- **Recent changes in medication doses:** decrease in glucocorticoids, Addisonian crisis in people on long-term glucocorticoids (p.232), failure to take thyroid replacement (p.237), or recent increase in opioids, sedatives, antidepressants, anticonvulsants, or antiemetics.
- **Fever:** sources of infection including meningitis (p.252), encephalitis (including primary herpetic infections in the immunocompromised), or renal/respiratory tract sepsis (p.126, p.282) causing systemic shutdown. People on long-term glucocorticoids who become septic need to have urgent adrenal replacement.
- **History of diabetes:** consider hypoglycaemia especially if oral intake is variable and hypoglycaemic agents have continued without dose revision (p.226) or careful monitoring. Consider hyperglycaemia (p.228) (ketoacidosis, hyperosmolar coma) as a cause of an acute deterioration.
- **Oxygen therapy:** carbon dioxide retention may cause a decreased level of consciousness as carbon dioxide levels rise in people with hypoxic respiratory drive.

Subacute onset (1–3 days) of decreased levels of consciousness and ...

- **Severe hepatic dysfunction:** hepatic encephalopathy can cause progressive obtundation (p.177).
- **Anuria or decreased urinary output:** prerenal causes include dehydration, renal causes are often associated with drug toxicity, and postrenal causes include obstruction of the urinary tract (intraluminal, extraluminal) (p.286).
- **Dehydration:** people with decreased oral intake may have severe prerenal impairment. High output stomas or fistulae, especially involving the small bowel, can rapidly lead to dehydration.
- **History of diminishing function** consistent with an expected death as the body closes down from a life-limiting illness.
- **Space-occupying lesion:** consider focal impaired awareness seizures in the differential diagnosis (p.249).
- **Vascular disease or atrial fibrillation:** consider transient ischaemic attack or stroke as a cause.
- In a person with known mediastinal disease consider **superior vena cava (SVC) obstruction** where the first presentation may be with a decreased level of consciousness (p.122).
- In a person with cancer (solid/haematological) this may be a presentation of **hypercalcaemia** (p.215). Consider other

paraneoplastic phenomena such as SIADH (p.220), cerebellar degeneration, or encephalitis.

Insidious onset (days to weeks) of decreased level of consciousness

- **History of frailty and dementia:** consider **subdural haematoma** (p.256) although a history of falls or head trauma may not be forthcoming.
- **History of a space-occupying lesion:** an increase in the size of the lesion may lead to diminishing consciousness.

Can you modify anything contributing to the symptom?

Subdural bleeds need to be treated in people where contributing pathology, such as coagulopathy, can be reversed. Intracranial and subarachnoid bleeds are likely to have much worse outcomes in people with a life-limiting illness.

Medications: new medications, medications with recent dose changes, and medications that may accumulate need to be reviewed carefully. People taking non-prescribed medications or people who have had prescriptions from multiple professionals need to have thorough histories taken. The use of transdermal medications, including opioids, may be overlooked in people with a decreased level of consciousness.

Sepsis can generally be treated and even in people with a very poor prognosis may be the best way to palliate the symptoms of sepsis.

Obstructive hydrocephalus needs neurosurgical review especially if the person has otherwise been functioning well.

Epilepsy (p.249) can be treated, and if it is the cause of changed consciousness or mentation this is likely to improve the person's function considerably.

Dehydration contributing directly to decreased levels of consciousness can be treated with the judicious use of parenteral hydration. In the absence of identifiable causes of decreased level of consciousness, hydration alone is unlikely to make a substantial difference.

Hyponatraemia may be amenable to therapy in someone who is functioning reasonably well (p.219).

Carbon dioxide retention should be treated with a decrease in supplemental oxygen and optimizing respiratory function.

Hypercalcaemia (p.215), especially at first presentation, is usually reversible with bisphosphonates and gentle hydration.

Hypoglycaemia (p.226) and **hyperglycaemia** (p.228) can be corrected even late in disease.

What underlying factors cannot be improved?

Without an ability to reverse the underlying catabolic state, **cachexia** cannot be reversed.

Intracranial and **subarachnoid bleeds**, especially in late-stage disease, are not likely to be operable given the overall circumstances of the person.

Symptomatic treatment

Non-pharmacological intervention

A calm peaceful environment is important. Even though people with a decreased level of consciousness may not be able to respond, there are data that demonstrate that they can still hear familiar voices and feel familiar touch. Supporting families to continue to spend time and have conversations with the person is important.

In a person with impaired consciousness, speech therapist review of swallowing may put in place a plan to lessen difficulties with oral intake or medications being aspirated. People with impaired consciousness should not take anything by mouth until this assessment is done.

Pharmacological intervention

If the person has already been on symptom control medications, these should be continued by an appropriate route of administration (SL, rectal, transdermal, or SC).

Further reading

Bates D (2020). The unconscious patient (Chapter 24.5.5). In: *Oxford Textbook of Medicine*, 6th ed. Oxford: Oxford University Press. Available at: https://doi.org/10.1093/med/9780198746690.003.0579

Ko D et al. (2021). Withholding and withdrawing life-sustaining treatment (including artificial nutrition and hydration) (Chapter 19.7). In: *Oxford Textbook of Palliative Medicine*, 6th ed. Oxford: Oxford University Press. Available at: https://doi.org/10.1093/med/9780198821328.003.0111

Agitation

Onset of symptom

Acute onset (<24 h) of agitation

- **Unrelieved physical symptoms** especially pain and nausea, urinary retention, or constipation.
- **History of a psychiatric disorder:** delirium, agitated depression, or hypomania can manifest with agitation.
- **Recent bad news:** the person with the life-limiting illness may have had bad news or the immediacy of dying may have started to have an impact in a very specific way. Fears which are often difficult to articulate, anxiety, frustration, or recurrent nightmares may all contribute to agitation. Previous experience of other people close to them dying may influence how they see their own death.
- **Medications known to cause agitation** including drugs with dopaminergic effects that can cause akathisia (including metoclopramide and haloperidol) or those which may occasionally cause paradoxical agitation such as opioids and benzodiazepines.
- **Withdrawal** from prescribed and illicit medications, alcohol, nicotine, or even caffeine can cause marked agitation. Consider benzodiazepines (some of which have a very long half-life) and opioids. Have medications inadvertently not been charted (especially transdermal medications)?
- **Acute confusional state**, with any of its causes (p.29).
- **Impaired ability to communicate:** unable to verbalize, especially in the setting of an expressive or receptive aphasia.
- **Metabolic causes** including **hypoxaemia**, **hypoglycaemia** (p.226), **uraemia** (p.208), or **hyponatraemia** (p.219).
- **Cerebral metastases** especially with withdrawal of glucocorticoids, an acute bleed, or the emergence of obstructive hydrocephalus.

Subacute onset (1–3 days) of agitation

- **Fevers, hypothermia, or hypotension:** sepsis can present as agitation, especially occult urinary (p.282) or respiratory tract infections (p.126).

Insidious onset (days to weeks) of agitation

With a history of anxiety: anxiety states (p.270) may cause agitation and be exacerbated by evidence of disease progression or loss of function. Depression (p.266) and anxiety often coexist. Adjustment disorders may also have a component of agitation. Long-term schizophrenia may have an element of low-grade agitation.

Can you modify anything contributing to the symptom?

An open discussion about agitation is key. Eliciting fears in a supportive way while respecting how difficult it is to talk about many of these issues may be very helpful.

Medications causing extrapyramidal side effects can usually be stopped or a substitute found. For example, domperidone can be substituted for metoclopramide for nausea because domperidone does not cross the blood–brain barrier.

Acute psychiatric problems need adequate assessment. Even late in the course of illness, treating psychiatric problems is important. In someone acutely depressed, assess risk for suicide (p.264). (Does the person wish to hasten death? Has the person thought about how they would end their life? Has the person ever attempted suicide before? Have they made actual plans to end their life? What support do they have from family, friends, or health professionals?)

What underlying factors cannot be improved?

Often there are limited choices in replacing or withdrawing key medications that are maintaining function or comfort.

Symptomatic treatment

Non-pharmacological intervention

What does this person think is causing their agitation? Do they have insight into the agitation and its possible causes? Naming the person's agitation and listening to their concerns is the cornerstone of working with them.

Pharmacological intervention

There is a place for the short-term use of appropriate anxiolytics. This may include a benzodiazepine such as lorazepam.

SSRIs have a specific role to play in panic attacks. This may be while underlying causes of the agitation are reversed or in the clinical setting where no reversible causes are found.

Restless legs, independent of the factors already outlined, can be an entity in themselves, worse at night, and very distressing. Treatment should include:

- stopping excess intake of stimulants
- replacing electrolyte, iron, and vitamin deficiencies
- considering a trial of dopaminergic agents (bromocriptine, pergolide), or in mild cases, benzodiazepines (clonazepam).

Further reading

Voltz R, Lorenzi S (2021). Neurological disorders other than dementia (Chapter 15.5). In: *Oxford Textbook of Palliative Medicine*, 6th ed. Oxford: Oxford University Press. Available at: https://doi.org/10.1093/med/9780198821328.003.0093

Constipation

Onset of symptom

Constipation is defined as highly subjective change in the frequency of the passage of stools **or** difficulty with evacuation of stools. Other associated symptoms may include hard stools, straining, sensation of anorectal blockage, incomplete evacuation, abdominal discomfort, or bloating.

Acute onset (days)

- **Acute change in bowel habits** with few other symptoms occurs with medication changes, a change in usual routine such as travel, decreased oral intake, or an acute change in mobility.
- **Cramping abdominal pain, associated with altered bowel habits** (constipation progressing to obstipation, nausea, and vomiting) may be due to GIT obstruction (p.163), severe underlying impaction, adhesions, tumours, strangulated hernia, volvulus, or gallstone ileus.

Subacute onset (weeks) of change in bowel habits

- Cancer or cancer-related causes: colorectal cancer, dehydration, intestinal radiation, tumour compression of large intestine, peritoneal metastases, chemotherapy.
- Endocrine causes: hypothyroidism, diabetes, hyperparathyroidism, (pan)hypopituitarism.
- GIT disorders: diverticulosis, megacolon, pelvic floor dysfunction, rectoceles, strictures.
- Metabolic causes: hypercalcaemia, hypocalcaemia, hypokalaemia, hypomagnesaemia, uraemia.
- Neurological causes: autonomic neuropathy, dementia, multiple sclerosis, muscular dystrophies, Parkinson's disease, spinal cord lesions, stroke, dementia.
- Pain secondary to anal fissures or haemorrhoids.
- Psychological causes: anxiety, depression, eating disorders.
- Lack of privacy or time.
- Myopathies (dermatomyositis, polymyositis, inclusion body myositis).

Chronic (months or years)

- Primary or idiopathic chronic constipation is the result of long-standing dysfunction of the anorectal neuromuscular structures leading to three subtypes (Table 1.2).

Table 1.2 Subtypes of constipation

Subtype	Estimated frequency in constipated adults	Description
Slow transit constipation	5%	Prolonged transit of colonic contents neuropathy or myopathy
Dyssynergic defecation	30%	Uncoordinated abdominal and pelvic muscles resulting in difficulty with passing stool
Normal transit constipation	65%	Infrequent or difficulty passing stool together with abdominal pain or discomfort

Can you modify anything contributing to the symptom?

What is the duration of symptoms? The longer the duration of constipation, the more intractable it is likely to be.

A rectal examination will identify local problems: haemorrhoids or faecal impaction. This also assesses anal tone and the pelvic floor. Decreased anal tone is a late sign of spinal cord compression.

Assess hydration clinically and, if appropriate, with electrolytes, urea, and creatinine (EUC), calcium and magnesium levels.

Plain abdominal X-rays can help to exclude bowel obstruction. Studies of colon transit time and pelvic floor assessments are not routine in palliative care but, if clinically indicated when a patient is well enough, may help guide treatment in consultation with a gastroenterologist.

What underlying factors cannot be improved?

There are predisposing conditions that are difficult to modify. Older people and those who are bedridden are at a greater risk of problems. Changes associated with progressive disease such as cachexia leading to muscle loss are important contributing factors.

Symptomatic treatment

Non-pharmacological intervention

Where appropriate, non-pharmacological strategies are important and include regular physical activity, adequate fluid intake, establishing routines, and advice on toileting posture.

Constipation can be a difficult topic to talk about for both patients and health professionals with embarrassment acting as a barrier to proper assessment and management.

Pharmacological intervention

Many medications contribute to secondary constipation with polypharmacy strongly correlating with laxative use. Review existing prescriptions and if possible, reduce or switch to alternative therapies with fewer anticholinergic effects (p.68).

All people commenced on opioids should receive information about constipation along with recommendations for treatment. There is little evidence to support the superiority of one simple laxative over others. If problems persist, increase laxatives doses, consider an opioid switch, or commence one of the options of the mu-opioid receptor antagonist naloxone.

Along with dietary recommendations and supportive counselling, the initial agent of choice for managing functional constipation is polyethylene glycol. However, people are likely to have symptoms for prolonged periods and the more intractable problems are likely to be. Discussion with a gastroenterologist is recommended.

Further reading

Larkin PJ (2021). Constipation and diarrhoea (Chapter 8.3). In: *Oxford Textbook of Palliative Medicine*, 6th ed. Oxford: Oxford University Press. Available at: https://doi.org/10.1093/med/978019 8821328.003.0054

Orme S, Harari D (2020). Bladder and bowels (Chapter 6.9). In: *Oxford Textbook of Medicine*, 6th ed. Oxford: Oxford University Press. Available at: https://doi.org/10.1093/med/9780198746 690.003.0060

Diarrhoea

Onset of symptom

Secretory diarrhoea (compared with non-secretory diarrhoea) persists even with fasting and is characterized by high-volume, watery diarrhoea. Causes include *Vibrio cholerae* and *Escherichia coli*, *Shigella*, *Campylobacter* species, and viral infections, medications (methylxanthines), and hormone-secreting tumours (serotonin, calcitonin, gastrin, and vasoactive intestinal peptide).

Acute onset (<24 h) of diarrhoea
- **Influenza-like symptoms:** viral gastroenteritis is the most common cause of acute diarrhoea. Other infectious agents include *Giardia lamblia* and *Clostridium difficile*, especially with a recent history of antibiotics causing pseudomembranous colitis (p.153). Pseudomembranous colitis can occur with exposure to any antibiotic. Consequently, frequently used antibiotics cause most cases, but risk is highest when lincosamides or monobactams are used.

Subacute onset (1–3 days) of diarrhoea
- **Recent radiotherapy** (involving bowel directly in the field of therapy) can present with increasing severity of diarrhoea (p.150).
- **Recent chemotherapy**, especially with 5-fluorouracil, methotrexate, or doxorubicin.
- Over-zealous use of **aperients** (probably the most common cause) and other medications (antibiotics, NSAIDs, antacids, glutamate).
- **Colonic and rectal tumours**.
- **Enterocolonic fistula** (p.180) in a person with known malignancy, past history of surgery, or radiotherapy.

Insidious onset (days to weeks) of diarrhoea
- **History of constipation** with faecal overflow.
- **History of inflammatory bowel disease:** consider whether people are not tolerating routine medications for IBD, such as people with uncontrolled vomiting or late-stage anorexia.
- **History of pancreatic disease** with steatorrhoea.
- **Previous GIT surgery** with short bowel or blind loop syndrome or bile salt diarrhoea because of a previous ileal resection.
- **History of diabetes mellitus** with autonomic neuropathy.
- **Thyroid replacement therapy** that has not been adjusted as the person loses weight.
- **Neuroendocrine tumours including carcinoid** (especially towards the end of the dose for long-acting octreotide).
- **AIDS** from organisms including cryptosporidium, *Mycoplasma avium–intracellulare* (MAI), *Giardia lamblia*, *Cytomegalovirus*, or herpes simplex virus.

Can you modify anything contributing to the symptom?

Hydration status should be assessed and managed.

Viral gastroenteritis requires support; for most people oral rehydration should be sufficient. Rarely, specific electrolyte problems will need parenteral support.

Check recent use of **antibiotics** (*Clostridium difficile* toxin can be identified in stools and treated with oral vancomycin 125 mg every 6 h. Check for recent overseas travel.

Exclude **constipation** with faecal overflow with physical examination.

In **pancreatic insufficiency**, use pancreatic enzyme replacement with food.

People with **ileal resection** may benefit from cholestyramine (4 g three times daily).

Corticosteroids and mesalazine (500 mg orally three times daily) should be used to treat **inflammatory bowel disease**.

Chemotherapy may be of significant benefit in managing neuroendocrine tumours.

Regular octeotide (100 micrograms SC three times daily) may be of benefit in people with **radiation-induced diarrhoea** to reduce fluid loss and the length of any hospital admission.

Review current medications used for **constipation** and reduce if necessary.

What underlying factors cannot be improved?

In shortened bowel (surgery, fistula formation), controlling long-term frequent loose bowel motions can be difficult. Failure to do so may lead to numerous adverse consequences, including dehydration, malnutrition, electrolyte imbalance, and impaired immune function.

Symptomatic treatment

Non-pharmacological intervention

Fluid support is the mainstay of non-pharmacological intervention. Bulking agents such as ispaghula husks can be of benefit to decrease frequency of diarrhoea and improve continence control.

Pharmacological intervention

Identify infective causes and treat vigorously even late in the course of a life-limiting illness.

Opioids (morphine 5 mg orally or 2.5 mg SC, as required/every 4 h) can be used for diarrhoea.

Oral cholestyramine (4 g three times daily) can be used to manage diarrhoea secondary to shortened ileum.

Octreotide (start with 100 micrograms three times daily) may be of use in truly refractory diarrhoea (*Cryptosporidium*, carcinoid, Zollinger–Ellison syndrome, high-output ileostomy).

Add 5-hydroxytryptamine type 3 (5-HT$_3$) antagonists (ondansetron 4 mg SL/IV/SC) in Zollinger–Ellison syndrome.

Further reading

Larkin PJ (2021). Constipation and diarrhoea (Chapter 8.3). In: *Oxford Textbook of Palliative Medicine*, 6th ed. Oxford: Oxford University Press. Available at: https://doi.org/10.1093/med/978019 8821328.003.0054

Orme S, Harari D (2020). Bladder and bowels (Chapter 6.9). In: *Oxford Textbook of Medicine*, 6th ed. Oxford: Oxford University Press. Available at: https://doi.org/10.1093/med/9780198746 690.003.0060

Nausea (and vomiting)

Be sure that this person has nausea rather than anorexia as they may be used interchangeably.

Nausea is the unpleasant sensation of wanting to vomit. It is a feared symptom.

Onset of symptom

Acute onset (<24 h) of nausea

- **A history of new medications including recent chemotherapy**.
  Always consider that the new medication may be crucial to symptom
  control and other medications with which they may be interacting
  can be ceased. Medications often blamed include opioids, antibiotics,
  cytotoxic agents, digoxin, and iron supplements. Always ask about non-
  prescribed medications.
- **Epigastric discomfort:** consider gastritis, peptic ulcer disease, gastric
  outlet obstruction, and intestinal obstruction. Gastritis is more common
  with NSAIDs (especially if co-prescribed with glucocorticoids), or
  recent upper abdominal radiotherapy.
- **Known cerebral metastases:** consider an acute increase in
  intracranial pressure including acute intracranial bleed (p.256),
  ventricular obstruction causing acute hydrocephalus, tumour
  progression, leptomeningeal malignant infiltration, or cerebellar
  metastases.
- **Fever, rigors, hypotension, or hypothermia:** consider sepsis as
  a cause for acute-onset nausea. Occult sites include the urinary tract
  (especially with the presence of hydronephrosis) (p.282), cholecystitis
  (p.172), or atypical chest infections (p.126).
- **Unrelieved pain** may lead to nausea.

Subacute onset (1–3 days) of nausea

- **Nausea associated with movement**. Consider cerebellar
  metastases, irritation of the vestibular apparatus, or gastroparesis
  (secondary to opioids or ascites).
- **Worsening renal failure** can present as worsening nausea. Consider
  ureteric obstruction (p.286) or medication toxicity (aminoglycosides or
  anti-inflammatory agents).
- **Worsening hepatic failure** can present as worsening nausea.
  Consider drug toxicity (including paracetamol) or Budd–Chiari
  syndrome (hepatic vein thrombosis) for hepatic failure (p.177).
- **Evidence of sepsis:** consider less typical sites if there is clear evidence
  of sepsis and no obvious site (infective endocarditis (p.108), non-
  bacterial meningitis, abscess formation including a cerebral abscess).
  The elderly and immunocompromised have less florid presentations of
  sepsis.
- **Anxiety and fear**.
- **Electrolyte abnormalities** (hypercalcaemia (p.215), hyponatraemia
  (p.219)).
- **Gastric compression** from hepatomegaly, ascites, or peritoneal
  disease may cause nausea and early satiety.

Insidious onset (days to weeks) of nausea
- **Any of the causes of nausea already mentioned:** can have a more protracted onset.
- **Eating** (often at the insistence of well-meaning family) despite anorexia/cachexia syndrome.
- **Cerebral disease**.
- **Anxiety:** the diagnosis of anticipatory nausea, or fear and anxiety causing nausea, is one of exclusion but should be considered in a person with difficult-to-control nausea.
- **Constipation:** should not by itself cause vomiting but it can cause significant nausea.

Can you modify anything contributing to the symptom?

Advice about not eating when the person is not hungry is crucial to controlling nausea for many people with advanced disease.

Medications contributing directly to nausea (e.g. antibiotics) or specific toxicity (e.g. anti-inflammatories causing gastritis) should be stopped and a therapy causing less nausea should be substituted.

Reduce cerebral oedema for any cause of raised intracranial pressure. Use glucocorticoids (oral dexamethasone 8 mg in the morning and at midday) to try to reduce cerebral oedema.

Drainage of tense ascites may reduce nausea and allow oral intake.

What underlying factors cannot be improved?

As nausea is often a manifestation of underlying pathology, without an ability to change the course of the life-limiting illness, a symptomatic approach is needed. People with leptomeningeal spread of cancer or rapidly worsening renal function often have nausea that is difficult to treat.

Symptomatic treatment

Non-pharmacological intervention

Many people with nausea at the end of life have heightened sensitivity to smell, linked with substantial changes in tastes. Ensuring minimal exposure to the smell of food cooking is important.

Refocus oral intake on preferred foods, in preferred amounts, at preferred times (rather than a 'balanced' diet where people eat what they think that they need at set times).

Check hydration status (tissue turgor, tachycardia, hypotension) and carefully reverse any deficit.

Pharmacological intervention

Choose medications to treat nausea by considering the underlying pathophysiology.

For metabolic causes of nausea, haloperidol (0.5–3.0 mg orally or SC at night regularly).

CNS causes may respond to dexamethasone (4–8 mg orally or SC daily).

Evidence of gastroparesis should be treated with metoclopramide (10 mg orally or SC four times daily). If there is any suspicion of GIT obstruction, pro-peristaltic agents such as metoclopramide or domperidone should be avoided. Aperients should also be stopped completely.

Cytotoxic-induced nausea and vomiting should be pre-emptively managed with antiemetics prior to treatment (dexamethasone 4–8 mg immediately, lorazepam 0.5–1.0 mg SL immediately), during treatment (5-HT$_3$ antagonists/dexamethasone, aprepitant (selective NK-1 antagonist), metoclopramide), and after therapy (dexamethasone, metoclopramide).

Medications such as chlorpromazine or levomepromazine may be useful in people with nausea not responding to other therapies.

Further reading

Dorman S (2021). Nausea and vomiting (Chapter 8.2). In: *Oxford Textbook of Palliative Medicine*, 6th ed. Oxford: Oxford University Press. Available at: https://doi.org/10.1093/med/978019 8821328.003.0053

Unheralded vomiting

Onset of symptom

Vomiting is the forceful expulsion of the gastric contents through the mouth and is feared.

Acute onset (<24 h) of vomiting

- **History of new medications:** check that new pro-peristaltic agents (metoclopramide or domperidone, sennosides) have not been added in someone with the potential of a bowel obstruction (p.163).
- **Epigastric discomfort:** consider pre-pyloric ulceration secondary to anti-inflammatories or glucocorticoids (especially if the person is on both).
- **Known cerebral metastases or leptomeningeal disease:** consider an acute increase in intracranial pressure including acute intracranial bleed, ventricular obstruction causing acute hydrocephalus, or a rise in pressure due to tumour progression. There is often no preceding nausea, and vomiting can occur at any time.
- **Bowel obstruction:** the more proximal the bowel obstruction, the more likely the person is to have unheralded vomiting. The obstruction does not need to be a total obstruction and so the person may still be passing flatus and stool (p.163).

Subacute onset (1–3 days) of unheralded vomiting

- **Nausea associated with movement:** consider cerebellar metastases or irritation of the vestibular apparatus.
- **Ascites or gross hepatomegaly:** squashed stomach can lead to unheralded vomiting that worsens as the pressure crushing the stomach worsens (p.166).

Can you modify anything contributing to the symptom?

In upper GIT obstruction, advice about having small volumes of clear fluids frequently is crucial for minimizing vomiting for many people with advanced disease. The volume of gastric secretions can be reduced using a H_2 receptor antagonist (ranitidine 300 mg orally twice daily or 50 mg SC four times daily). Proton pump inhibitors (PPIs) reduce the volume of upper GIT secretions to a lesser extent.

Reducing cerebral oedema with any cause of raised intracranial pressure is important. Use of glucocorticoids (oral dexamethasone 8 mg in the morning and at midday) may help to reduce cerebral oedema while the underlying exacerbating causes are defined.

In someone who is not cachectic, consider other methods of providing nutrition if vomiting is only related to an inoperable obstruction.

With raised intracranial pressure, exclude an undiagnosed subdural haematoma. With cerebral metastases, consider dexamethasone and whole brain radiotherapy. With obstructive hydrocephalus in someone who is otherwise well, consider a neurosurgical opinion for the insertion of a ventriculoperitoneal (VP) shunt.

What underlying factors cannot be improved?

Bowel obstruction, especially multilevel obstruction from malignant peritoneal seeding, will rarely be amenable to stenting, surgical bypass, or a defunctioning ileostomy.

A squashed stomach will continue to be symptomatic for most people.

Symptomatic treatment

Non-pharmacological intervention

Oral intake for squashed stomach relies on changing oral intake to small frequent snacks.

In bowel obstruction, oral fluids will continue to be tolerated unless the obstruction includes the jejunum, duodenum, or stomach.

Pharmacological intervention

If there is any suspicion of GIT obstruction, pro-peristaltic agents such as metoclopramide or domperidone should be avoided. Aperients should also be stopped completely in suspected GIT obstruction.

In addition to regular ranitidine, hyoscine butylbromide 20 mg SC every 4 h regularly is likely to help with any colicky pain.

If an obstruction is not settling, there is little to be gained by adding octreotide. If a short trial is considered, octreotide 100–200 micrograms SC three times daily regularly may help to reduce frequency and volume of vomiting in some people.

Further reading

Dorman S (2021). Nausea and vomiting (Chapter 8.2). In: *Oxford Textbook of Palliative Medicine*, 6th ed. Oxford: Oxford University Press. Available at: https://doi.org/10.1093/med/9780199 8821328.003.0053

Watson M et al. (eds) (2019). Gastrointestinal symptoms (Chapter 9). In: *Oxford Handbook of Palliative Care*. 3rd ed. Oxford: Oxford University Press. Available at: https://doi.org/10.1093/med/9780198745655.003.0009

Fever

Symptoms of sepsis with a very acute onset are much more likely to be either bacterial or viral infections.

In people with progressive life-limiting illnesses, elderly people, and those on long-term immunosuppression (including glucocorticoids), signs of sepsis may be muted.

Fever may also be due to non-infectious causes.

Onset of symptom

Acute onset (<24 h) of fever and ...

- **Recent cytotoxic chemotherapy:** although some agents are less likely to cause neutropenia, check differential neutrophil counts in all people who have recently had chemotherapy (p.184). (Busulphan, melphalan, and procarbazine cause late myelosuppression (6–8 weeks after administration).)
- **Epidural or intrathecal lines:** consider both meningitis and epidural abscess in people with long-term lines.
- **Lymphoedema, severe peripheral oedema, or peripheral skin damage including tinea:** consider cellulitis which may present with very subtle changes initially.
- **Cough or shortness of breath:** community-acquired pneumonia or an infective exacerbation of long-term obstructive lung disease needs to be treated (p.126). A new pulmonary embolus may also present with fever, shortness of breath, and chest pain. Fever is likely when a pleural infarct has occurred (p.119).
- **Guarding or rebound tenderness on abdominal examination:** frequently encountered causes include diverticulitis, cholecystitis, and appendicitis.
- **Urinary frequency, urgency, or dysuria:** any of these symptoms requires further investigation. In unilateral complete ureteric obstruction, urine analysis may not demonstrate any abnormality (p.282).
- **Myalgias and arthralgias:** these symptoms suggest a systemic viral infection or the constitutional symptoms of any severe sepsis.
- **Stents:** biliary or ureteric stents can harbour infection which may be difficult to treat without changing the stent.
- **Vascular devices:** check cannulae or central lines including peripherally inserted central catheter lines. Always attempt to take a set of blood cultures when the person is febrile through central lines if the person has one.
- **Known or suspected valvular heart disease:** always have a high index of suspicion for this being the source of sepsis or a 'sanctuary' site in the presence of recurrent sepsis (p.108).
- **Presence of ascites:** consider spontaneous bacterial peritonitis (or damaged bowel if there has been a recent drainage procedure) (p.166).
- **Recent or ongoing blood transfusion:** this may be a transfusion reaction. An incorrect cross-match is a medical emergency where the person develops fever and anaphylaxis.

- **Medications:** drug reactions may occur soon after commencing medications or months after ceasing a medication. This is often a diagnosis of exclusion.
- **Severe pain:** secondary to major insults such as bone fractures, a myocardial infarction, or gut ischaemia may precipitate fever.

Subacute onset (1–3 days) of fever

- **General influenza-like symptoms:** people with severe immunocompromise may develop symptoms and signs of sepsis over several days.
- **A palpable purpuric rash** suggests meningococcal septicaemia or a systemic vasculitis (p.92).
- **Disseminated malignancy:** fever may represent progressive disease, new liver metastases, or a paraneoplastic phenomenon.

Insidious onset (days to weeks) of fever

- **History of B symptoms:** the person with an established history of sweats, particularly at night, lethargy, and weight loss suggests lymphoma and may mask underlying sepsis.
- **Previous treatment for sepsis:** the person may not have had an adequate length of treatment or had a poor choice of antibiotics, and recrudescence of infection is likely in this setting. Areas of infection that may also have a poor blood supply (such as head and neck cancers) may require longer courses of antibiotics. The other major cause for inadequate treatment is that there is an underlying fungal infection which has not been identified. CNS and respiratory tract infections are sites to consider. Any foreign substances (stents, valves, central venous catheters) need to be considered as sanctuary sites.
- **Endocrine disturbances:** hyperthyroidism may present with fever, tachycardia, and sweating. This may be a complication from a recent iodine load from radiological contrast (p.235).

Can you modify anything contributing to the symptom?

Life expectancy will be cut short by failure to recognize neutropenic sepsis. Urgently establish IV access, commence fluid resuscitation, and, having taken blood cultures (including from any central venous catheters), commence broad-spectrum antibiotics. Combinations include an aminoglycoside (with levels monitored every other day) and an anti-pseudomonal lactam (ticarcillin–clavulanate or piperacillin–tazobactam) or ceftazidime.

Sepsis, even late in disease, should be treated with the aim of improving the person's comfort or function (including cognition).

In the late stages of a life-limiting illness, treating sepsis is rarely with the aim of changing prognosis but with the focus on achieving good symptom control. In the terminal phase (the last hours or days of life before this infection), treatment is symptomatic.

Neoplastic fevers may respond to either dexamethasone 4 mg daily or an NSAID (naproxen 750–1000 mg daily). Sometimes benefit will be gained from oral cimetidine 400 mg twice daily. Prior to commencing dexamethasone, it is important to exclude infection as the cause of fever.

Fevers from bone fractures, infarcts, or ischaemia may settle with management of the underlying problem. Regular paracetamol may be of benefit.

What underlying factors cannot be improved?

Recurrent or untreatable sepsis may occur in the setting of irreversible pathology. Infection distal to large airway obstruction or in obstructed urinary or biliary systems may be difficult to treat in the presence of continued obstruction. Systemic sepsis should be controlled, but recurrence is highly likely in these settings.

Symptomatic treatment

Non-pharmacological intervention

Fever should be actively treated with paracetamol (1 g three times daily orally or 500 mg three times daily rectally) in people in the terminal stages who cannot swallow and are febrile.

Pharmacological intervention

- Sepsis with an absolute neutrophil count of $<1.0 \times 10^9$/L (febrile neutropenia):
  - Empirical broad coverage including *Pseudomonas aeruginosa*.
  - Gentamicin 4–6 mg/kg daily IV plus ceftazidime 1 g every 8 h IV or ticarcillin 3g/clavulanate 0.1 g every 6 h IV.
  - Add vancomycin 1 g IV every 12 h if person is severely shocked or known to be colonized with methicillin-resistant *Staphylococcus aureus* (MRSA).
- CNS sepsis—intrathecal line:
  - Cover must include staphylococci until Gram stain or cultures are available.
  - Vancomycin 500 mg IV every 6 h plus ceftriaxone 2 g IV every 12 h.
- CNS—epidural abscess:
  - Cover for *S. aureus*.
  - Flucloxacillin 2 g IV every 6 h plus gentamicin 4–6 mg IV daily.
- Lower urinary tract sepsis:
  - Cover for *Escherichia coli*, *Staphylococcus saprophyticus*:
    - first choice: oral trimethoprim 300 mg daily for 3 days
    - second choice: oral amoxicillin 500 mg + clavulanate 125 mg every 12 h for 5 days.
  - Additional cover for *P. aeruginosa*: oral norfloxacin 400 mg every 12 h for 3 days.
- Upper urinary tract infection:
  - Ampicillin 1 g IV every 6 h plus gentamicin 4–6 mg/kg IV daily in someone with normal renal function.
  - In penicillin hypersensitivity, use aminoglycoside alone or ceftriaxone 1 g daily IV.
- Lower respiratory tract sepsis:
  - Cover for *Streptococcus pneumoniae*, *Mycoplasma pneumoniae*, *Chlamydia pneumoniae*, and *Legionella* species:
    - first choice: benzylpenicillin 1.2 g IV every 6 h plus oral roxithromycin 300 mg daily for 7 days (plus gentamicin if Gram-negative bacilli seen on sputum stain)
    - second choice: with a history of reaction to penicillin, ceftriaxone 1 g IV daily or, with immediate hypersensitivity to penicillin, oral moxifloxacin 400 mg daily for 7 days.

- Empyema:
  - Cover for *Streptococcus pneumoniae/milleri/anginosus*:
    - first choice: ticarcillin 3 g + clavulanate 0.1 g IV every 6 h.
  - Cover for *S. aureus*:
    - first choice: dicloxacillin 2 g IV every 6 h.
  - Cover for MRSA: vancomycin 1 g IV every 12 h.
- Cellulitis:
  - Cover for *Streptococcus pyogenes* and *S. aureus* (especially with pre-existing wounds):
    - first choice: dicloxacillin 2 g IV every 6 h
    - second choice (penicillin hypersensitivity): cephazolin 1 g IV every 8 h
    - second choice (immediate penicillin hypersensitivity): clindamycin 450 mg IV every 8 h.
- Suspected infective endocarditis:
  - Broad-spectrum cover until cultures available. Contact cardiothoracic surgery and infectious diseases as soon as possible. Consider interventions in the light of prognosis before this episode of sepsis:
    - first choice: benzylpenicillin 1.8 g IV every 4 h plus dicloxacillin 2 g IV every 4 h plus gentamicin 4–6 mg/kg daily in normal renal function
    - second choice (history of sensitivity to penicillin): vancomycin 1 g IV every 12 h plus gentamicin 4–6 mg/kg IV daily.
- Biliary tree sepsis:
  - Cover: usually Gram-negative sepsis:
    - first choice: ampicillin 2 g IV every 6 h plus gentamicin 4–6 mg/kg IV (plus metronidazole 500 mg IV every 12 h if there has been previous biliary tract surgery)
    - second choice: ceftriaxone 1 g IV daily if previous hypersensitivity to penicillin.
- Spontaneous bacterial peritonitis:
  - Cover: usually Gram-negative bacilli *E. coli*:
    - first choice: ceftriaxone 1–2 g IV daily.

Further reading

Cohen J, Khatamzas E (2020). Infection in the immunocompromised host (Chapter 8.2.4). In: *Oxford Textbook of Medicine*, 6th ed. Oxford: Oxford University Press. Available at: https://doi.org/10.1093/med/9780198746690.003.0072

Ryan R, Casey R (2021). Endocrine and metabolic complications of advanced cancer (Chapter 14.9). In: *Oxford Textbook of Palliative Medicine*, 6th ed. Oxford: Oxford University Press. Available at: https://doi.org/10.1093/med/9780198821328.003.0084

Care in the last hours of life

Diagnosing dying

This is a diagnosis that clinicians must make actively.

The diagnosis of dying for most people with a life-limiting illness is a diagnosis of an expected event. If there are unexpected changes in condition, clinicians need to exercise careful clinical judgement in the assessment of any easily reversible causes for the deterioration.

For most people with a life-limiting illness, the terminal phase of their illness is a progression of the systemic pathology—a final common pathway characterized by increasing fatigue and lethargy, anorexia, and weight loss.

This is a catabolic state in which there are few bodily reserves for unexpected insults such as infection. Once established, the cachexia syndrome cannot be reversed without addressing the underlying cause(s) of the life-limiting illness.

Progressive cachexia is seen in all life-limiting illnesses (cancer, end-stage organ failure, neurodegenerative diseases, or AIDS). Most obviously, this process is reflected in the rate of change of functional status—systemic change not related to the sites of symptoms or underlying pathology.

At first, the rate at which decline can be noted is measured over months, but this gradually accelerates so that the time period during which change can be recognized shortens. As this decline is noticed, ensure that long-term medications are reviewed and that the goal of each of these medications is known. Continuation of long-term medications should only be to prevent likely and immediate symptomatic problems as a person's condition starts to deteriorate (p.81).

The time period for change is also an estimate of future life expectancy. If function is declining by the week, prognosis is probably measured in weeks unless there is a clearly reversible cause for the deterioration.

The person who is dying from cachexia spends more time in bed, and is increasingly dependent on help with activities of daily living. The last hours or days of life are generally associated with:

• profound lethargy
• decreasing periods of wakefulness
• decreasing peripheral perfusion, often with progressive hypotension and hypoxaemia
• increasing clouding of consciousness or drowsiness.

What underlying factors can be improved?

Up to one in three people who are dying are likely to experience distressing symptoms including **pain**, **breathlessness**, or **agitation**. The person dying and their family will be distressed by uncontrolled symptoms. Continue with symptom control medications at the doses that the person has required until this time.

History

Although a person is dying, a careful assessment of the likely causes of **pain** is required which includes a review of the person's past experiences of pain and requirements for good analgesia.

Breathlessness is a feared symptom in the terminal phase of a life-limiting illness. Consider the person's history of lung disease, comorbidities, and current frailty. Many people will develop noisy respirations sometimes referred to as the 'death rattles'. While the evidence is sparse, this is more likely in people who have previously required medications that administer a high anticholinergic load (p.68), people who are ventilated, and those with primary lung cancers, CNS malignancy, respiratory infections, or pulmonary oedema.

Agitation, with or without confusion, is prevalent and can be very distressing. Identified risk factors for developing delirium include male sex, progressive frailty, hearing or visual impairment, and CNS malignancy.

Physical examination

An unsettled or uncomfortable dying person is a clinical emergency. Physical examination is targeted to exploring easily reversible cause(s).

Investigations and management

Investigations are very rarely indicated at this time.

Ensure that all medications for **pain** are continued appropriately.

Check pulse oximetry. With low-flow oxygen, try and maintain saturation above 90%.

Symptomatic treatment

Non-pharmacological intervention

Ensure that the person is positioned for comfort. This includes avoiding putting someone with pleural effusion on the side with the unaffected lung in a dependent position or positioning the person to avoid painful areas (sacral pressure sores, known bony metastases).

Given **increasing immobility**, place the person on an air mattress whenever possible. This limits the number of times the person needs to be repositioned and helps with skin care in dependent areas.

Involvement of family/carers: if it is the dying person's wish, ensure that the people important in this person's life are aware that time is now measured in hours to days. Encourage people to continue to talk to the person and continue to hold and touch them, even if there appears to be little response.

Privacy: ensure an environment which balances privacy for the person and their family with excellent attention to detail in nursing care. Ensure that when the person is no longer able to check that they are adequately clothed or covered, caring health professionals attend to modesty.

Good mouth care: keeping the mouth moist, especially if the person is mouth breathing, can involve both family and staff. This intervention will help to lessen the sensation of thirst.

Noisy respirations: if the secretions have pooled in the pharynx, provide the person with 30° head elevation. Reassure family and friends that noisy respirations in someone with a diminished level of consciousness are unlikely to cause distress to the dying person.

Breathlessness: check pulse oximetry and use oxygen only if the person has an oxygen saturation that is <90%. Ensure careful positioning to maximize respiratory function.

Acute confusional state (delirium): ensure a quiet and softly lit environment. Minimize noise from visitors. Ensure that visitors and staff provide quiet reassurance. Exclude pain, breathlessness, urinary retention, or constipation as a cause of agitation.

Fear or anxiety: this can be an overwhelming feeling at times for people at the end of life, even in the last hours of life if existential issues are at the forefront of their mind. Allow the person, if able, to describe their fears rather than provide false or glib reassurance.

Pharmacological interventions

The route of administration of medications may need to change as oral intake diminishes. Always use the simplest route of administration (e.g. SL) and avoid unnecessary use of infusion pumps. (People do *not* need to have an infusion pump to be comfortable as they die.)

Noisy respirations: ensure that this is not simply cardiac failure or iatrogenic fluid overload. Use hyoscine butylbromide 20 mg SC every 4 h regularly if there has been a response. Even with adequate treatment, noisy respiratory secretions can continue to be a problem. If cardiac failure/fluid overload is contributing to the problem, administer frusemide 20–40 mg SC immediately and apply a glycerol trinitrate 25 mg patch. Reduce or cease any parenteral fluid input.

With **breathlessness**, consider the use of regular opioids. For opioid-naïve people, start with 2.5mg morphine subcutaneously every 4 h. If previously on opioids, increase the dose by 25%. For those with known renal impairment or in the frail elderly, reduce the frequency of dosing to every 6-8 h. Evidence to support the use of other opioids for breathlessness is sparse.

Acute confusional states increase in frequency and severity as death approaches for many people. Agitated people at risk of harm to themselves or others may require a regular dose of a long-acting benzodiazepine such as oral lorazepam 1 mg every 12 h or clonazepam 0.5 mg SL every 12 h. Ensure that 'as-needed' subcutaneous midazolam is available (2.5–5.0 mg every 2–3 h). If a person is very distressed in the last hours or days of life, consider haloperidol 0.5–2.5 mg SC daily. In younger, less cachectic people (e.g. with primary CNS malignancies) higher doses may be needed. Olanzapine wafers can be used.

Fear or agitation: having excluded easily reversible causes and treated any delirium, consider a regular dose of a long-acting benzodiazepine such as oral lorazepam 1 mg every 12 h or clonazepam 0.5 mg SL every 12 h. Ensure that breakthrough SC midazolam is available (2.5–5.0 mg 2- to 3-hourly).

Further reading

Kite S, Hurlow A (2020). Care of the dying person (Chapter 7.4). In: *Oxford Textbook of Medicine*, 6th ed. Oxford: Oxford University Press. Available at: https://doi.org/10.1093/med/978019 8746690.003.0066

Watson M et al. (eds) (2019). The terminal phase (Chapter 30). In: *Oxford Handbook of Palliative Care*. 3rd ed. Oxford: Oxford University Press. Available at: https://doi.org/10.1093/med/9780198745655.003.0030

Catastrophic terminal events

History

While catastrophic terminal events such as haemorrhage or airway obstruction are very uncommon, the risk is real and causes anxiety and distress for the person who is dying, their family, and staff. Some events are unexpected but consider if there are risk factors: fungating wounds close to major airways or arteries, lung or head and neck cancers obstructing airways, or clotting disorders.

Physical examination

This should not delay the administration of medication. If the cause of the acute event is not immediately obvious, physical examination is indicated as this may point to the underlying problem. For example, a gut perforation will be associated with a rigid abdomen.

Investigations and management

Investigations at the time of such an event are very rarely indicated. However, when considering the risk of such an event, having previously reviewed available, relevant imaging may help to plan care.

Forewarning families of the possibility of such an event can be challenging. However, if a home death is planned for a person at risk of a catastrophic event, the family need to be advised of this with this discussion including providing the family with strategies to address the event should it occur, including non-pharmacological measures such as green towels in the event of haemorrhage.

While the evidence that informs management of such events is limited, qualitative reports highlight that experienced palliative care nurses have stressed the importance of **remaining with the person who is dying**, always ensuring that they are not left alone.

Such events are acknowledged as very distressing for all involved. This reiterates that families are offered support and counselling after the event. Similarly, health professional team debriefings should be organized.

Crisis medications

In such a crisis, it is important to ensure that the person does not suffer. On such occasions in opioid- and benzodiazepine-naïve people, one would use a crisis order such as morphine 10 mg IV and midazolam 5 mg IV. **Do not** use the SC route in this setting.

The issue becomes more complex when people are using opioids, benzodiazepines, or both. In such cases there would need to be at least a 50% increase in the background dose of their medication.

It is imperative that these medications are made immediately available to ensure the comfort of the person and to acknowledge that the comfort of those around them—their family and friends—is equally important. Leaving doses drawn up at the bedside is the best way to ensure this.

Further reading

Watson M et al. (eds) (2019). The terminal phase (Chapter 30). In: *Oxford Handbook of Palliative Care*, 3rd ed. Oxford: Oxford University Press. Available at: https://doi.org/10.1093/med/9780198745655.003.0030

Implantable defibrillators

History

The number of people affected by heart failure is increasing. This in turn has led to an increase in the use of implantable cardioverter defibrillator (ICD) devices. Such devices can not only extend life by preventing cardiac arrest by treating life-threatening cardiac arrhythmias but also improve quality of life. However, when people are dying, it is unlikely that the defibrillator will contribute to a quality of death. Estimates have suggested that at least one-third of people in the last 24 h of life will experience one or more painful shocks, a situation that may be distressing for the person, their family, and health professionals.

Investigations and management

While the use of defibrillators is increasing, previous investigations suggest that may people are not engaged in discussions regarding deactivation of the device at the time of insertion of the ICD or even later in the disease.

Ideally, discussions regarding the benefits of deactivating the defibrillator should be prompted earlier in the disease trajectory and not the final stages of life. Triggers for these crucial conversations include:

- at the time of insertion of the ICD
- when 'not for resuscitation' orders are placed
- in the presence of refractory heart failure symptoms despite maximal therapy
- advancing cachexia
- the presence of other progressive comorbid illnesses.

The decision to deactivate an ICD needs to be made collaboratively by the person (or their proxy decision-maker) and the healthcare team involved in the person's care. Information about the device should be sought from the centre where it was implanted, including details regarding the most appropriate technician to contact. If the person's prognosis is very limited, every healthcare facility should have access to a bar or clinical ring magnet which will temporarily deactivate the defibrillator. This may be taped in place if needed.

Further reading

Pantilat S et al. (2021). Advanced heart disease (Chapter 15.3). In: *Oxford Textbook of Palliative Medicine*, 6th ed. Oxford: Oxford University Press. Available at: https://doi.org/10.1093/med/9780198821328.003.0091

Making a request for organ donation

History

Organ transplantation is a highly effective treatment for advanced organ failure but, worldwide, the number of people who would benefit from transplantation far outweighs the numbers of donations. This continues despite strategies to address the issue. One strategy to improve the rates of organ donations is encouraging health professionals to identify potential donors. If a person is identified as a potential candidate, it is imperative that they are provided with the same high-quality care as any other person. The quality of care received by people before their death is one significant factor that strongly influences their family's decision to proceed to organ donation.

Investigations and management

The most important step is to consider whether a dying person might be a suitable candidate for donation and then alerting the transplant coordinators in a timely way. There are few medical contraindications to organ donation with the exception of malignancy (although corneas can still be donated), infectious diseases, and evidence that a transplanted organ is unlikely to function. With regard to infectious diseases, syphilis, HIV, hepatitis B virus, West Nile virus, encephalitis of unknown cause, Creutzfeldt–Jakob disease, malaria, and tuberculosis (TB) are of major concern. While organs from people <50 years of age are likely to be more successfully transplanted as the demand for organs continues to climb, more older people are becoming organ donors.

Even when people have identified that they wish to be organ donors, it is still imperative that the relatives of the dying person are engaged. Despite the fact that many countries have adopted systems where universal consent for organ donation is implied by failure to opt out, one of the most common reasons that organ donation does not proceed is family refusal. This observation highlights the need for well-trained staff to work with the person who is dying and their family. Other factors that improve engagement with families include a pause between the communication that their family member is not likely to survive and the approach by a clinician who is part of the transplant team (while not dressed in surgical garb).

Further reading

Einav S et al. (2021). Palliative medicine in the intensive care unit (Chapter 3.3). In: *Oxford Textbook of Palliative Medicine*, 6th ed. Oxford: Oxford University Press. Available at: https://doi.org/10.1093/med/9780198821328.003.0013

Specific clinical presentations

Specific clinical presentations

Chapter 2

Clinical pharmacology

Medications with a narrow therapeutic index 60

Medications with non-linear pharmacokinetics 61

Medications that interact with warfarin 62

Medications that are contraindicated when on a monoamine oxidase inhibitor 64

Washout times for antidepressants 65

Serotonin syndrome 66

Anticholinergic load 68

Malignant hyperthermia 70

Palliative medications that require dose modification in renal failure 71

Palliative medications that require dose modification in hepatic failure 73

Medications that are highly protein bound 74

Medications that are metabolized by cytochrome P450 75

Deprescribing (for comorbid disease) 81

Medications with a narrow therapeutic index

Many medications have a relatively narrow therapeutic index and, as such, need monitoring of plasma levels of free drug. Careful monitoring is needed to avoid toxicity and to ensure adequate therapeutic effect. These medications include:

- antibiotics: gentamicin, amikacin, tobramycin, vancomycin
- anticoagulants: warfarin
- antiarrhythmics: digoxin, lidocaine, procainamide, quinidine, amiodarone, perhexiline
- mood stabilizers: lithium, clozapine
- immunosuppressants: ciclosporin, tacrolimus
- antiepileptics: carbamazepine, phenytoin, sodium valproate, phenobarbitone, primidone
- other agents: theophylline, levothyroxine.

Other agents with relatively narrow therapeutic indices for which routine direct plasma level testing is not available include oral hypoglycaemic agents, most cytotoxic chemotherapies, disopyramide, monoamine oxidase inhibitors (MAOIs) (p.64), and insulin.

Further reading

Miles R et al. (2021). Principles of drug therapy (Chapter 7.5). In: *Oxford Textbook of Palliative Medicine*, 6th ed. Oxford: Oxford University Press. Available at: https://doi.org/10.1093/med/9780198821328.003.0038

Medications with non-linear pharmacokinetics

Most medications are eliminated by a *constant fraction* for each unit of time. The half-life in this model is constant at all times (first-order elimination). Elimination is exponential and a true half-life can be established.

When initiating therapy, a steady state will have been reached within five half-lives in this model. As medications are discontinued, within five half-lives there will be approximately 2% of the medication left in the body (assuming a single-compartment model of drug distribution).

A small number of medications have non-first-order (zero-order) elimination where a *constant amount* of the medication is eliminated for each unit of time. This is seen when a substance is metabolized by a specific enzymatic pathway that becomes saturated. In this model, the rate of clearance fails to increase with increasing concentrations. Clearance is linear, and a true half-life cannot be established as the half-life increases as plasma concentration increases.

This means that a small increase in dose (e.g. 10%) may lead to a very large increase in plasma level (e.g. 100%). Conversely, drug clearance will appear to accelerate at lower levels.

In palliative practice, medications that have non-first-order pharmacokinetics include:
- phenytoin
- theophylline
- salicylates
- ethanol.

Further reading

O'Shaughnessy K (2020). Principles of clinical pharmacology and drug therapy (Chapter 2.6). In: *Oxford Textbook of Medicine*, 6th ed. Oxford: Oxford University Press. Available at: https://doi.org/10.1093/med/9780198746690.003.0012

Medications that interact with warfarin

Warfarin interferes with vitamin K-dependent clotting factors (factors II, VII, IX, and X), and with protein C and protein S production.

There are several ways that warfarin levels can be affected including:
• modified drug metabolism (cytochrome P450 (CYP) pathways CYP3A4, CYP2C, and CYP1A2) (p.75)
• those medications that displace warfarin from plasma albumin (p.74)
• changes in vitamin K metabolism, especially with changes to gut flora with antibiotic use
• hypothyroidism may reduce degradation of anticoagulation factors.

Any change in medication (or a substantial change in diet) warrants close monitoring of the anticoagulant activity of warfarin. There are multiple simultaneous pathways that unpredictably affect the level of anticoagulation (Tables 2.1–2.3).

Antibiotics likely to reduce vitamin K-producing gut flora sufficiently to increase the effect of warfarin are:
• broad-spectrum penicillins (piperacillin–tazobactam, ticarcillin)
• second- and third-generation cephalosporins
• clindamycin.

When choosing antibiotics, consider narrow-spectrum agents with less chance of changing gut flora: penicillin, amoxicillin, ampicillin, dicloxacillin, first-generation cephalosporins, and tetracycline.

Table 2.1 Medications causing increased anticoagulation when on warfarin

Symptom control	
Analgesics	Paracetamol, dextropropoxyphene
Antidepressants	SSRIs, venlafaxine
Anticancer therapy	
Hormone therapies	Tamoxifen
HIV/AIDS	
Antivirals	Ritonavir
Intercurrent illnesses	
Oral hypoglycaemic agents	Glibenclamide
Antiarrhythmics	Propranolol, amiodarone, quinidine
Antibiotics	Co-trimoxazole, erythromycin, clarithromycin, isoniazid, metronidazole, ciprofloxacin, tetracycline
Antifungals	Fluconazole, itraconazole, ketoconazole, miconazole
Antiepileptics	Phenytoin
Other agents	Alcohol (with liver disease), allopurinol, statins, methylphenidate, thyroxine, cimetidine, omeprazole, piroxicam

Further reading

Keeling D (2020). Therapeutic anticoagulation (Chapter 16.16.2). In: *Oxford Textbook of Medicine*, 6th ed. Oxford: Oxford University Press. Available at: https://doi.org/10.1093/med/978019 8746690.003.0376

Table 2.2 Medications causing decreased anticoagulation when on warfarin

Intercurrent illnesses	
Antibiotics	Dicloxacillin
Antifungals	Griseofulvin
Antiepileptics	Phenobarbital, carbamazepine
Other agents	Vitamin K, sucralfate

Table 2.3 Medications with unpredictable effects on anticoagulation

Symptom control	
Glucocorticoids	Prednisolone
Anticancer therapy	
Cytotoxic therapy	Cyclophosphamide
Intercurrent illnesses	
Antiepileptics	Phenytoin
Other agents	Cholestyramine, ranitidine, statins, propylthiouracil

Medications that are contraindicated when on a monoamine oxidase inhibitor

There are two groups of MAOIs: irreversible inhibitors (phenelzine, tranylcypromine, isocarboxazid) which block type A (deaminates nor-epinephrine and serotonin) and type B monoamine oxidases (deaminates dopamine and tyramine), and reversible inhibitors (moclobemide) which reversibly block type A monoamine oxidases.

Non-reversible blockade of MAOIs can cause problems with:

- pethidine (hypertension, sweating)
- tramadol (serotonergic syndrome)
- dextromethorphan
- other opioids including morphine—use with caution (isolated case reports of hypotension, drowsiness)
- selegiline
- ephedrine (in cough/cold preparations—hypertension)
- amphetamines (hypertension)
- methylphenidate (hypertension)
- clomipramine
- venlafaxine
- SSRIs (serotonergic syndrome)
- oral hypoglycaemic agents (enhanced hypoglycaemic effects)
- insulin (enhanced hypoglycaemic effects)
- tricyclic antidepressants (serotonin syndrome)
- modafinil
- cheeses/aged meats/brewed beers.

Further reading

Cowen PJ (2020). Psychopharmacology in medical practice (Chapter 26.4.1). In: *Oxford Textbook of Medicine*, 6th ed. Oxford: Oxford University Press. Available at: https://doi.org/10.1093/med/9780198746690.003.0625

Washout times for antidepressants

- Tricyclic antidepressants (amitriptyline, clomipramine, imipramine, nortriptyline, dothiepin, doxepin, trimipramine): taper dose by 25% per day and then allow 2–4 days before commencing another antidepressant.
- SSRIs (citalopram, escitalopram, fluvoxamine, paroxetine, sertraline): taper gradually (25% per day). Allow 2–4 days before commencing another antidepressant.
- Fluoxetine: allow 1 week before starting another antidepressant, except for MAOIs, when 5 weeks of washout should be allowed.
- Venlafaxine: taper by 25% per day and allow 1–2 days before starting a new antidepressant.
- Mirtazapine and mianserin: withdraw gradually (25% per day) and then wait 2–4 days before starting a new antidepressant.
- Moclobemide: no withdrawal reported. Allow 1–2 days before starting a new antidepressant.
- Non-reversible MAOIs (phenelzine, tranylcypromine): gradually taper to minimize withdrawal side effects. Observe a 1-week washout period when changing to another antidepressant, except for fluoxetine (5 weeks) or another MAOI (2 weeks). Continue a 3-week restriction on diet and other medications after discontinuation (p.64).

Symptoms associated with antidepressant withdrawal

With SSRIs, mirtazapine, mianserin, or venlafaxine, people may experience fatigue, myalgia, diarrhoea, nausea, light-headedness, dizziness, agitation, headache, or insomnia if long-term administration is stopped abruptly.

With tricyclic antidepressants, people may experience a syndrome of cholinergic rebound characterized by increased saliva, runny nose, diarrhoea, or abdominal cramping and insomnia.

Further reading

Cowen PJ (2020). Psychopharmacology in medical practice (Chapter 26.4.1). In: *Oxford Textbook of Medicine*, 6th ed. Oxford: Oxford University Press. Available at: https://doi.org/10.1093/med/9780198746690.003.0625

Serotonin syndrome

Serotonin syndrome is the consequence of sufficient exposure to medications with serotonergic properties (Box 2.1).

Box 2.1 Causes of serotonin syndrome

- Tricyclic antidepressants and (any of) clonazepam, alprazolam, lithium, SSRIs, or thioridazine.
- MAOIs and (any of) L-tryptophan, dextromethorphan, SSRIs, pethidine, or clonazepam.
- Single agent or combinations involving SSRIs, serotonin and norepinephrine reuptake inhibitors (SNRIs), tramadol, sumatriptan, buspirone or carbamazepine.

History

Clinically, this syndrome may manifest with:
- changed mood (anxiety, agitation, restlessness, and hypomania)
- an acute confusional state, or
- neurological changes.

Serotonin syndrome is a diagnosis of exclusion (given the wide range of aetiologies for the clinical presentation).

Physical examination

- Changes in affect may include:
  - anxiety
  - hypervigilance
  - pressured speech.
- Neurological dysfunction may include:
  - tremor, myoclonus
  - increased tone
  - hyper-reflexia
  - poor coordination
  - horizontal ocular clonus.
- Autonomic dysfunction may include:
  - tachycardia
  - labile blood pressure
  - tachypnoea
  - sweating
  - increased bowel sounds in moderate to severe manifestations
  - increased temperature (a sign of more severe manifestation)
  - sialorrhoea.

Investigations and management

Serotonergic syndrome is a diagnosis of exclusion. Ensure that there are no infectious or metabolic causes for these symptoms and establish a temporal relationship with the introduction of a serotonergic medication.

Poor prognostic factors include:
- raised temperature (>41°C)
- raised creatinine kinase or myoglobinuria, or
- any evidence of rhabdomyolysis especially if associated with worsening renal function.

Other complications with a poor prognosis include disseminated intravascular coagulation (DIC) (p.196) and seizures (p.249).

A serotonergic syndrome is usually self-limiting and settles in <7 days.
- Stop the offending medication(s).
- Use anticonvulsants for seizures, agitated behaviour, or neuromuscular dysfunction.
- Use benzodiazepines for any rigidity.
- Use dantrolene for hyperthermia along with non-pharmacological cooling measures.

Further reading

Caraceni A et al. (2021). Neurological problems in advanced cancer (Chapter 14.8). In: *Oxford Textbook of Palliative Medicine*, 6th ed. Oxford: Oxford University Press. Available at: https://doi.org/10.1093/med/9780198821328.003.0083

Anticholinergic load

Many medications have a level of anticholinergic activity. When taken together, they generate an 'anticholinergic load'.

Introducing an additional medication with anticholinergic activity can cause a patient to manifest anticholinergic symptoms, with blame placed on the medication most recently introduced. Most often, anticholinergic load is the cumulative effect of all the medications being taken with anticholinergic activity. If the most recently introduced medication is important for symptom control, it is worth considering a review of other medications that could be ceased to reduce the anticholinergic load and allow the medication for symptom control to continue.

Clearance of many medications that have anticholinergic activity decreases with age.

The **most common classes** associated with moderate to marked anticholinergic activity are:
• antipsychotics
• antidepressants
• medications to improve urinary continence
• antihistamines.

Medications **marketed for their anticholinergic activity** include glycopyrrolate, oxybutynin, benztropine, and propantheline.

Symptom control medications widely used in palliative care with a high anticholinergic load include (but are not limited to) all opioids, dexamethasone, benzodiazepines, prochlorperazine, promethazine, and loperamide.

Medications for comorbid conditions that are widely encountered in palliative care clinical practice include (but are not limited to) frusemide, warfarin, digoxin, fluticasone–salmeterol, prednisolone, famotidine, ranitidine, nifedipine, and diltiazem.

History

Clinically, try to establish a relationship between the onset of symptoms and the introduction of a medication that may have worsened the person's anticholinergic load.

Clinical manifestations of anticholinergic side effects typically can include:
• dry mouth and dry eyes
• vomiting
• constipation
• reduced sweating
• flushing
• tachycardia and arrythmias
• dizziness
• difficulty concentrating
• acute cognitive impairment/delirium/agitation/seizures
• urinary retention
• dilated pupils
• blurred vision
• precipitating narrow-angle glaucoma.

Physical examination

Symptoms due to an increased anticholinergic load need to be considered, especially when investigating delirium (p.246) that has no other obvious cause.

Carefully examine cardiovascular and ocular systems. Evaluation of cognition, especially for loss of executive function or fluctuations in function, is important.

Investigations and management

Treat any symptomatic manifestations directly.

Review all medications and consider medications that may not be necessary in the short to medium term. (Many medications for symptom control have significant anticholinergic load and their use may take precedence over medications for long-term comorbidities that are not active.)

If a medication cannot be ceased, is there another medication that could be reduced or ceased to lessen the anticholinergic load? Can a medication with a lower anticholinergic load be substituted to achieve the same (or similar) therapeutic benefit?

Malignant hyperthermia

Malignant hyperthermia is almost always caused by exposure to anaesthetics (fluranes, halothane, or succinylcholine). Rare causes in people with susceptibility include a viral illness or exposure to statins.

It is characterized by a rapidly rising temperature, muscle rigidity and/or spasms, tachycardia or tachyarrhythmias, and tachypnoea.

History

The disorder is transmitted through an autosomal dominant gene.

With a family history and previous exposure to anaesthetic agents without harms, still consider malignant hyperthermia as its manifestation may be idiosyncratic.

Physical examination

Look for:
- tachycardia or tachyarrhythmia
- tachypnoea
- sweating and mottled skin
- increased muscle tone.

Investigations and management

In evaluating the person's tachypnoea, there may be evidence of a rapid deterioration in blood oxygenation (and rising carbon dioxide if it is measured).

Check creatinine kinase—rising levels may reflect a degree of rhabdomyolysis.

Except in someone who is already in the terminal stages of their illness, consider active supportive measures including the following:
- Dantrolene (2.5 mg/kg rapid IV bolus) repeated as necessary helps to reduce the release of calcium into muscles.
- Cool the person's body.
- Administer oxygen to maintain adequate saturations.
- Establish IV access and ensure adequate hydration.

Further reading

Hilton-Jones D, Edwards R (2020). Metabolic and endocrine disorders (Chapter 24.19.4). In: *Oxford Textbook of Medicine*, 6th ed. Oxford: Oxford University Press. Available at: https://doi.org/10.1093/med/9780198746690.003.0611

Palliative medications that require dose modification in renal failure

In most clinical settings, medications in established but stable renal impairment can be adjusted by either reducing the dose or increasing the dose interval in accordance with the degree of renal impairment. In elderly patients, renal excretion of medications tends to decrease. (The volume of distribution also tends to increase in elderly patients as muscle is replaced by increased adipose tissue.)

Renal elimination of a medication relies on glomerular filtration tubular excretion, or tubular resorption.

Medications that can worsen renal failure need to be stopped, if possible, if renal function is deteriorating.

Analgesics

Morphine and codeine are metabolized to morphine-3-glucuronide and morphine-6-glucuronide which are renally cleared. Dextropropoxyphene's metabolite, norpropoxyphene, can also accumulate in renal impairment, with reports of cardiac toxicity. (Fentanyl and buprenorphine do not require dose adjustment in renal impairment.)

Although glucuronide and sulphide metabolites of paracetamol are renally excreted, the dose is not usually adjusted in renal failure.

NSAIDs cause a reversible decrease in glomerular filtration rate in people with pre-existing renal impairment which may severely compromise renal function and cause hyperkalaemia. Indomethacin and diflunisal are renally excreted. Sulindac in equipotent doses may inhibit the cyclooxygenase pathway less than other NSAIDs.

Benzodiazepines

Diazepam metabolites can accumulate in severe renal impairment (glomerular filtration rate (GFR) <10 mL/min). Nitrazepam, temazepam, and midazolam can be used.

Medications for frequently encountered comorbidities

Digoxin levels need to be carefully followed with changing renal function, with lower loading and maintenance doses. Amiodarone doses should be reduced for GFR <20 mL/min. Diuretics (especially potassium-sparing diuretics such as spironolactone, triamterene, and amiloride) and angiotensin-converting enzyme inhibitors should be reviewed carefully in people with worsening renal function at the end of life.

Antibiotics

Caution is needed with aminoglycosides and vancomycin in renal failure, with careful monitoring of trough levels on a regular basis.

For people with GFR <20 mL/min, adjust dose down by a percentage for the following: amoxicillin–clavulanic acid (50%), benzyl penicillin (maximum of 20 mU/day), trimethoprim (50%), piperacillin–tazobactam (50%), and ceftazidime (75%).

Anticoagulants

Low molecular weight heparins need dose reduction in people with renal impairment. Monitor warfarin as it may be less protein bound. Hypoalbuminaemia leads to increased sensitivity to warfarin.

CNS medications

- Lithium doses need to be carefully monitored.
- Phenothiazines and butyrophenones do not need dose adjustment.
- Reduce doses for vigabatrin and gabapentin.
- Valproate and carbamazepine doses can be given unchanged.
- Protein binding of phenytoin decreases in renal failure and more free drug may be found in plasma, requiring a dose reduction.

Oral hypoglycaemic agents

Gliclazide, glipizide, and gliquidone are the safest sulphonylureas to use but must be adjusted down if GFR is <10 mL/min. Biguanides (e.g. metformin) should not be used if GFR is <20 mL/min because of a prolonged half-life.

Bisphosphonates

Bisphosphonates can still be used in renal impairment, especially if hypercalcaemia is contributing to poor renal function. Use doses at the lower end of the range, and in people with significant renal impairment (<20 mL/min) infuse pamidronate at a maximum of 20 mg/h.

Further reading

Watson M et al. (2019). Renal failure (Chapter 18). In: *Oxford Handbook of Palliative Care*, 3rd ed. Oxford: Oxford University Press. Available at: https://doi.org/10.1093/med/9780198745655.003.0018

Palliative medications that require dose modification in hepatic failure

Hepatic function does not correlate well with changes in drug metabolism, plasma estimates, or potential toxicity. Medications that rely on hepatic metabolism in people with severe hepatic impairment may need to have another medication substituted or, if that is not possible, the dose should be adjusted accordingly (Table 2.4).

Table 2.4 Medications which require dose reduction in severe hepatic impairment

Symptom control	
Antidepressants	Amitriptyline, clomipramine (increased sedation)
Analgesic	Codeine,[a] morphine,[a] paracetamol[b]
Antiemetics	Metoclopramide
Benzodiazepines	Clonazepam,[a] diazepam[a]
Anticancer therapy	
Antineoplastic agents	Cyclophosphamide, cytarabine, doxorubicin, methotrexate[b]; vinblastine, vincristine
HIV/AIDS	
Antivirals	Indinavir, lopinavir, ritonavir (reduce in moderate hepatic impairment), saquinavir, zidovudine
Intercurrent illnesses	
Antibiotics	Amoxicillin + clavulanic acid (increased risk of cholestasis), clindamycin, doxycycline, metronidazole
Anticoagulants	Warfarin, heparin[c]
Antiepileptics	Carbamazepine,[c] phenobarbital, phenytoin
Immunosuppressants	Azathioprine, ciclosporin
Hypoglycaemics	Glibenclamide, metformin (withdraw)
Antihypertensives	Nifedipine, propranolol, verapamil
Antipsychotics	Chlorpromazine
Other agents	Allopurinol, theophylline, medroxyprogesterone, promethazine, ranitidine

[a] Avoid or titrate more carefully than usual in order to avoid precipitating encephalopathy or coma.
[b] Dose-related toxicity.
[c] Reduce in severe hepatic dysfunction.

Paracetamol (especially in the setting of chronic alcohol use, when glutathione stores may be depleted) may lead to unexpected toxicity.

Drugs bound to albumin may have a greater risk of toxicity due to decreased protein production (p.74).

In severe hepatic impairment, or in cases of a porto-systemic shunt, decreased first-pass metabolism may allow increased bioavailability, leading to toxicity.

When considering anticoagulants, not only can clearance of warfarin be reduced in liver disease but clotting factor production can also be reduced.

Medications that are highly protein bound

Medications that are highly protein bound will compete with other highly protein-bound medications. Displacement of a medication can lead to rapid rises in plasma concentrations because so little drug is normally free in the plasma.

Binding can occur to albumin, β-globulin, or α_1-acid glycoprotein. Renal failure, inflammation, fasting, and malnutrition will tend to displace medications from protein binding. (The proportion of a medication that is bound to protein can be considered to have no biological effect.)

Medications that are highly plasma bound and can displace each other include:
- warfarin
- aspirin
- phenytoin
- diazepam
- propranolol.

Medications that are metabolized by cytochrome P450

CYP is a family of haemoproteins responsible for metabolism, including many medications. Although predominantly found in the liver, they are also present in the wall of small intestines, kidneys, and lung.

Induction of enzyme pathways by drug A lowers the available levels of drug B (subtherapeutic levels) and may take as long as weeks to become clinically apparent. The same time frame is required for effects to disappear once the relevant medication has been stopped.

Inhibition of CYP enzymatic pathways by drug A mean that more of drug B will be available (toxicity); this develops over days.

CYP3A4 accounts for the metabolism of >50% of all medications (Table 2.5). In order, the next most important pathways are CYP2D6 (Table 2.6), CYP1A2 (Table 2.7), CYP2C/9/10/19 (Table 2.8), and CYP2B6 (Table 2.9).

Table 2.5 CYP3A4 isoenzyme (>50% of all medications are metabolized through this pathway)

Substrates	
Symptom control	
Analgesics	Alfentanil, paracetamol, dextromethorphan, methadone
Antidepressants	Amitriptyline, imipramine, mirtazapine, sertraline, venlafaxine, fluvoxamine
Steroids	Cortisol, prednisolone
Antiepileptics	Carbamazepine
Benzodiazepines	Alprazolam,[a] clonazepam, diazepam, midazolam, triazolam
Other hypnotics	Zopiclone
Anticancer therapy	
Antineoplastic agents	Cyclophosphamide, paclitaxel, vinblastine, etoposide, imatinib
Hormonal agents	Tamoxifen, testosterone, progesterone, flutamide, oestrogen
HIV/AIDS	
Antivirals	Saquinavir, ritonavir, indinavir
Antifungals	Miconazole, ketoconazole, fluconazole, itraconazole
Intercurrent illnesses	
Anticoagulants	Warfarin

(Continued)

Table 2.5 (Contd.)

Antibiotics	Clarithromycin, erythromycin
Antiarrhythmics	Amiodarone, digoxin, quinidine, lidocaine
Immunosuppressants	Ciclosporin, tacrolimus
Antipsychotics	Haloperidol, risperidone, ziprasidone, olanzapine, quetiapine, chlorpromazine
Antihypertensives	Amlodipine, diltiazem, verapamil, disopyramide, enalapril, felodipine, nifedipine
Other agents	Statins, cisapride, omeprazole, terfenadine, loratadine
Inducers	
CYP3A4	Carbamazepine, phenytoin, barbiturates, modafinil, oral contraceptives, ciclosporin, ritonavir, nevirapine, efavirenz
Antiepileptics	Carbamazepine, phenytoin, phenobarbital
Glucocorticoids	Dexamethasone, prednisolone
Other agents	Modafinil, ciclosporin, ritonavir, nevirapine, efavirenz
Inhibitors	
Analgesics	Propoxyphene
Antidepressants	Fluoxetine, fluvoxamine, paroxetine, sertraline
Antibiotics	Clarithromycin, erythromycin, metronidazole, norfloxacin
Antifungals	Fluconazole, itraconazole, ketoconazole, miconazole, clotrimazole
Antiarrhythmics	Quinidine
Antihypertensives	Diltiazem, verapamil, nifedipine
Antiretrovirals	Indinavir, ritonavir, saquinavir
Antineoplastic agents	Imatinib
Other agents	Cimetidine, grapefruit juice

* Not available in the *British National Formulary*.

NB: the CYP3A4 isoenzyme's activity decreases with age—lower doses will be needed for the same clinical effect (CYP2D6 function does not appear to change with age).

Table 2.6 CYP2D6 isoenzyme (25% of all medications are metabolized by this pathway)

Substrates	
Symptom control	
Analgesics	Codeine, oxycodone, morphine, methadone, hydrocodone, pethidine, tramadol, dextromethorphan
Antidepressants	Amitriptyline, nortriptyline, doxepin, desipramine, imipramine, citalopram, fluoxetine, fluvoxamine, paroxetine, venlafaxine
Antiemetics	Ondansetron
Anticancer therapy	
Antineoplastic agents	Paclitaxel, vinblastine
Hormonal agents	Tamoxifen, testosterone
HIV/AIDS	
Antivirals	Saquinavir, ritonavir, indinavir
Intercurrent illnesses	
Antiarrhythmics	Propranolol, metoprolol, labetalol, mexiletine, flecainide, quinidine, lidocaine
Immunosuppressants	Ciclosporin, tacrolimus
Antipsychotics	Chlorpromazine, haloperidol, trifluperidol, risperidone, olanzapine, clozapine
Antihypertensives	Captopril
Other agents	Methylphenidate, dexamphetamine, omeprazole, loratadine, perhexiline
Inducers	
Antiepileptics	Carbamazepine, phenytoin, phenobarbital
Antivirals	Ritonavir
Inhibitors	
Analgesics	Methadone
Antidepressants	Citalopram, clomipramine, desipramine, fluoxetine, paroxetine, fluvoxamine, sertraline, moclobemide
Antiarrhythmics	Amiodarone, quinidine
Antipsychotics	Haloperidol, thioridazine
Other agents	Cimetidine

NB: the CYP2D6 isoenzyme has genetic polymorphism. Two per cent of the population have multiple copies, leading to very rapid substrate metabolism.

Table 2.7 CYP1A2 isoenzyme (>15% of all medications are metabolized by this pathway)

Substrates	
Symptom control	
Analgesics	Paracetamol, methadone, phenacetin
Antidepressants	Amitriptyline, clomipramine, desipramine, fluvoxamine, imipramine, mirtazapine
Benzodiazepines	Diazepam
Antiemetics	Ondansetron
Anticancer therapy	
Antineoplastic agents	Procarbazine
Hormonal agents	Tamoxifen, flutamide
HIV/AIDS	
Antivirals	Ritonavir
Intercurrent illnesses	
Anticoagulants	Warfarin
Antibiotics	Clarithromycin
Antipsychotics	Haloperidol, olanzapine, clozapine
Antiarrhythmics	Lidocaine
Antihypertensives	Verapamil
Other agents	Theophylline, caffeine
Inducers	
Antiepileptics	Phenytoin, phenobarbital
Antivirals	Ritonavir
Acid suppressants	Omeprazole
Other agents	Cigarette smoke, cruciferous vegetables
Inhibitors	
Antidepressants	Fluvoxamine, paroxetine
Antibiotics	Clarithromycin, erythromycin, ciprofloxacin, norfloxacin
Antifungals	Ketoconazole
Other agents	Grapefruit juice, cimetidine, omeprazole

Table 2.8 CYP2C9, -10, and -19 isoenzymes

Substrates	
Symptom control	
Analgesics	NSAIDs
Antidepressants:	Tricyclic antidepressants, fluoxetine (CYP2C9), citalopram (CYP2C19), moclobemide (CYP2C19)
Antiepileptics	Sodium valproate, phenytoin, phenobarbital (CYP2C19)
Other agents	Tetrahydrocannabinol, diazepam (CYP2C19)
Anticancer therapy	
Antineoplastic agents	Cyclophosphamide, paclitaxel
Hormonal agents	Tamoxifen, testosterone, progesterone
Intercurrent illnesses	
Anticoagulants	Warfarin
Antiarrhythmics	Amiodarone, propranolol
PPIs	Omeprazole, lansoprazole
Other agents	Glibenclamide (CYP2C9), fluvastatin (CYP2C9)
Inducers (CYP2C9/10 only)	
Antiepileptics	Carbamazepine (CYP2C19 also), phenobarbital
Glucocorticoids	Dexamethasone
Other agents	Ethanol
Inhibitors	
Antidepressants:	Fluoxetine, fluvoxamine, sertraline (all CYP2C9/19), paroxetine (CYP2C9)
Antibiotics	Clarithromycin, erythromycin, metronidazole, norfloxacin
Antifungals	Fluconazole, ketoconazole (CYP2C9/10)
Antiarrhythmics	Amiodarone (CYP2C9/19)
Antivirals	Ritonavir
Other agents	Cimetidine, omeprazole (CYP2C9/10), clopidogrel (CYP2C9), bupropion (CYP2C9), modafinil (CYP2C19)

NB: the CYP2C19 isoenzyme has genetic polymorphism.

Table 2.9 CYP2B6 isoenzymes

Substrates	
Symptom control	
Analgesics	Methadone
P450 enzymatic pathway inducers	
Antiepileptics	Phenobarbital

NB: the CYP2B6 isoenzyme has genetic polymorphism.

Further reading

Miles R et al. (2021). Principles of drug therapy (Chapter 7.5). In: *Oxford Textbook of Palliative Medicine*, 6th ed. Oxford: Oxford University Press. Available at: https://doi.org/10.1093/med/9780198821328.003.0038

O'Shaughnessy K (2020). Principles of clinical pharmacology and drug therapy (Chapter 2.6). In: *Oxford Textbook of Medicine*, 6th ed. Oxford: Oxford University Press. Available at: https://doi.org/10.1093/med/9780198746690.003.0012

Deprescribing (for comorbid disease)

Many people with a life-limiting illness have comorbid conditions.

Is that comorbidity still active (or likely to become active if the medication were ceased)?

Evaluating all of a person's medications is a constant role for clinicians and, ideally, should involve a pharmacist.

Therapeutic goal of prescribing

Why was a medication commenced?

Has the person had a sufficient therapeutic trial (dose and duration)?

Consider whether a medication was commenced for primary, secondary, or tertiary prevention.

- If for primary prevention, almost all medications can be ceased late in the course of a life-limiting illness.
- If for secondary or tertiary prevention, weigh up the benefits and risks for each medication in light of the burden of each comorbid disease and its likely clinical path. Generally, medications for established disease that is active (or is likely to become active relatively quickly) should be ceased with caution, and then only late in the course of a life-limiting illness.

The potential to cease a medication

What are the likely risks from ceasing a medication? If there are risks, in what time frame will these occur?

Is there a known withdrawal syndrome if the medication is ceased? If so, does the dose need to be tapered?

Equally, what is the risk of a medication being continued, especially as a person's health deteriorates with a life-limiting illness? For example, continuing antihypertensives as a person loses weight may expose them to the risk of symptomatic hypotension, with the potential for falls or syncope.

Further reading

Ahmed E (2021). The contribution of the clinical pharmacist in palliative care (Chapter 4.12). In: *Oxford Textbook of Palliative Medicine*, 6th ed. Oxford: Oxford University Press. Available at: https://doi.org/10.1093/med/9780198821328.003.0027

Chapter 3

Dermatological problems

Severe cutaneous adverse reactions (SCARs) 84
Hypersensitivity reactions 87
Angio-oedema 90
Cutaneous vasculitis 92
Warfarin-induced skin necrosis 94
Chemotherapy-induced acral erythema 95
Skin reactions to targeted antineoplastic agents and
    immunotherapy 96

Severe cutaneous adverse reactions (SCARs) :☠:

SCARs refer to a group of clinical presentations that include Stevens–Johnson syndrome (SJS)/toxic epidermal necrolysis (TEN), drug reaction with eosinophilia and systemic symptoms (DRESS), acute generalized exanthematous pustulosis (AGEP), and generalized bullous fixed drug eruptions (GBFDE).

Each SCAR has characteristic cutaneous presentations, causative medications, clinical courses, and treatments (Table 3.1).

Table 3.1 SCARs

Type	Description	Causes
SJS/TEN	Mucosal erosions or ulcers with variable extents of skin detachment 1–4 weeks after commencing index medication Skin lesions are usually flat and target-shaped on the trunk, often becoming confluent and blistered Systemic symptoms may develop, which include fever, general malaise, flu-like symptoms, and, at times, other organ involvement SJS is classified as skin detachment involving <10% of body surface area compared with TEN where it is >30%. For those involving 10–30%, they are classified as SJS/TEN overlap	Anticonvulsants Sulfa-containing drugs Antibiotics NSAIDs Uric acid-lowering agents
DRESS	Severe systemic hypersensitivity drug reaction characterized by widespread rash, facial oedema and systemic symptoms including fever, hypotension, lymphadenopathy, evidence of visceral organ involvement, and often eosinophilia	Anticonvulsants Anti-infectious agents (antibiotics, antiviral, drugs for TB) Sulfonamides Uric acid-lowering medications
AGEP	1–11 days after commencing the index medication. Sudden onset of multiple non-follicular pustules on oedematous erythema These may be accompanied by facial swelling and blisters	Pristinamycin Ampicillin/amoxicillin Quinolones Hydroxychloroquine Anti-infective sulfonamides Terbinafine Diltiazem

History

SJN, TEN, and SJN–TEN are variants of the same problem. It manifests 4–28 days after drug exposure. People present with **fever** and malaise, cough, myalgia, arthralgia, increasing breathlessness (pneumonitis), rhinorrhoea, and conjunctivitis or conjunctival ulceration. The skin lesions are typically **'target' lesions** with three rings: bright red or pink inner ring, a lighter middle ring, and a dark outer ring. These will blister and desquamate. People may develop mouth or genital ulcers. GIT involvement causes diarrhoea.

DRESS syndrome presents 2–8 weeks after starting the index medication. People present with non-specific fever and rashes but may also have hepatitis, pneumonitis, and colitis.

AGEP presents as a burning, itchy scarlatiniform erythematous rash with semi-small pustules occurring abruptly 1–4 days after commencing antibiotics.

Physical examination

- SJN/TEN/SJN–TEN:
  - Target **lesions which confirm the diagnosis**.
  - Examine the mouth and genitalia for ulcers.
  - Examine the abdomen for right upper quadrant tenderness (associated hepatitis).
  - Evaluate the person's hydration status as there may be considerable fluid loss through the blistered lesions and diarrhoea. This is further complicated if the person has difficulty in swallowing due to lesions in the mouth and upper GIT.
  - Ensure careful evaluation of the eyes.
- DRESS syndrome:
  - Urticarial and maculopapular eruptions.
  - Vesicles, bullae, pustules, purpura, and target lesions may be present.
  - Examine for facial oedema.
  - Most common visceral problems include myocarditis, pericarditis, hepatitis, pneumonitis, nephritis, and colitis. Visceral pathology is the major cause of morbidity and mortality.
- AGEP:
  - Examine for pustules in axillary and inguinal folds.
  - Examine the mouth for oral mucosa involvement.

Investigations and management

Prognosis measured in hours to days prior to the onset of this problem (symptom control)

- The emphasis of care of these patients is supportive, regardless of prognosis.
- Immediately cease the causative medication, despite limited prognosis.
- If patients have loose bowel actions, consider octreotide (100 micrograms SC three times daily).

- Hydrate parenterally. This may require IV hydration with extensive skin damage. Extensive skin or mucosal lesions may be painful, and adequate analgesia must be available. If skin damage is severe, use sterile paraffin for open areas.
- Treat conjunctivitis with proactive eye care.

Prognosis measured in weeks prior to the onset of this problem (in addition to symptom control)

- **Cease medication(s)** that may be responsible.
- Check **full blood count** (FBC) for neutrophilia to suggest superimposed infection, and **serum EUC** for renal function given large fluid losses.
- Check **hepatic function** as hepatitis may be present.
- If there are extensive blisters or the person is febrile, consider superimposed infections of the skin and collect blood cultures.
- An urgent dermatological consult should be sought.

Prognosis measured in months to years prior to the onset of this problem (in addition to the above)

Seek dermatological advice as those with extensive disease require transfer to a high dependency unit for management similar to extensive burns.

The following investigations and treatments must be initiated while transfer is organized:

- Rehydrate with 0.9% NaCl IV.
- Check serum EUC (prerenal failure), LFTs (hepatitis), amylase (pancreatitis), arterial blood gases (respiratory failure), blood cultures, FBC, and coagulation studies (coagulopathy).
- Commence deep vein thrombosis (DVT) prophylaxis (enoxaparin 40 mg daily).
- Commence a PPI (omeprazole 40 mg IV daily).
- Provide analgesia with patient-controlled analgesia (PCA).

Seek urgent advice regarding the specific treatment which may include corticosteroids, immunoglobulins, ciclosporin, or plasmapheresis.

The mortality rates of SJS/TEN and DRESS worsen with the age and extent of skin involved.

Further reading

Walsh S (2020). Cutaneous reactions to drugs (Chapter 23.16). In: *Oxford Textbook of Medicine*, 6th ed. Oxford: Oxford University Press. Available at: https://doi.org/10.1093/med/978019 8746690.003.0565

Hypersensitivity reactions ☠

A pathological interaction of an allergen with the immune system generates a hypersensitivity reaction (Table 3.2).

Table 3.2 Types of hypersensitivity reaction

Types	Common types
Type I	
Immediate reaction mediated by immunoglobulin (Ig) E leading to mast cell degranulation, releasing histamine and other inflammatory mediators	Within 1 h of exposure to allergen people present with asthma, food allergy, allergic conjunctivitis, anaphylactic shock
Type II	
Cytotoxic reactions mediated by IgG and IgM antibodies, leading to the complement system activation, and cell damage or lysis	Within 2–24 h of exposure to allergen, people present with anaemia, thrombocytopenia, renal failure, myasthenia gravis or Graves' disease depending on the autoantibody target
Type III	
Immune complex reactions mediated by IgG, IgM, and sometimes IgA, leading to complement system activation and tissue damage	Within 4–10 days of exposure to allergen people present with serum sickness, post-streptococcal glomerulonephritis, systemic lupus erythematosus (SLE), farmers' lung (hypersensitivity pneumonitis), or rheumatoid arthritis
Type IV	
Delayed-type mediated by T cells or macrophages which are activated secondary to cytokine release, leading to tissue damage	After exposure to an allergen, people will present with either contact dermatitis, drug fever, granulomatous response, or drug-induced hypersensitivity syndrome

History

- **Type I:** seek exposure to allergens including foods (e.g. shellfish, nuts, soy, wheat, eggs), animal sources (e.g. insect bites, cats, dogs, rats and other vermin) environmental factors (e.g. mould, dust mites, pollen, latex). Check for a history of atopic conditions such as dermatitis or asthma, and previous allergic reactions, previous wheezing, pruritus, or abdominal pain.
- **Type II:** check for a history of blood transfusions (incompatible blood), or recent medications.
- **Type III:** history will depend on the route of entry of the allergen. For example, a local injection may result in a necrotizing skin lesion while an inhaled allergen may lead to hypersensitivity pneumonitis.

- **Type IV:** after a variable period of time after skin contact with the allergen, dermatitis will occur. Check clothing, preservatives or industrial chemicals, people's daily activities, occupation, and hobbies.

Physical examination

- **Type 1:** the most severe type I reaction is anaphylaxis characterized by widespread rash, hypotension, tachycardia, audible wheeze, and impaired cognition.
  - In less severe cases, examine for widespread rash, rhinorrhoea, and periorbital oedema.
- **Type II:** physical examination depends on the reaction. Excessive destruction of red cells may lead to jaundice as opposed to thrombocytopenia where people may demonstrate widespread petechiae, bruising, or bleeding gums.
- **Type III:** examine the skin for changes of autoimmunity such as a malar rash.
  - Examine for joint tenderness suggestive of synovitis or swelling suggestive of arthritis.
- **Type IV:** examine for scaly, erythematous rash suggestive of contact dermatitis. Some people may develop much more serious skin changes such as SJS/TEN.
  - Check for a fever.

Investigations and management

Prognosis measured in hours to days prior to the onset of this problem (symptom control)

The most acute, life-threatening hypersensitivity reaction is anaphylaxis.

If there is a clear temporal relationship between the onset of the skin changes and systemic symptoms, then the management is clear. Even at the very end of life, consider administering:

- adrenaline 1:1000 (0.3–0.5 mL) intramuscular (IM)/SC, and
- dexamethasone 8 mg SC or hydrocortisone 100–300 mg IV, and
- cyclizine 12.5–25 mg SC, and
- salbutamol 0.5 mg SC.

These medications have been selected as they can be given SC and are available in palliative care units. The aim is to alleviate wheeze and respiratory distress due to laryngeal oedema.

Simultaneously, abdominal pain should be managed with opioid analgesia and sedation provided for respiratory distress. Oxygen may improve comfort in the presence of hypoxaemia.

Prognosis measured in weeks prior to the onset of this problem (in addition to symptom control)

Ensure IV access and start fluid hydration to maintain the blood pressure. Give:

- adrenaline 1:1000 IM (0.3–0.5 mL) immediately and repeated in 5 min, and
- diphenhydramine IV 25–50 mg, and
- ranitidine 50 mg IV immediately and then three times daily, and

- hydrocortisone 100–300 mg IV immediately, and
- inhaled salbutamol 2.5–5.0 mg four times daily if bronchospasm present.

It is important to keep these people under close observation as there may be a second phase of reaction 8–24 h later.

Prognosis measured in months to years prior to the onset of this problem (in addition to the above)

If the diagnosis is not clear, these people require an electrocardiogram (ECG) and measurement of cardiac enzymes, FBC, serum histamine, and tryptase levels.

Further reading

Klenerman P (2020). Adaptive immunity (Chapter 4.3). In: *Oxford Textbook of Medicine*, 6th ed. Oxford: Oxford University Press. Available at: https://doi.org/10.1093/med/9780198746 690.003.0040

Angio-oedema ☼

- Angio-oedema is the clinical presentation of either a genetic or acquired deficiency of the C1 inhibitor (Table 3.3).
- Angio-oedema describes the physical symptom of a circumscribed swelling of the skin, respiratory tract, or GIT.

Table 3.3 Causes of angio-oedema

Congenital angio-oedema	Acquired angio-oedema
Hereditary angio-oedema type I	B-cell malignancies (multiple myeloma, Waldenström's macroglobulinaemia, B-cell lymphoma, chronic lymphocytic leukaemia)
Hereditary angio-oedema type II	
Oestrogen-dependent angio-oedema	
	Medications (angiotensin-converting enzyme (ACE) inhibitors), beta-lactam antibiotics, NSAIDs

History

People present with recurrent episodes of **circumscribed swelling (angio-oedema)** but without urticaria. This is not itchy and is more likely to be described as burning rather than painful. This swelling may be found over any body surface.

Other problems include **GIT problems** (nausea, vomiting, diarrhoea, abdominal pain) and respiratory problems (wheeze, shortness of breath, chest tightness).

Triggers to the attack include infections, medications (ACE inhibitors, oestrogen-containing medications), procedures, stress, and menstruation. A history of previous attacks or changes to medications must be sought.

Physical examination

- Episodes of **angio-oedema** may affect any part of the body, but often involve the extremities and the face. Typically the swelling is not red.
- The **abdomen may be tender** with guarding. People may be **dehydrated** due to fluid sequestered into the bowel.
- The voice may be hoarse indicating laryngeal oedema.
- An audible wheeze may be present. Breathless and frightened people with an audible wheeze, using accessory muscles of respiration, are a medical emergency. Seek immediate assistance.

Investigations and management

Prognosis measured in hours to days prior to the onset of this problem (symptom control)

People known to have hereditary angio-oedema who develop laryngeal oedema may still be more comfortable at this stage of life with administration of **C1 inhibitor replacement** (500 U if <50 kg, 1000 U if 50–100 kg, and 1500 U if >100 kg) IV infusion. Despite administering the concentrate, crisis medications (p.53) must still be available in the case of acute respiratory distress as the onset to effect may be as long as 1 h.

If there is no laryngeal oedema, this group should receive analgesia and gentle fluid replacement.

People who present with angio-oedema *de novo* (in the absence of systemic symptoms or urticaria to suggest an allergic response) should not undergo further investigations. These people require analgesia, gentle fluids, and crisis medications (p.53) on hand with the onset of respiratory distress.

Prognosis measured in weeks prior to the onset of this problem (in addition to symptom control)

People who present with their first episode of angio-oedema should be investigated for **complement levels** (C4, C2). The aim of diagnosing hereditary angio-oedema in people at this late stage of life is so that, if necessary, they can receive C1 inhibitor replacement with any subsequent episodes. People with acquired angio-oedema have antibodies to the C1 receptor, so they do not respond to replacement therapy. These people must have crisis medications (p.53) available as the risk of another acute episode of laryngeal oedema remains.

People with cutaneous swelling in the absence of laryngeal and gut mucosal involvement do not require intervention.

Prognosis measured in months to years prior to the onset of this problem (in addition to the above)

Acute onset of angio-oedema with laryngeal oedema should be considered a **medical emergency**. These people require transfer to a high dependency unit for stabilization of their airway, fluid management, analgesia, and investigations.

In people with hereditary C1 inhibitor deficiency, if C1 inhibitor replacement is not available or the diagnosis has not yet been established, intubation and tracheotomy may have to be performed with severe respiratory compromise. Once these people have been stabilized, investigations should be initiated. This should also occur in people who present with milder episodes.

Additional investigations include:
- HIV, T-lymphotropic viruses, and hepatitis serology
- LFTs, LDH, EUC, FBC, and thyroid function tests (TFTs).

An immunology consultation is required.

Further reading

Shpadaruk V, Harman KE (2020). Cutaneous vasculitis, connective tissue diseases, and urticaria (Chapter 23.7). In: *Oxford Textbook of Medicine*, 6th ed. Oxford: Oxford University Press. Available at: https://doi.org/10.1093/med/9780198746690.003.0556

Cutaneous vasculitis ☼

- Numerous vasculitic conditions present with cutaneous involvement (Box 3.1).
- When the skin is involved, **palpable purpura** help make the clinical diagnosis.
- Cutaneous vasculitis should prompt consideration of systemic vasculitis, especially in the presence of arthralgia, arthritis, haematuria, nausea, vomiting, diarrhoea, fatigue, or fever.

Box 3.1 Frequent causes of vasculitis

- **Infections:** bacterial (meningococcal, streptococcal, staphylococcal in particular), viral, fungal, parasitic.
- **Inflammatory disease:** SLE, rheumatoid arthritis, Behçet's disease, inflammatory bowel disease, ANCA-associated vasculitis, polyarteritis nodosa.
- **Drugs:** penicillins, sulphonamides, allopurinol, amiodarone, streptokinase, thiazides, and warfarin.
- **Paraneoplastic** (especially breast cancer).
- **Idiopathic**.

History

People present with **purpura** although they may also have papules, vesicles, bullae, pustules, ulcers, or urticaria. These may all be painful, itchy, or both.

The associated **systemic symptoms** may include fevers, arthralgia, myalgias, haemoptysis, cough, wheezing, sinusitis, numbness and tingling of the extremities, abdominal pain, haematuria, testicular pain, weight loss, night sweats, or painful red eyes.

Onset may be **catastrophic** with an acute abdomen (bleed, rupture, ischaemia), acute shortness of breath (pleural effusion, pulmonary bleed, myocardial ischaemia), or anuria (acute kidney injury).

Physical examination

- Examine the skin for **palpable purpura** and other skin lesions. Examine the mouth for ulcers.
- The eyes may be red and irritable (uveitis, conjunctivitis, retinitis).
- Palpate for tender sinuses.
- Inspect and palpate the hands and feet for joint deformities or digital infarcts.
- Auscultate the chest for a wheeze, fine crackles (fibrosis), or a pleural effusion. Check pulse oximetry.
- Examine for signs of heart failure (myocardial necrosis secondary to coronary artery inflammation).
- Examine the abdomen for tenderness and exclude an acute abdomen (pancreatitis, mesenteric angina or infarction, ruptured aneurysm, GI bleeding or gut oedema, intussusception).

Investigations and management

Prognosis measured in hours to days prior to the onset of this problem (symptom control)

- This is a clinical diagnosis and further investigations are not indicated.
- People who develop purpura without major systemic problems do not require intervention.
- For people with systemic manifestations, it is likely that vasculitis will hasten death.

Prognosis measured in weeks prior to the onset of this problem (in addition to symptom control)

This group requires consideration of the precipitating factors. Interventions depend on clinical severity:

- Mild cases may not require further treatments.
- More extensive cutaneous problems, without systemic symptoms require topical corticosteroids and antihistamines (promethazine 25 mg daily or twice daily).
- For severe cases, attention to symptoms and systemic corticosteroids is indicated (hydrocortisone 100 mg IV daily in a reducing dose).
- Treat hypertension if present.

Prognosis measured in months to years prior to the onset of this problem (in addition to the above)

This group requires investigations and treatment:

- FBC, serum EUC, LFTs.
- **Urinalysis** spun for active sediment.
- **Immunological screen** (complement levels, antinuclear antibodies, erythrocyte sedimentation rate (ESR), C-reactive protein (CRP), rheumatoid factor, antineutrophilic cytoplasmic antibodies).
- **Skin biopsy**.
- **Chest X-ray (CXR)** if there is clinical suspicion of infection or a pleural effusion.
- If there is no response to corticosteroids, other immunosuppressive treatments may be necessary and immunology/dermatology consults must be sought urgently.

Further reading

Shpadaruk V, Harman KE (2020). Cutaneous vasculitis, connective tissue diseases, and urticaria (Chapter 23.7). In: *Oxford Textbook of Medicine*, 6th ed. Oxford: Oxford University Press. Available at: https://doi.org/10.1093/med/9780198746690.003.0556

Warfarin-induced skin necrosis ⚙️

This is a rare but devastating complication of oral anticoagulant therapy.

It has been linked to people with hypercoagulable states (protein C or protein S deficiency, factor V Leiden, antiphospholipid antibodies, cancer, people who have had heparin-induced thrombocytopenia).

History

There is onset of numbness and tingling in well-circumscribed areas of the skin 3–7 days after commencing warfarin. Although this is the expected time of onset, the disorder has been noted in people years after commencing warfarin.

Following the sensory changes, erythematous skin lesions occur, which may be very painful. This is most likely to occur over the breasts, anterior thighs, and buttocks in women. Men have no particular pattern of skin involvement.

Physical examination

Initially, the physical examination may be unremarkable. Then, **erythematous lesions** surrounded by oedema may appear. These later develop into **haemorrhagic bullae**, which indicate full skin-thickness injury. Later an eschar forms, resulting in deep scarring.

Investigations and management

Prognosis measured in hours to days prior to the onset of this problem (symptom control)

- Warfarin should be discontinued and vitamin K 10 mg IM/IV administered.
- Commence LMWH as the aim is to prevent a hypercoagulable state.
- Once bullae appear, the process is irreversible.
- Adequate analgesia must be administered.

Prognosis measured in weeks prior to the onset of this problem (in addition to symptom control)

- Adequate analgesia must be available.
- It is unlikely these people will be well enough for surgical debridement and so good wound care is essential.

Prognosis measured in months to years prior to the onset of this problem (in addition to the above)

It is likely these people will require surgical debridement and skin grafting of the deeper scars. An early dermatological consultation should be sought. Options for long-term anticoagulation should be discussed with a haematologist.

Further reading

Keeling D (2020). Therapeutic anticoagulation (Chapter 16.16.2). In: *Oxford Textbook of Medicine*, 6th ed. Oxford: Oxford University Press. Available at: https://doi.org/10.1093/med/978019 8746690.003.0376

Chemotherapy-induced acral erythema ①

Acral erythema is a dose-dependent complication of chemotherapy that presents as painful, erythematous changes that affect the skin of the hands and feet (Table 3.4). It is also known as palmar–plantar erythrodysaesthesia, toxic erythema of the palms and soles, or hand–foot syndrome.

Table 3.4 Causes of acral erythema

Commonly implicated medications	Less commonly implicated medications
Doxorubicin	Bleomycin
Cytarabine	Cisplatin
Docetaxel	Cyclophosphamide
Capecitabine or infusional 5-fluorouracil	Daunorubicin
	Doxifluridine
	Etoposide
	Fludarabine
	Gemcitabine
	Hydroxyurea
	Idarubicin
	Ixabepilone
	Methotrexate
	Mitotane
	Paclitaxel
	Vinorelbine

History

Prior to visible skin changes, people will describe dysaesthesia of the palms and soles. This is followed by a painful, well-demarcated erythema which may progress to desquamation, erosion, and ulceration.

Investigations and management

Prognosis measured in hours to days prior to the onset of this problem (symptom control)

- This is a clinical diagnosis.
- Cease chemotherapy and apply topical, alcohol-free emollients.
- Actively manage wound care.
- Adequate analgesia including a medication for any neuropathic pain.

Prognosis measured in weeks prior to the onset of this problem (plus symptom control)

As above and, if tolerated, elevate the most affected area.

Prognosis measured in months to years prior to the onset of this problem (in addition to the above)

As above, and immediately discuss with medical oncology colleagues whether medication substitution or dose modification is required.

Skin reactions to targeted antineoplastic agents and immunotherapy ①

Targeted therapies and immunotherapies are associated with a wide range of dermatological adverse events resulting from common signalling pathways involved in malignant behaviour and normal homeostatic functions of the epidermis and dermis (Table 3.5).

Table 3.5 Causative systemic agents for skin changes in newer cancer therapies

Agents	Skin changes
Inhibitors of epidermal growth factor receptor inhibitor (EGFRI)	Acneiform rash
	Dry skin
	Widespread pruritis
	Dry mouth
	Photosensitivity
	SJS/TEN (very rarely)
BCR–ABL tyrosine kinase inhibitors	Maculopapular eruption
	Photosensitivity
	Periorbital oedema
	DRESS syndrome
	SJS/TEN
Vascular endothelial growth factor receptor (VEGFR)/platelet-derived growth factor receptor (PDGFR) inhibitors	Hand–foot syndrome
	Alopecia
	Dry skin
	Photosensitivity
	Keratoacanthoma
BRAF inhibitor-induced toxicities	Squamous cell carcinomas
	Changes in melanocytic lesions
	Hand–foot syndrome
	Maculopapular 'hypersensitivity-like' rash
BRAF plus MEK inhibitors	Acneiform rash
	Dry mouth
	Widespread pruritis
PI3K inhibitors	Maculopapular rash
	SJS/TEN
	DRESS syndrome
JAK inhibitors	Non-melanoma skin cancers
CDK inhibitors	Alopecia
	Maculopapular rash
	Pruritus

Table 3.5 (Cntd.)

Agents	Skin changes
CCR4 inhibitor	Psoriasis-like plaques
	Folliculitis
	SJS/TEN
Immune checkpoint inhibitors	Non-specific maculopapular rash
	Eczema-like or psoriatic lesions
	Lichenoid dermatitis
	Bullous pemphigoid
	SJS-like eruptions

History

Skin lesions are common adverse effects of targeted and immunotherapy. Skin lesions associated with these novel agents typically present 3–4 weeks after starting treatment. While for many people the skin changes are mild, for some, skin changes may impact quality of life and capacity to continue treatment.

A minority of people may develop more severe drug reactions such as hand–foot syndrome, SJS/TEN, or DRESS syndrome (p.84).

Physical examination

- There are many described skin toxicities that range from mild to life-threatening.
- Physical examination is important to define the extent and severity of skin changes.
- Exclude superimposed infection.

Investigations and management

Prognosis measured in hours to days prior to the onset of this problem (symptom control)

- Skin toxicity related to cancer treatments are a clinical diagnosis.
- It is most appropriate to cease treatments currently.
- If the changes are mild, no treatment is likely to be required.
- If changes are severe and distressing, systemic corticosteroids and analgesia may be required.
- If there are changes consistent with SJS/TEN, DRESS syndrome (p.84), or hand–foot syndrome (p.95), manage as previously outlined.

Prognosis measured in weeks prior to the onset of this problem (plus symptom control)

In addition to the management outlined for people with very limited prognosis, check for any signs of superimposed infection and, if present, consider antibiotics.

Prognosis measured in months to years prior to the onset of this problem (in addition to the above)

In addition to the urgent assessment and stabilization of the person, discuss with medical oncology whether medication substitution or dose modification is required.

Chapter 4

Cardiovascular problems

Acute cardiac decompensation *100*
Cardiac tamponade *104*
Pericarditis *106*
Infective endocarditis *108*
Thoracic aortic dissection *110*
Bleeding abdominal aortic aneurysm *112*
Cutaneous arterial bleed *114*
Acute limb ischaemia *116*
Venous thromboembolic disease *119*
Superior vena cava obstruction *122*

Acute cardiac decompensation ☠️

- This is the clinical presentation of cardiac output failing to match tissue perfusion needs (Table 4.1).
- Characterize acute cardiac decompensation as predominantly left- or right-sided.
- Most acute changes will be associated with left-sided systolic failure.
- Most people with acute cardiac decompensation will have known pre-existing pathology.

Table 4.1 Causes of acute cardiac decompensation in people with known pump failure

	Frequently encountered causes	Less frequently encountered causes
Cancer	People with previous treatment with anthracyclines	Arrhythmias associated with direct myocardial irritation by tumour
Intercurrent illnesses	Acute myocardial infarction Anaemia Alcohol Cardiac arrhythmias Fluid overload Mitral valve rupture	Beriberi Viral cardiomyopathy Poorly controlled diabetes

History

- **Left-sided cardiac failure** is predominantly characterized by (in order) exertional breathlessness, breathlessness at rest, orthopnoea, and paroxysmal nocturnal dyspnoea (often associated with audible wheeze for the first time in this person's life).
- **Right-sided failure** is characterized by oedema, ascites, anorexia, and nausea.
- Remember that the most severe left-sided cardiac failure may present with right-sided signs.
- **Silent myocardial ischaemia**, especially in elderly people or people with diabetes, needs consideration when someone has unexplained cardiac compromise.
- **High-output failure** can be caused by anaemia or thyrotoxicosis, especially in people who have had an iodine load (IV radiological contrast or use of amiodarone) or sepsis.
- At the end of life, even **small parenteral fluid** loads administered for 'comfort' can precipitate acute cardiac decompensation.
- **Cerebral impairment** results from decreased perfusion and oxygenation.
- Distinguish acute cardiac decompensation from the clinical presentations of abnormal water and sodium retention or hypovolaemia causing shock.

Physical examination

- These people will look very unwell, tired with breathlessness at rest or on minimal exertion.
- **Tachycardia** is frequently present with pulsus alternans (strong and weak pulses alternating).
- **Hypotension** may be the predominant finding in acute cardiac failure.
- **Decreased pulse pressure** and cyanosis highlight severe decompensation.
- On auscultation, third or fourth heart sounds may be heard.
- **Mid to late inspiratory crackles may be heard at the lung bases**, which may also be dull to percussion from pleural effusions.
- **Ascites, congestive hepatomegaly** (pulsatile in tricuspid regurgitation), and **dependent oedema** may be demonstrated. This may be worsened in the palliative setting because of hypoalbuminaemia.
- In chronic heart failure, **cachexia** may be the predominant finding.

Investigations and management

Prognosis measured in hours to days prior to the onset of this problem (symptom control)

People require rest, elevation of the head of the bed, and management of their symptoms. They do not require further investigations.

Morphine 2.5 mg IV/SC may be given as required for chest pain or breathlessness.

If there is chest pain, administer glyceryl trinitrate 600 micrograms SL immediately. If there is ongoing chest pain suggestive of cardiac ischaemia, commence regular opioids (morphine 2.5 mg SC every 4 h if opioid naïve, or increase the background dose by 25% and titrate to comfort) and topical nitrates (glyceryl trinitrate patch 25 mg daily).

It is possible to manage cardiac failure when people are no longer able to swallow:
- Furosemide 20–40 mg SC daily.
- Topical or SL nitrates.
- SC morphine.
- Oxygen may provide relief if a person is hypoxaemic.

People who are peripherally shut down may require IV rather than SC medications.

Prognosis measured in weeks prior to the onset of this problem (in addition to symptom control)

In this group, investigations are directed to establish the cause of acute decompensation:
- IV access must be established.
- ECG obtained to define cardiac rate, rhythm, and reflect a recent infarct.
- CXR will demonstrate enlargement of the heart chambers concerned. Distended pulmonary veins with redistribution of blood to the apices reflects acute left-sided cardiac failure. The lateral film may show right

ventricular enlargement in the retrosternal window suggesting fluid overload.
- Blood tests include **FBC** (anaemia, infection), **EUC** (renal failure, electrolyte abnormalities), **cardiac enzymes**, **TFTs**, and **LFTs** (congestive hepatic dysfunction).

The best management is to treat the cause:
- Anticoagulation (aspirin and LMWH) for acute myocardial infarction (exclude cerebral metastases, previous GIT bleeding, or recent surgery).
- Treat arrhythmias if they are causing the cardiac failure.
- Transfusion for anaemia.
- Carbimazole and beta-blockade for thyrotoxicosis.

Further management includes the following:
- **Rest, oxygen, and careful use of diuretics** (furosemide 40 mg daily or twice daily if not on diuretics or the addition of a second agent such as spironolactone 50 mg twice daily if already on diuretics).
- **ACE inhibitors** (lisinopril 2.5–5.0 mg twice daily) or **angiotensin receptor blockade** (irbesartan 75 mg daily). Start with low doses as these people are likely to be frail and may be at higher risk of adverse effects.
- **Vasodilators, topical nitrates** (25–50 mg daily), or **oral nitrates** (isosorbide 30–60 mg daily) may decrease breathlessness by reducing the preload. Monitor for headaches or postural hypotension.
- **Digoxin** is of value in cardiac failure. In this group, it is probably not necessary to reach therapeutic levels rapidly with a loading regimen. Ensure that renal function and electrolytes are normal and commence the person on an oral dose of 125 micrograms per day. Repeat drug levels in 7–10 days. Monitor blood pressure, heart rate, and the onset of unexplained nausea carefully.

Prognosis measured in months to years prior to the onset of this problem (in addition to the above)
- **Echocardiography** is useful in determining chamber size, cardiac function throughout the cardiac cycle, and valve function.
- **Hypotension** (systolic blood pressure <100 mmHg) indicates carcinogenic shock. This requires urgent transfer to a high dependency unit for inotrope support.
- **Hypertension** (systolic blood pressure >180 mmHg) may indicate hypertensive cardiac failure. Examine for encephalopathy. Organize immediate transfer to a high dependency unit for IV labetalol. (Do not give SL nifedipine as this may cause an uncontrollable drop in blood pressure.)
- **Acute myocardial infarction** must prompt immediate referral to cardiology for consideration of thrombolysis or angioplasty with stenting.
- **Acute valve dysfunction** secondary to ischaemia must also prompt immediate referral for consideration of surgery or a percutaneous procedure if appropriate.
- Presentation with cardiac failure and no obvious cause has a median prognosis of 6 months.

Further reading

Pantilat S et al. (2021). Advanced heart disease (Chapter 15.3) In: Oxford Textbook of Palliative Medicine, 6th ed. Oxford: Oxford University Press. Available at: https://doi.org/10.1093/med/9780198821328.003.0091

Ramrakha P, Hill J (eds) (2012) Heart failure (Chapter 7). In: Oxford Handbook of Cardiology, 2nd ed. Oxford: Oxford University Press. Available at: https://doi.org/10.1093/med/9780199643219.003.0007

Cardiac tamponade ☠

- In someone with unexplained breathlessness or hypotension, consider cardiac tamponade (Table 4.2).
- Its onset is often insidious with vague non-specific symptoms.
- The primary compromise is due to a rise in intrapericardial pressure leading to decreased ventricular filling and subsequent decreased cardiac output.

Table 4.2 Causes of pericardial effusion

	Frequently encountered causes	Less frequently encountered causes
Cancer	Malignant pericardial effusions (most often primary lung)	
End-stage organ failure	Uraemia	
Intercurrent illnesses	Acute viral pericarditis Pneumonia Trauma	Dissecting aortic aneurysm Myocardial infarction (Dressler syndrome, wall rupture) People with pericarditis treated with anticoagulants for other reasons Following thoracic surgery/invasive procedures Tuberculosis Hypothyroidism Inflammatory connective tissue diseases

History
- People often describe **breathlessness** and **tachypnoea** on exertion that worsens to air hunger at rest.
- **Postural symptoms** may predominate in people with hypotension.
- People may present **obtunded** or with a decreased level of consciousness.
- Other symptoms may include new-onset anorexia, dysphagia, or cough.

Physical examination
Physical findings need to be interpreted with care as findings are rarely 'classic'. A high index of suspicion is needed.
- Neck veins and veins in the forehead, scalp, and ocular fundi may be distended.
- Jugular venous pressure (JVP) may be elevated with a **positive Kussmaul's sign** (rise in JVP with inspiration). In rapidly developing tamponade, venous pulsations may be exaggerated because filling time is reduced.
- **Tachycardia** is frequent, although bradycardia may be seen, with uraemia or hypothyroidism as the underlying cause of tamponade.

- **Hypotension** with obvious shock and peripheral cyanosis are encountered late. **Pulsus paradoxus** (a drop of >10 mmHg of systolic pressure on inspiration) may be demonstrable. This will not be seen with severe compromise to cardiac output.
- An apex beat may still be palpable.
- Auscultation of the heart may reveal **muffled heart sounds** and a **pericardial rub**.

Investigations and management

Prognosis measured in hours to days prior to the onset of this problem (symptom control)

Investigations are not indicated. This is a clinical diagnosis. Treat breathlessness with opioids and anxiolytics (p.26). The presyncopal feeling as blood pressure gradually falls can be very frightening for people, and sedation may be necessary.

Prognosis measured in weeks prior to the onset of this problem (in addition to symptom control)

- **CXR** may show an enlarged, globular heart.
- An **ECG** may disclose alternating polarity for any waves, most typically the QRS complex, and at times the P wave (electrical alternans).
- **Echocardiography** may disclose the volume of the effusion, the chambers of the heart whose filling is affected by increased pericardial pressures, and whether there is loculation of the effusion. An echocardiograph may also disclose the septa moving to the left on inspiration and to the right on expiration. Chamber collapse is likely first on the right side of the heart and subsequently the left. Low-pressure tamponade relates to right-sided changes, has few classic signs, and occurs at pressures as low as 6–12 mmHg.
- Despite the limited prognosis of this group, a **pericardial drainage** should be considered.
- Ensure close monitoring while arranging a pericardiocentesis.
- Ensure that a large-bore intravenous cannula is in place.
- Check blood pressure frequently as circulatory collapse may occur without warning.
- Check **coagulation studies and platelet count** while arranging definitive treatment. **Discontinue anticoagulants**.
- In people with uraemic pericardial disease that is not causing critical haemodynamic compromise and who are already on dialysis, intensification of dialysis may control the effusion.

Prognosis measured in months to years prior to the onset of this problem (in addition to the above)

In people with probable bleeding or clot in the pericardium, or in whom there is likely to be effusive constrictive pericarditis, a surgical approach is required through a subcostal incision to create a pericardial window, having drained the contents of the pericardial sac.

Further reading

Ramrakha P, Hill J (eds) (2012). Cardiovascular emergencies (Chapter 17). In: *Oxford Handbook of Cardiology*, 2nd ed. Oxford: Oxford University Press. Available at: https://doi.org/10.1093/med/9780199643219.003.0017

Pericarditis ⚙

- Pericarditis is a local inflammatory response in both layers of the pericardium which may later lead to adhesions (Table 4.3).
- Normal intrapericardial pressure is negative but may became positive in the presence of inflammation, leading to impaired diastolic filling.

Table 4.3 Causes of pericarditis

	Frequently encountered causes	Less frequently encountered causes
Cancer	Primary or secondary lung cancer	Mesothelioma post-radiotherapy
End-stage organ failure	Renal failure	
Intercurrent illnesses	Idiopathic Viruses (Coxsackie B, Epstein–Barr, mumps, varicella, HIV) Myocardial infarction (acute, Dressler syndrome) Post-cardiothoracic surgery	Bacterial (tuberculous, pneumonia, rheumatic fever) Connective tissue diseases (rheumatoid arthritis, SLE) Hypothyroidism

History

People most often present with **sharply localized chest pain** that worsens with respiration. Often, the most comfortable position for the person is sitting forward. Pain may radiate to the epigastrium, the left shoulder, or the trapezius ridge. Fever may or may not be present. Occasionally, breathlessness or palpitations may be the prominent symptom. Non-specific symptoms may include hiccoughs or nausea and vomiting.

Physical examination

- A **friction rub** is often heard transiently in late expiration with the person sitting forward. The rub is described as a scratching or high-pitched grating.
- Evaluate for evidence of **cardiac tamponade**: cardiac decompensation including tachycardia, hypotension, elevated JVP, and muffled heart sounds (p.104).

Investigations and management

Prognosis measured in hours to days prior to the onset of this problem (symptom control)

Parenterally administered **anti-inflammatory agents** (ketorolac 10 mg SC four times daily or dexamethasone 4–8 mg SC daily, or parecoxib 20–40 mg IV twice daily) will help to reduce pain.

Prognosis measured in weeks prior to the onset of this problem (in addition to symptom control)

- An **ECG** shows widespread 'saddle-shaped' ST elevation with upright T waves early in the course of pericarditis, reflecting sub-pericardial inflammation. T waves may subsequently flatten and then invert over time. Over days to weeks, the ECG will normalize.

- **Echocardiography** demonstrates the volume of fluid and any cardiac compromise.
- **CXR** may show cardiomegaly. This only occurs in large effusions.
- **ESR** or **CRP** may be raised. Myocardial injury may be reflected with raised **creatine kinase-MB** or **troponin**.
- Other investigations include **FBC**, **EUC**, **TFTs**, and **blood cultures** if febrile.
- If there is cardiac compromise secondary to a large effusion, symptoms may be improved by drainage.
- **Colchicine** (0.5–1 mg daily for 3 months) and **NSAIDs** (tapered on resolution of symptoms) are the first-line treatment. Glucocorticoids such as **prednisolone** 0.2–0.5mg/kg/day can be considered where there is a contraindication to NSAIDs. Ensure concurrent administration of a PPI.
- Discuss with the cardiology service.

Prognosis measured in months to years prior to the onset of this problem (in addition to the above)

- In high-income countries, pericarditis is almost always due to a virus. If there is a concern for other aetiologies, investigations should include viral serology, blood and fungal cultures, and autoantibodies.
- People with renal failure-induced pericarditis usually require **dialysis**.
- Ensure that **myocardial ischaemia** has been excluded as a cause of pericarditis.
- 15–30% of people will experience recurrent pericarditis especially in the setting of cancer or connective tissue disease. Recurrent disease should prompt investigation for a non-viral aetiology if the cause is unknown.
- A small number of people will develop **cardiac tamponade**.
- **Constrictive pericarditis** may occur as a long-term complication. This may present as cardiac failure.
- If there is associated calcification, the treatment is pericardiectomy.

Further reading

Ramrakha P, Hill J (eds) (2012). Cardiovascular emergencies (Chapter 17). In: *Oxford Handbook of Cardiology*, 2nd ed. Oxford: Oxford University Press. Available at: https://doi.org/10.1093/med/9780199643219.003.0017

Infective endocarditis :O:

- Infective endocarditis occurs when sterile vegetations within the heart become infected (Table 4.4).
- If infective endocarditis is untreated, mortality is high.
- There is a high likelihood of sudden changes in condition, especially if heart valves or papillae are affected.
- In someone with a known valve lesion, fever, and sudden cardiac decompensation, urgently evaluate for infective endocarditis.

Table 4.4 Causes of infective endocarditis

	Frequently encountered causes
Cancer	Neutropenic sepsis after chemotherapy
End-stage organ failure	Structural heart disease—valvular (particularly prosthetic valve), hypertrophic disease, congenital changes, implantable cardiac devices
	Post-dental work or poor dentition
	Injectable drug use
	Post-procedure (urinary catheterization, cystoscopy)
	Respiratory, skin, gallbladder infections
	Unexplained recurrent sepsis
	Haemodialysis

History

- **Fever** is common and tends to be higher with acute presentations and more pathogenic organisms. In people with an advanced life-limiting illnesses, fever may be totally absent.
- **Myalgia** is also frequently encountered.
- Presentations of chronic infective endocarditis include anorexia, weight loss, fatigue, and night sweats—all symptoms often found in late-stage cachexia.
- **Embolic events** and **mycotic aneurysms** account for most complications in infective endocarditis—CNS, splenic, renal, or hepatic compromise, or gut ischaemia.

Physical examination

A new cardiac murmur (85%) in the presence of fevers must raise the question of infective endocarditis.

Peripheral manifestations
- Common: petechiae (20–40%), 'splinter' haemorrhages (non-specific), clubbing (long-standing disease), and signs of anaemia.
- Rare: retinal haemorrhages (Roth spots), nodules on digital pads (Osler's nodes), and nodular haemorrhages on palms and soles (Janeway lesions).
- Cardiac murmurs are almost always present except with early disease or tricuspid valve involvement.

- **Splenomegaly**, **petechiae**, or **clubbing** represent long-standing disease. Embolic events most frequently cause neurological deficits but may result in abscess formation (brain, heart, kidney, spleen, GIT, and lungs).

Investigations and management

Prognosis measured in hours to days prior to the onset of this problem (symptom control)

Even late in life, treatment with **appropriate antimicrobials** is an important palliative intervention in order to avoid painful peripheral emboli or sudden new neurological deficits. The need for this is because the rate of embolic events rapidly diminishes after the initiation of appropriate antimicrobial therapy.

Prognosis measured in weeks prior to the onset of this problem (in addition to symptom control)

- **Echocardiography** (including a transoesophageal approach in people with normal transthoracic studies) and blood cultures are needed for the diagnosis.
- **ECG** may show new atrioventricular, fascicular, or bundle branch block. In people with new ECG conduction defects, monitor until stable and exclude perivalvular abscess.
- Check **FBC** (with differential), **ESR** or **CRP**, **renal function**, and **urine analysis**.
- Continuing long-term anticoagulation in infective endocarditis should be carefully weighed against the risk of haemorrhage at the site of emboli or mycotic aneurysms.

Prognosis measured in months to years prior to the onset of this problem (in addition to the above)

Consult cardiothoracic surgery early; there is decreased mortality in people who can tolerate surgery, with early surgery for perivalvular disease or ongoing sepsis despite appropriate therapy. If left untreated, infective endocarditis has very high mortality rates, especially with virulent pathogens.

Further reading

Ramrakha P, Hill J (eds) (2012). Infective endocarditis (Chapter 4). In: *Oxford Handbook of Cardiology*, 2nd ed. Oxford: Oxford University Press. Available at: https://doi.org/10.1093/med/978019 9643219.003.0004

Thoracic aortic dissection ☠

- Thoracic dissections may involve one or more aortic segments (aortic root, ascending aorta, arch, or descending aorta). The most common site is the aortic root and ascending aorta.
- Ascending dissections are considered the most serious because of the possibility of impaired coronary and cerebral circulation, pericardial bleeding with subsequent tamponade, or acute aortic valve damage (Table 4.5).

Table 4.5 Causes of thoracic dissection

	Frequently encountered causes	Less frequently encountered causes
Intercurrent illnesses	Widespread atherosclerosis	Marfan or Turner syndrome
	Hypertension	Aortic arteritis
	Bicuspid aortic valves	Syphilis
	Chronic aortic dissection leading to aneurysm formation	
	Trauma	

History

These people may be asymptomatic prior to the presentation of a dissection (blood splits the aortic media) or rupture.

Most commonly, these people present with **severe chest and back pain**. The pain is often described as ripping or tearing. Pain that extending caudally suggests distal propagation of the dissection. Other symptoms may include limb pain or weakness (secondary to limb ischaemia or spinal cord ischaemia) and abdominal pain (mesenteric ischaemia).

Occasionally, these people may present with any one or more of the following:

- Increasing shortness of breath.
- Congestive cardiac failure.
- Acute myocardial ischaemia.
- Mass effect on large airways.
- Increasing dysphagia (pressure effect on the oesophagus).
- Back pain and hoarse voice.

Physical examination

- People will look **distressed and unwell**.
- They will be **hypertensive** and have **unequal arm pulse and blood pressure readings**. However, the clinical finding of hypotension as a symptom has higher positive predictive value.
- People may develop a new murmur of **aortic incompetence** (soft A2, high-pitched diastolic murmur occurring immediately after the second heart sound).
- Physical examination must include a full **neurological examination** (cerebral ischaemia, spinal artery ischaemia) and abdominal examination (mesenteric ischaemia).

Investigations and management

Prognosis measured in hours to days prior to the onset of this problem (symptom control)

This is a clinical diagnosis but is highly unlikely to occur in the last days of life, unless predisposing conditions are already apparent. No further investigations are indicated.

If the dissection involves the proximal aorta, this is likely to be a terminal event. People with distal dissections who survive the acute event still have a poor prognosis and remain at risk for subsequent dissections and rupture of a secondary aneurysm.

Regardless of the poor prognosis, treat any **hypertension**. This will help prevent propagation of the dissection and rupture of the aorta. Initially the management should include labetalol 50 mg IV over 1 min, followed by a vasodilator (transdermal glyceryl trinitrate 25–50 mg daily). **The vasodilator must not be instituted first; if it is, reflex catecholamine secretion will occur, worsening the blood pressure control and increasing the risk of rupture.**

These people are likely to be distressed and anxious. **Pain** must be addressed with parenteral opioids and **agitation** with benzodiazepines (diazepam 5 mg IV immediately, or midazolam 2.5–5.0 mg SC immediately, followed by either clonazepam 0.5 mg SL/SC twice daily or midazolam 10 mg via SC infusion over 24 h). Oxygen may help with breathlessness if they are hypoxaemic.

Prognosis measured in weeks prior to the onset of this problem (in addition to symptom control)

This person is unlikely to be a surgical candidate, and further investigations are not warranted. The exception is when endovascular stenting procedures are available. Seek an urgent surgical consultation. If this procedure is available, further investigations and management will include:

- **insertion** of an **IV cannula**
- **blood pressure control** (as above)
- **ECG**
- check **FBC**, **EUC**, and **coagulation** studies
- organize an **urgent chest/abdomen CT** or **MRI** scan to define level and extent
- **analgesia**.

Prognosis measured in months to years prior to the onset of this problem (in addition to the above)

These people require simultaneous treatment and investigations, while organizing an urgent surgical consultation.

Surgical intervention must be considered in people with a proximal dissection except when they have suffered a neurological event. In this situation, anticoagulation may cause an ischaemic event to haemorrhage, leading to severe neurological compromise.

There is an estimated 30% mortality for proximal dissections and 10% for distal dissections.

Further reading

Ramrakha P, Hill J (eds) (2012). Cardiovascular emergencies (Chapter 17). In: *Oxford Handbook of Cardiology*, 2nd ed. Oxford: Oxford University Press. Available at: https://doi.org/10.1093/med/9780199643219.003.0017

Bleeding abdominal aortic aneurysm ☠

- An untreatable symptomatic aortic aneurysm may be the reason for referral to a palliative care service. For others, risk factors reflect vascular risk factors (Table 4.6).
- The 1-year mortality in untreated aortic aneurysms >6 cm in diameter is 50%.
- The risk of bleeding from an aortic aneurysm increases with its size: risk increases from a diameter of 4 cm, and increases rapidly from a diameter of 6 cm.

History

Table 4.6 Causes of abdominal aortic aneurysms

	Frequently encountered causes	Less frequently encountered causes
Intercurrent illnesses	Widespread atherosclerosis	Connective tissue diseases (Marfan syndrome, Ehlers–Danlos syndrome)
	Age	Chronic infection (tuberculosis)
	Hypertension	Acute infections (brucellosis, salmonellosis)
	Hyperlipidaemia	
	Smoking	

For most people, an **aneurysm is asymptomatic prior to rupture**. Pain is the presenting symptom of a ruptured aortic aneurysm. It typically occurs in the periumbilical region and radiates to the back, both the iliac fossa, and the groin.

There are a number of patterns of rupture:

- Rupture into the peritoneal cavity presenting as severe pain and shock, and sudden death.
- People have severe pain that has a biphasic nature, reflecting a small first bleed into the retroperitoneal region that is usually followed by a more substantial bleed. Following the larger bleed, these people appear critically unwell.
- Rupture into the duodenum (fistula between the aorta and the duodenum) will cause massive GI bleeding that is a terminal event.
- Rupture into the vena cava. These people present with pain, gross lower limb oedema, and high-output cardiac failure.

Physical examination

- These people will be shocked and unwell.
- A pulsatile abdominal mass may be palpable.
- The abdomen may be **rigid, with guarding**.
- **Bowel sounds may not be audible**.
- Following a rupture into the caval system, a continuous loud murmur will be heard over the abdomen.

Investigations and management

Prognosis measured in hours to days prior to the onset of this problem (symptom control)

- These people must have **adequate analgesia**. If they are shocked, IV administration of medications is the most reliable route.
- People who are bleeding are often **anxious**. Prescribe benzodiazepines.
- A **very agitated person** will require benzodiazepines plus a major tranquillizer (chlorpromazine 25–50 mg IM if shocked or levomepromazine 25–50 mg SC).

Prognosis measured in weeks prior to the onset of this problem (in addition to symptom control)

The main differential diagnosis is acute pancreatitis. Check serum lipase and amylase. It is unlikely that the person will recover from a ruptured aneurysm but may stabilize from acute pancreatitis with supportive measures including hydration and analgesia.

Prognosis measured in months to years prior to the onset of this problem (in addition to the above)

This is a surgical emergency. Seek immediate surgical advice. Immediate investigations and management include:

- **CT or MRI** will delineate the extent of local bleeding. If not available, plain abdominal X-ray (75% of people with an abdominal aortic aneurysm will have calcification visible)
- **abdominal ultrasound** will demonstrate the extent of most abdominal aortic aneurysms
- ensure **adequate venous access**
- **keep systolic blood pressure at 100 mmHg**, initially with colloid and then blood as soon as it is available
- **urgent** cross-match, FBC, EUC, and coagulation studies
- **ECG**.

These people should be transferred to the operating suite as soon as possible

The options currently available are operatively replacing the aneurysmal section of the aorta or placing a vascular stent. Both carry significant morbidity and potential mortality even in the setting of skilled clinicians.

Prognostic risk factors to predict mortality in ruptured aneurysms have been identified as:

- age >75 years
- creatinine >190 μmol/L
- haemoglobin (Hb) <9 g/dL
- loss of consciousness
- ECG changes consistent with ischaemia.

Three or more factors are associated with 100% mortality from rupture. Two factors carry a mortality of 48% and one factor carries a mortality of 28%. Even if there is none of these risk factors, there is still a mortality risk of 18%.

Further reading

Powell J, Davies A (2020). Peripheral arterial disease. In: *Oxford Textbook of Medicine*, 6th ed. Oxford: Oxford University Press. Available at: https://doi.org/10.1093/med/9780198746 690.003.0371

Cutaneous arterial bleed ☠

- Arterial bleeding is a feared complication of many end of life illnesses (Table 4.7).
- Although a sentinel bleed may occur, there needs to be a high index of suspicion for people with head and neck cancers, or extensive soft tissue involvement from sarcomas or melanomas.

Table 4.7 Causes of major bleeding

	Frequently encountered causes	Less frequently encountered causes
Cancer	Erosion of the carotid artery in squamous cell carcinomas of the head and neck Intercurrent illness Infection Anticoagulation Coagulopathy	Bleeds into any active tumour beds including cerebral tumours, cutaneous tumours, and sarcomas

History

- **Head and neck cancers**.
- **Sentinel bleeds** can also occur from the mouth, nose, or ear. Severe local infection can increase the risk of bleeding.
- Any **cutaneous tumour**.
- Local trauma, recent anti-tumour therapy such as radiotherapy or chemotherapy (which may destroy a tumour that is stopping bleeding), or a coagulopathy all increase the risk of bleeding.

Physical examination

- Look for **local signs of sepsis** including erythema, swelling, and tenderness.
- For a potential cutaneous bleed, examine for local factors including evidence of compromise distal to the affected blood vessel.
- In head and neck cancer, palpate the carotid arteries and listen for bruits.
- Examine neurologically for any new evidence of ipsilateral Horner's syndrome, or lesions of cranial nerves IX or X.

Investigations and management

Prognosis measured in hours to days prior to the onset of this problem (symptom control)

It is highly likely that an acute bleed in this situation will be a terminal event. **Crisis medications** (p.53) for sedation must be readily available and may need to be administered IV. The aim is to ensure the person has no pain or memory of this episode if they survive. Address the fear that arterial bleeding engenders for the person bleeding, their family and friends, and clinical staff.

Red or dark green linen will help to reduce the visual impact of arterial bleeding. Apply gentle pressure to the bleeding site and ensure that the person is nursed in a single room.

Prognosis measured in weeks prior to the onset of this problem (in addition to symptom control)

- If a sentinel bleed occurs, ensure that all **medications that may exacerbate bleeding are discontinued** (NSAIDs, heparin, warfarin).
- Check for a coagulopathy and correct if necessary (vitamin K 10 mg IV/oral, platelets, fresh frozen plasma (FFP)).
- **Treat infection**.
- Commence oral tranexamic acid (1 g four times daily) if there is no history of venous thromboembolic disease or haematuria.

If actively bleeding, decide whether this is a life-threatening situation. If it is life-threatening, what should be done in the light of the known disease burden and overall condition? For example, in advanced head and neck cancer in someone with advanced cachexia in whom anticancer treatment is already exhausted, an eroded carotid artery is a terminal event and, for most, even the need for sedation is rapidly superseded by death. For a person with a smaller bleed, provide local pressure (with epinephrine-soaked gauze) and establish urgent venous access. Consider blood collection for cross-matching, FBC, and coagulation studies.

Prognosis measured in months to years prior to the onset of this problem (in addition to the above)

If a sentinel bleed occurs, radiotherapy or angiography and selective embolization may be of benefit. Even in this group of people, catastrophic bleeding is almost certainly a terminal event.

Further reading

Hulme B et al. (2021). Assessment and management of bleeding complications in the medically ill (Chapter 12.5). In: *Oxford Textbook of Palliative Medicine*, 6th ed. Oxford: Oxford University Press. Available at: https://doi.org/10.1093/med/9780198821328.003.0070

Watson M et al. (eds) (2019). Palliation of head and neck cancer (Chapter 14). In: *Oxford Handbook of Palliative Care*, 3rd ed. Oxford: Oxford University Press. Available at: https://doi.org/10.1093/med/9780198745655.003.0014

Acute limb ischaemia ☠

- Total limb ischaemia is a surgical emergency because without treatment the limb will be irrevocably compromised within 6 h. Amputation then becomes the only definitive treatment. People at the end of life are often unable to tolerate amputation.
- Limb ischaemia may be due to thrombosis, emboli, graft occlusion, or trauma (Table 4.8).

Table 4.8 Causes of acute limb ischaemia

	Frequently encountered causes	Less frequently encountered causes
Cancer		Pathological fracture (tibia)
		Extensive venous thrombosis
		Direct vascular invasion
		Malignancy-induced DIC (particularly when associated with acute lymphoblastic leukaemia)
End-stage organ failure	Peripheral arterial disease	Infective endocarditis
	Atrial fibrillation with large arterial embolus	Aortic dissection
		Cholesterol embolus
	Aneurysm	Arterial cannulation (aortic balloon pump, angioplasty)
	Left ventricular thrombus	
Intercurrent illnesses		Pneumococcal or meningococcal sepsis
		Intra-arterial drug administration
		Pelvic surgery (cystectomy or anterior resection where pelvic collaterals compensate for aorto-iliac disease)
		Thoracic outlet syndrome
		Coronavirus disease 2019 (COVID-19) infection

History

People often complain of the sudden onset of **severe pain** in the affected limb with altered sensation. Sometimes paralysis may occur. At times, the onset may mimic Raynaud's phenomenon.

Physical examination

- Early in the process, on observation, the affected limb (usually the leg) may have **blue digits**. When severe, the limb may be marble white, evolving over hours into a blue or purple mottled appearance as deoxygenated blood fills the skin. The skin will blanch on pressure. Darker mottling suggests local coagulation which will severely limit

salvage of the limb. Fixed staining, blistering, or liquefaction indicate a limb that cannot be salvaged.
- On palpation, the presence of peripheral pulses does not exclude significant vascular injury. However, an absent pulse suggests complete limb ischaemia.
- An acutely swollen and painful limb raises the possibility of extensive venous thrombosis.

Investigations and management

Prognosis measured in hours to days prior to the onset of this problem (symptom control)

This is a painful condition for most people. **Adequate parenteral analgesia is crucial.** If already on opioids, increase the dose by at least 25–50% of their current dose. There may be a significant neuropathic component from nerve damage. In this situation, add clonazepam (start with 0.5 mg SC/SL twice daily), amitriptyline 25 mg nocte, or gabapentin 100 mg three times daily and titrate as tolerated.

Consider **epidural/intrathecal analgesia** early in complete, untreatable lower limb ischaemia.

Prognosis measured in weeks prior to the onset of this problem (in addition to symptom control)
- These people require **urgent surgical consultation**.
- Ensure venous access and **regular limb observations**.
- **Check coagulation studies**, **FBC**, and **EUC**.
- **Doppler ultrasound** will demonstrate current arterial flow rates most accurately.
- The definitive study is angiography but should only be performed in people well enough to tolerate any subsequent interventions.
- Incomplete limb ischaemia in the setting of a life-limiting illness can only be treated with anticoagulation and supportive measures. Complete ischaemia from an embolus needs urgent treatment if the person is well enough to tolerate it. This may include **surgical embolectomy**, **thrombolysis** (streptokinase or tissue plasminogen activator), and **fasciotomy** for compartment syndrome. If there is established ischaemia, consider **amputation**.
- In people too unwell to tolerate surgery, **percutaneous lumbar sympathectomy** under computed tomography (CT) guidance may be useful. Following injection of the sympathetic plexus, some people achieve increased distal perfusion and reduced pain. Success is <50%. Some people get worse pain.
- With severe venous thrombosis, **elevate** the limb, **heparinize**, and **provide analgesia** (parenteral opioids). This is an extremely painful condition. In the group of people in whom no intervention is planned, consider spinal (epidural or intrathecal) analgesia early.

Prognosis measured in months to years prior to the onset of this problem (in addition to the above)

This is a **medical emergency**. Seek an urgent surgical opinion. Arrange angiography and either local thrombolysis or open embolectomy. Once surgically stable, anticoagulate and investigate the source of the embolus. Post-embolectomy mortality is 10–20% because of the comorbid conditions that predispose to acute limb ischaemia and reperfusion injuries (compartment syndrome, muscle infarction, acidosis, hyperkalaemia, and myoglobinaemia).

People unsuitable for surgical intervention require consideration of sympathectomy. Combined discussions with surgical, anaesthetic, and radiology specialists will help create a care plan.

Further reading

Powell J, Davies A (2020). Peripheral arterial disease (Chapter 16.14.2). In: *Oxford Textbook of Medicine*, 6th ed. Oxford: Oxford University Press. Available at: https://doi.org/10.1093/med/9780198746690.003.0371

Venous thromboembolic disease ☠

- Venous thromboembolic disease is often without symptoms or has non-specific symptoms. Risk factors should raise the possibility of venous thromboembolic disease (Table 4.9).
- Venous thromboembolic disease is very poorly tolerated in people with other cardiorespiratory compromise.
- There is a need for a high index of suspicion as it is estimated that 7–10% of hospital deaths are related to pulmonary emboli, with 70–90% of these people having no prior symptoms.
- The majority of fatal pulmonary emboli are identified postmortem.

Table 4.9 Causes of venous thromboembolic disease

	Frequently encountered causes
Cancer	Any cancer
	Acute myeloid leukaemia (AML; M5 has higher incidence)
	DIC
Intercurrent illnesses	Protein C deficiency; protein S deficiency; factor V Leiden; antithrombin III deficiency; antiphospholipid antibodies
	Recent surgery
	Prolonged bed rest
	Recent CVA or AMI

History

People with a thrombosis arising in the deep veins of the legs (rarely arms, and then mostly in the presence of a central venous catheter) may present with **swelling and pain of the affected limb**. Symptoms rarely occur until thrombus arising distally affects proximal veins.

Up to 50% of people with an established DVT and no respiratory symptoms will have evidence of pulmonary emboli on perfusion imaging.

People with pulmonary emboli may present with **acute onset of distressing breathlessness** and associated pleuritic chest pain. 10% of symptomatic pulmonary emboli cause death within 1 h.

Physical examination

- **DVT** may cause pain, swelling, discoloration, and redness of the affected limb. Superficial venous dilatation may be seen.
- **Pulmonary emboli** may cause tachycardia, tachypnoea, and hypotension. People may be cyanotic with increased respiratory effort (but its absence does not exclude a pulmonary embolus).
- When increased respiratory effort occurs, individuals are often very distressed and frightened.
- Findings of **right-sided heart strain** (elevated JVP, distended neck veins, loud pulmonary component of second heart sound) or hypotension suggest serious haemodynamic compromise.

- **Pleural effusion and pleuritic rubs** are late manifestations of a
  pulmonary infarct associated with pleural inflammation.

Investigations and management

Prognosis measured in hours to days prior to venous emboli (symptom control)

Pain is a problem in many people with DVTs. Compression stocking use
should be delayed until collateral vessels have an opportunity to open.
Elevation will help to minimize pain. Arterial compromise due to massive DVTs requires extreme leg elevation. Despite the short prognosis,
anticoagulation with LMWH should be commenced (enoxaparin either
1 mg/kg twice daily or 1.5 mg/kg daily) to reduce swelling, improve pain,
and reduce the risk of fatal pulmonary emboli. Check the most recent renal
function tests and calculate creatinine clearance. If creatinine clearance
<30 mL/min, reduce the dose by half.

People at the end of life who develop a pulmonary embolus may have
distressing breathlessness. Investigations are not indicated. Focus on
symptom reduction. Commence opioids (p.26) and oxygen (aim to keep
oxygen saturation >92% to reduce breathlessness and chest pain by reducing pulmonary vascular resistance). NSAIDs are useful for pleuritic pain.
Sedation may be necessary if the person is distressed or frightened. Crisis
medications (p.53) must be available.

*Prognosis measured in weeks prior to venous emboli (in addition to symptom
control)*

Arrange **venous Doppler imaging**. The person should then be commenced on **LMWH** as above or directly acting oral anticoagulants
(apixaban, rivaroxaban, dabigatran). Warfarin is inferior to LMWH. Prior
to commencing anticoagulation, **EUC, FBC,** and **coagulation studies**
should be checked. As noted above, anticoagulation aims to reduce the risk
of fatal pulmonary emboli.

Acute onset of breathlessness in this group should be investigated with a
CXR, arterial blood gases (especially in the presence of long-standing
respiratory disease to guide oxygen supplementation), and the definitive
examination of a **computed tomography pulmonary angiogram
(CTPA)**.

*Prognosis measured in months to years prior to venous emboli (in addition
to the above)*

If this is the first venous thromboembolic event, check levels of **protein
C, protein S, antithrombin III, antiphospholipid antibodies, and
factor V Leiden**. Also collect blood for **FBC, coagulation studies,
and EUC (calculate creatinine clearance)**. This group requires aggressive interventions.

People with a high probability of pulmonary emboli without shock should
undergo a **CTPA** and an assessment of right ventricular function. If the
ventricular function is not impaired, heparin (IV unfractionated heparin at
80 U/kg immediately, then infused at 18 U/kg/h to maintain the activated
partial thromboplastin time (APTT) at 1.2–2.5 normal or LMWH; check
with local haematology guidelines).

Thrombolysis should not be considered in a person who is clinically stable. Thrombolysis has the best evidence in people with haemodynamic instability (low systolic blood pressure).

Consider embolectomy in people with shock and failed thrombolysis.

Intermediate-risk pulmonary emboli create a clinical dilemma—the risks of thrombolysis may outweigh any benefits. Seek urgent advice from respiratory medicine.

Drainage of pleural effusions should only be considered if there are significant symptoms, given that anticoagulation must be suspended in order to perform drainage safely.

Haemodynamic compromise on presentation carries an acute mortality rate of 10%.

Further reading

Noble SIR et al. (2021). Assessment and management of thrombotic complications (Chapter 12.4). In: *Oxford Textbook of Palliative Medicine*, 6th ed. Oxford: Oxford University Press. Available at: https://doi.org/10.1093/med/9780198821328.003.0069

Ramrakha P, Hill J (eds) (2012). Cardiovascular emergencies (Chapter 17). In: *Oxford Handbook of Cardiology*, 2nd ed. Oxford: Oxford University Press. Available at: https://doi.org/10.1093/med/9780199643219.003.0017

Superior vena cava obstruction ⚠

- In superior vena cava (SVC) obstruction, decreased venous return from the upper half of the body causes a rise in central venous pressure.
- The obstruction may be due to external compression, thrombus inside the vessel, or direct vessel invasion by malignancy (Table 4.10).

Table 4.10 Causes of SVC obstruction

	Frequently encountered causes	Less frequently encountered causes
Cancer	Lung cancer (especially small cell or squamous cell)	Lymphoma Mediastinal metastases History of mediastinal radiotherapy
Intercurrent illness		Recently placed central venous catheter (vessel trauma) Benign mediastinal tumours Thoracic aortic aneurysms Thyroid enlargement SVC thrombus

History

- With an insidious onset of SVC obstruction, people may complain of neck and facial swelling, headache or 'fullness' on bending or lying down, and increasing shortness of breath.
- In acute-onset SVC obstruction, people often complain of dizziness and sudden onset of shortness of breath.
- Rarely, people may present obtunded due to cerebral oedema.

Physical examination

- On observation, **dilated veins** (neck, forehead, anterior chest wall) are often seen. Bloodshot conjunctiva may be present, with facial oedema.
- On occasion, there may be tachypnoea, proptosis, oedema of the arms and neck, and peripheral cyanosis. **Pemberton's sign** is elicited by putting their hands above their head and looking for facial flushing and hand veins that may not collapse.
- Assess airway patency as laryngeal oedema may cause life-threatening respiratory compromise.
- Assess cerebral function as cerebral oedema may be severe in the acute onset of an SVC obstruction.

Investigations and management

Prognosis measured in hours to days prior to the onset of this problem (symptom control)

- **Opioid analgesia** will be necessary for the relief of breathlessness or headache.
- Check oxygen saturations and use **supplemental oxygen** if the person is breathless. The head of the bed should be elevated to 30°.
- **Dexamethasone** (16 mg/day) may reduce oedema in a small group of people.
- These people may be anxious and are at risk of seizures.
- In acute airway compromise, **crisis medications** (p.53) for sedation must be available.

Prognosis measured in weeks prior to the onset of this problem (in addition to symptom control)

- **CXR** will be abnormal in 85% of people with a widened mediastinum and, at times, a right-sided pleural effusion. In the setting of gradual onset, there will be collateral venous circulation.
- **Chest CT** will demonstrate decreased or absent opacification of central venous structures and the probable cause of obstruction.
- Management of this group should include **a trial of dexamethasone**.
- If present, central venous catheters should be removed if possible.
- For extrinsic compression, **endovascular stenting** is the definitive treatment of choice. If thrombus is present, stenting can be combined with thrombolysis at the time of the procedure. Patency at 3 months is reported to be >80% with recurrence rates of 7–21%.
- The precise role of **anticoagulation** is uncertain but is considered where thrombus is the cause of the obstruction.

Prognosis measured in months to years prior to the onset of this problem (in addition to the above)

- Once the person has been stabilized, **radiotherapy** may be of benefit in a number of cancers but symptoms can flare during treatment and the maximum benefit can take weeks.
- **Chemotherapy** should be considered in early SVC obstruction in tumours that are exquisitely chemosensitive (small cell lung cancer or lymphoma with an expected symptomatic response rate of 60%). Median prognosis after the diagnosis of SVC obstruction is <3 months.
- In the event that a SVC obstruction is the presenting complaint of a new malignancy, urgent biopsy prior to the administration of disease-modifying therapy (radiotherapy, corticosteroids, chemotherapy) is usually a priority.

Further reading

Hoskin P (2021). Radiotherapy in symptom management (Chapter 14.3). In: *Oxford Textbook of Palliative Medicine*, 6th ed. Oxford: Oxford University Press. Available at: https://doi.org/10.1093/med/9780198821328.003.0078

Chapter 5

Respiratory problems

Pneumonia *126*
Pleural effusion *129*
Empyema *131*
Pneumothorax *133*
Tracheo-oesophageal fistula *135*
Mediastinitis *136*
Large-airway obstruction *138*
Haemoptysis *140*
Pneumonitis *142*
Lymphangitis carcinomatosis *144*

Pneumonia ☼

Pneumonia is defined as an acute infection of the pulmonary parenchyma.
Consider the genesis of the person's pneumonia:

* Community-acquired pneumonia (CAP): acquired outside of the hospital setting.
* Hospital-acquired pneumonia (HAP): acquired ≥48 h after admission to the hospital.
* Ventilator-associated pneumonia (VAP): acquired ≥48 h after endotracheal intubation.
* Aspiration pneumonia: acquired in any setting after inhalation of gastric contents.

Community-acquired pneumonia

Previously, most CAP was attributed to typical bacterial infections including *Streptococcus pneumoniae* and atypical bacterial infections such as *Mycoplasma* spp.

More recently, infections from respiratory viruses including rhinovirus, influenza, and, most recently, COVID-19 are increasing. There is a small but important risk of community-acquired MRSA as a cause of severe CAP in people with risk factors: previous MRSA infection or use of parenteral antibiotics in the previous 90 days.

History

Pneumonia may present with **sudden onset of fevers**, **purulent sputum**, and, at times, **pleuritic** pain. Less typical presentations include insidious onset of influenza-like symptoms (myalgias and arthralgias, headache, or fatigue) and dry cough. The degree of breathlessness varies widely. For many people, symptoms of sepsis dominate over respiratory compromise.

In someone with a life-limiting illness, clinicians need to distinguish between:

* an infection complicating an overall deterioration (often seen as a terminal event), and
* a pneumonic process in someone who is otherwise still relatively well.

Physical examination

Acutely, people may have **fever and tachycardia**, be hypotensive or obtunded when severely ill, and have **central cyanosis** (lips or ear lobes) with **significant respiratory compromise**.

On examination over the affected side, there may be decreased expansion, a dull percussion note, decreased vocal resonance, and reduced air entry with coarse crackles. Less typically, there may be few physical findings except for scattered rales or first onset of wheezing in an adult.

Investigations and management

Prognosis measured in hours to days prior to the onset of this problem (symptom control)

For a person at the end of life who intercurrently develops a pneumonia, keep them comfortable.

Symptom control is as for **breathlessness** (p.26) and any associated **confusion** (p.29). Reverse any symptomatic **hypoxaemia** with supplemental oxygen. **Treat fever** with paracetamol or NSAIDs (p.46). Ensure adequate hydration because of sepsis.

Prognosis measured in weeks prior to the onset of this problem (in addition to symptom control)

CXR will demonstrate pulmonary infiltrates in most people with pneumonia but their absence does not exclude pneumonia. Absence of infiltrates can occur early in the course of the infection or people with immune suppression. Multicentric infiltrates suggest haematogenous spread with diffuse infiltrates suggesting an atypical organism, including *Pneumocystis carinii* or a virus.

Cavitation can occur from oral anaerobes, *Staphylococcus aureus*, *Streptococcus pneumoniae*, *Mycobacterium tuberculosis*, *Nocardia*, and fungal infections including *Histoplasma capsulatum*, *Coccidiodes immitis*, and *Blastomyces dermatitidis*.

Fungal infections can cause hilar lymphadenopathy and pleural effusions. Chest CT is useful to further define pulmonary infiltrates:
- when there is a negative CXR but high clinical suspicion of pneumonia, or
- to exclude other possible diagnoses including pulmonary embolism.

Other investigations

In established pneumonia, leucopoenia and thrombocytopaenia are recognized as poor prognostic factors along with hypotension, hypothermia, uraemia, or confusion: ≥3 of these factors is associated with severe pneumonia as are septic shock or respiratory failure.

Treatment

Identifying underlying aetiologies is often not possible. Treatment remains largely empiric.
- For people with less severe pneumonia, short courses of therapy that address typical and atypical organisms are recommended. Mono- or combination therapy should be based on local recommendations.
- For those with severe pneumonia consider fluid and electrolyte resuscitation and oxygen therapy. Failure to respond within 24–48 h should shift the goal of care to comfort.

Prognosis measured in months to years prior to the onset of this problem (in addition to the above)

A clinical response is expected within 24–48 h after initiation of antibiotic therapy and other supportive measures. However, in those who worsen or fail to respond, consideration should be given to either a resistant or atypical organism. Other issues to consider include an alternative diagnosis or whether this person has developed a superimposed complication of their original disease such as an empyema. In this situation, it is strongly recommended that local algorithms are reviewed, and further consultation from the respiratory team is sought.

Other pneumonias
- HAP.
- VAP.
- Aspiration pneumonia.

HAP and VAP

Pathogenic organisms that are frequently encountered in HAP include Gram-negative bacilli, *Pseudomonas aeruginosa*, *Staphylococcus aureus*, and oral anaerobes.

The criteria to diagnose HAP and VAP include clinical suspicion and radiographic evidence of infiltrates. Check for hypotension, hypothermia, leucopenia, thrombocytopenia, uraemia, or confusion: ≥3 of these is associated with severe pneumonia as are septic shock or respiratory failure.

Check oxygenation, blood cultures, and respiratory fluid cultures. If no respiratory secretions are available, consider induced sputum in HAP or nasotracheal/endotracheal aspiration in VAP.

Treatment of HAP/VAP requires consideration of local algorithms including consideration of individual factors such as comorbidities, recent use of antibiotics, and results of previous cultures.

Pneumonia associated with aspiration

There are potentially three sources of aspiration: oral flora, food, or acidic gastric contents.

Aspiration pneumonia often develops insidiously. More than 50% of adults will normally have measurable microaspiration of upper aerodigestive tract contents while sleeping. This is worsened with gingival disease.

Oral flora that can cause lung infections include Gram-positive *Actinomyces* species, Gram-negative *Prevotella melaninogenica*, *Fusobacterium*, *Bacteroides* species other than *Bacteroides fragilis*, and anaerobic cocci including Gram-positive *Peptostreptococcus* and Gram-negative *Veillonella*.

For aspiration of oral contents, X-ray changes are most frequently in the basilar segments of the lower lobes if upright when aspirating or, if supine, in the posterobasilar segments of the upper lobe or the superior segment of the lower lobe.

Food is usually aspirated when consciousness is impaired or with dysphagia. A post-obstruction bacterial pneumonia can develop in people with a tumour obstructing the large airways. In people with dysphagia, the introduction of nasogastric (NG) feeds does **not** decrease risk of aspiration pneumonia.

Aspiration of gastric contents can cause a chemical pneumonitis, with diffuse changes on X-ray occurring rapidly after the aspiration.

Further reading

Chapman SJ et al. (2021). Respiratory infection (Chapter 41). In: *Oxford Handbook of Respiratory Medicine*, 4th ed. Oxford: Oxford University Press. Available at: https://doi.org/10.1093/med/9780198837114.003.0041

Lim WS (2020). Pneumonia in the normal host. In: *Oxford Textbook of Medicine*, 6th ed. Oxford: Oxford University Press. Available at: https://doi.org/10.1093/med/9780198746690.003.0403

Pleural effusion :☼:

- The majority of people with a pleural effusion are asymptomatic from the effusion and are most likely to have presented as a result of the disease that caused the effusion. Treat the person, not the imaging studies showing an effusion.
- The initial step includes comprehensive history and detailed physical examination as 75% of effusions can be attributed to heart failure, pneumonia, or malignancy.

History

Increasing shortness of breath on exertion is the most common presentation when the effusion is symptomatic with the size of the effusion poorly correlating with the severity of breathlessness.

Often people will note that they are unable to lie on the side *opposite* to the effusion. For most people the progression of symptoms with a pleural effusion is subtle.

Sudden onset of shortness of breath in the presence of a pleural effusion should flag exclusion of other pathology: pneumonia, pulmonary embolus, or large airway obstruction.

Physical examination

On observation, check for **central cyanosis** (tongue or ear lobes). Is the trachea deviated away from the side of the effusion?

Record respiratory and pulse rate.

When checking blood pressure check for evidence of pulsus paradoxus (drop of >10 mmHg in systolic blood pressure on inspiration). Given the risk of concomitant pericardial fluid, check for jugular venous engorgement. **Decreased expansion of the affected side may be seen together with dullness to percussion, decreased vocal resonance, and decreased or absent air entry**.

Investigations and management

Prognosis measured in hours to days prior to the onset of this problem (symptom control)

Pleural effusions are commonly encountered at the end of life. The only reason to consider bedside drainage is that the person had rapidly re-accumulating fluid and symptomatic benefit from previous drainage. If loculated, do not attempt to drain. At the bedside, check pulse oximetry. Oxygen may be of benefit in people with significant hypoxaemia.

Energy conservation should be used to minimize breathlessness.

People who are opioid naïve and are breathless may benefit from regular, low-dose morphine. People already on opioids should be offered a 25% increase of their baseline dose. Anxiety may benefit from relaxation techniques or anxiolytics.

Prognosis measured in weeks prior to the onset of this problem (in addition to symptom control)

In the community or in hospital, a **CXR** can define the effusion and any underlying lung pathology such as pneumonia or a wedge-shaped pulmonary infarct from an embolus. A **chest ultrasound** can define the size of the effusion, whether or not it is loculated, and provide direct guidance for drainage.

If symptomatic, consider drainage to a level that breathlessness is relieved. People occasionally experience re-expansion pulmonary oedema in the hours after evacuation of pleural fluid with sudden respiratory decompensation.

In the absence of metastatic cancer, bilateral pleural effusions are more likely to be a transudate (due to organ failure) rather than an exudate (due to infection or malignancy).

Prognosis measured in months to years prior to the onset of this problem (in addition to the above)
Thoracic CT **can better define underlying lung pathology**.

Diagnostic pleural tap
Perform a diagnostic tap and send pleural fluid for laboratory evaluation. **Pleural fluid** should be examined for **cell count** (>5000/µL suggests pulmonary embolism or neoplasm), **cytology** (ratio of pleural to serum levels >0.5 consistent with exudate), **protein levels** (ratio of pleural to serum levels >0.5 consistent with exudate), **lactate dehydrogenase** (ratio of pleural to serum levels >0.6 consistent with a transudate), **microscopy** (including seeking acid fast bacilli), and **culture** (including TB if the cause of the effusion is unknown) (Table 5.1).

Table 5.1 Causes of pleural effusions

Transudate	Exudate
Congestive cardiac failure	Pneumonia
Cirrhosis	Malignancy
Pulmonary embolism	Pulmonary embolism
Nephrotic syndrome	Collagen vascular disease

If the effusion is malignant, consider drainage through a chest tube, followed by pleurodesis if the cavity can be made dry. Consider a tunnelled pleural catheter as an acceptable alternative. Alternatively, a video-assisted thoracoscopy may be indicated. If the effusion is loculated (*de novo* or as a result of previous attempts at pleurodesis), use ultrasound guidance.

If the lung fails to re-expand, further drainage is not indicated.

Further reading

Chapman SJ et al. (2021). Pleural effusion (Chapter 35). In: *Oxford Handbook of Respiratory Medicine*, 4th ed. Oxford: Oxford University Press. Available at: https://doi.org/10.1093/med/978019 8837114.003.0035

Empyema :⚙:

- While pus in the pleural space may occur secondary to a para-pneumonic process, previous instrumentation of the pleural space, ruptured oesophagus, haematogenous spread, or as part of a subdiaphragmatic infection, the mechanisms underlying many empyemas are unclear.
- Long-term mortality associated with empyemas is significant, especially in people aged >65 years.
- Pus loculates rapidly and should be drained urgently, with or without adjuvant fibrinolysis.

History

The combination of a pleural effusion and/or a pneumonic process, fevers, or previous invasive procedures involving the pleural space should raise clinical suspicion of an empyema. This is particularly relevant in high-risk groups such those with poor oral hygiene, predisposition to aspiration, cardiovascular disease, diabetes, cirrhosis of the liver, or disseminated malignancy.

Physical examination
Physical findings will reflect the fluid within the pleural cavity.
Other findings might include hypotension, tachycardia, or hypoxaemia.

Investigations and management
Prognosis measured in hours to days prior to the onset of this problem (symptom control)
Treat fever with **paracetamol** or **NSAIDs**. Definitive treatment is not possible in people who are frail and near death. Other symptoms that may require care include cough, breathlessness, or chest pain.

Prognosis measured in weeks prior to the onset of this problem (in addition to symptom control)
Pleural fluid should be sent for urgent biochemistry, **microscopy**, and **culture**. **Turbid fluid**, **pH >7.2**, **polymorphs**, **low glucose,** and **high LDH** suggest empyema and need for surgical drainage.

Culture pleural fluid, including TB as yield is better if injected into culture bottles immediately. Aerobic and anaerobic organisms each account for 50% of empyemas. Aerobic organisms include *Streptococcus pneumoniae* and *Staphylococcus aureus*. Gram-negative bacilli include *Enterobacter*, *Klebsiella*, and *Proteus* species. Anaerobic organisms include *Actinomyces* species, *Prevotella melaninogenica*, *Fusobacterium*, *Peptostreptococcus*, and *Veillonella*.

Prognosis measured in months to years prior to the onset of this problem (in addition to the above)
Ensure adequate close monitoring while arranging for drainage of the chest cavity with a chest tube. Ensure that a large-bore cannula is in place. Commence empiric antibiotics based on local recommendations, presumed underlying aetiology, and whether this problem is likely to be community or hospital acquired.

If already loculated, consider use of intrapleural fibrinolytic and mucolytic agents in combination with saline washes. This should be managed jointly with the cardiothoracic services.

Further reading

Chapman SJ et al. (2021). Pleural effusion (Chapter 35). In: *Oxford Handbook of Respiratory Medicine*, 4th ed. Oxford: Oxford University Press. Available at: https://doi.org/10.1093/med/978019 8837114.003.0035

Pneumothorax ☼

- In people with a life-limiting illness, a pneumothorax is rarely a primary event. Secondary pneumothoraces may be spontaneous or traumatic (Table 5.2).
- A pneumothorax is a more significant problem in the palliative setting because of pre-existing lung compromise.

Table 5.2 Causes of a pneumothorax

	More frequently encountered causes	Less frequently encountered causes
Cancer	Any lung cancer, following lung biopsy or pleural aspiration	Pathological rib fracture, oesophageal rupture
End-stage organ failure	Chronic obstructive pulmonary disease (rupture of bullae)	Cystic fibrosis
Intercurrent illnesses	Placement of a central venous catheter	Mechanical ventilation, *Pneumocystis carinii* pneumonia

History

- Most people with a life-limiting illness have a pneumothorax found as an incidental finding on CXR. It is often not associated with chest pain or any other discomfort. If asymptomatic and stable, observation may be sufficient.
- People may initially experience some mild shortness of breath on exertion or pleuritic pain on deep inspiration.
- **If the person has respiratory symptoms, urgently exclude a tension pneumothorax**.

Physical examination

Tracheal **shift** away from the midline on the affected side suggests a tension pneumothorax with signs of respiratory and subsequent cardiac compromise (tachypnoea, tachycardia, hypotension, desaturation). Absent air entry **on the affected side supports this diagnosis**. Urgently decompress with a chest drain on the affected side.

Physical signs include reduced expansion on the affected side together with decreased air entry. Hyper-resonance is difficult to elicit. Vocal resonance may be increased.

In a pneumothorax secondary to instrumentation, physical signs may be absent or subtle. A high index of suspicion is needed.

Investigations and management

Prognosis measured in hours to days prior to the onset of this problem (symptom control)

Assess for respiratory compromise. **Supplemental oxygen** should be administered while the extent of the problem is being defined. **Anxiety and breathlessness can be prominent. Any significant pneumothorax is likely to be a terminal event in people already dying**.

Prognosis measured in weeks prior to the onset of this problem (in addition to symptom control)

A **CXR** will demonstrate the degree of lung collapse. It is also the crucial way to follow progress. A pneumothorax that is increasing in size needs to be followed closely. **Thoracic CT** will help to define any underlying pathology when the person has been stabilized.

When intrapleural pressure is above atmospheric pressure and there is free gas in the pleural space, the person has a **tension pneumothorax**. Impaired cardiac output and hypoxaemia rapidly cause death. The decision to treat will need to be made with the person who has a life-limiting illness.

A large-bore needle should be introduced into the pleural space urgently and replaced with an intercostal drain as soon as possible.

The other indication for a chest drain is if a pneumothorax is >30% or expanding.

In people with a small, post-biopsy pneumothorax, observation is usually sufficient. Air will be reabsorbed slowly from the pleural surface if the original leak is sealed. Simple aspiration is reserved for people with a primary spontaneous pneumothorax.

Prognosis measured in months to years prior to the onset of this problem (in addition to the above)

In someone where a chest tube is draining a pneumothorax and the lung (not tethered by scar tissue) has not re-expanded within a week, consider thoracoscopy.

Further reading

Chapman SJ et al. (2021). Pneumothorax (Chapter 37). In: *Oxford Handbook of Respiratory Medicine*, 4th ed. Oxford: Oxford University Press. Available at: https://doi.org/10.1093/med/978019 8837114.003.0037

Chapman SJ et al. (2021). Pneumothorax aspiration (Chapter 69). In: *Oxford Handbook of Respiratory Medicine*, 4th ed. Oxford: Oxford University Press. Available at: https://doi.org/10.1093/med/9780198837114.003.0069

Tracheo-oesophageal fistula ⓘ

Tracheo-oesophageal fistula (TOF) is a pathological connection between the trachea and the oesophagus which spills oral and GI secretions into the respiratory tree.

This is most commonly a complication of oesophageal or tracheal cancer related either to the disease or its treatment including radiation, surgery, and, more recently, bevacizumab. Other factors that have been associated with this problem include prolonged mechanical ventilation with an endotracheal or tracheostomy tube, chest trauma, infections of the mediastinum, ingestion of a foreign body, ingestion of a corrosive substance, or as a complication of stenting.

History

Aside from ventilated patients, the main symptoms that people are likely to experience are as the result of constant tracheal soiling. These include cough especially when swallowing liquid, aspiration leading to pneumonia, fever, chest pain, and haemoptysis.

Physical examination

The physical examination may be apparently normal in the presence of a small fistula.

In more established TOF, people are likely to be cachectic and may have abdominal bloating.

Investigations and management

Prognosis measured in hours to days prior to the onset of this problem (symptom control)

Stop oral intake and ensure adequate parenteral fluids. Consider an NG tube to empty gastric contents as a transient measure.

Adequate pain relief is required. For many people pain is the predominant symptom. Use maximal acid suppression with a PPI.

Prognosis measured in weeks prior to the onset of this problem (in addition to symptom control)

Although a **CXR** may show abnormalities, a **thoracic CT scan** is the best way to demonstrate free mediastinal or pleural air. A **Gastrografin®
swallow** will delineate the level of perforation. With a high index of suspicion, **oesophagoscopy** may also allow placing a stent to block the fistula in the same procedure. Most people with a life-limiting illness will not tolerate a definitive surgical procedure.

Check for evidence of local or systemic sepsis. Check the differential WCC and perform blood cultures if suspected. Cover with broad-spectrum antibiotics including oral anaerobes (p.128).

Prognosis measured in months to years prior to the onset of this problem (in addition to the above)

As TOFs are most frequently encountered in oesophageal cancer, explore all definitive options for treatment.

Further reading

Fitzgerald RC, di Pietro M (2020). Diseases of the oesophagus (Chapter 15.7). In: *Oxford Textbook of Medicine*, 6th ed. Oxford: Oxford University Press. Available at: https://doi.org/10.1093/med/9780198746690.003.0294

Mediastinitis :☠:

- Inflammation or infection within the mediastinal space is an event secondary to a small number of insults (Table 5.3).
- The onset of this may be sudden and present as a person who is *in extremis*.

Table 5.3 Causes of mediastinitis (rare clinical presentation)

	More frequently encountered causes	Less frequently encountered causes
Cancer	Perforation of an oesophageal cancer	Perforation during an upper digestive tract endoscopic procedure, insertion of a Blakemore tube, or during endoscopic oesophageal dilatation

History
People with mediastinitis are extremely ill.
Symptoms include pain and breathlessness. The pain will depend on which third of the mediastinum is affected. As the oesophagus runs through the posterior third, pain is often referred to the person's back, neck, arms, or shoulders. People may describe the pain as being 'constricting', akin to an acute coronary syndrome.

Post-surgically, people may present with acute sepsis or a purulent discharge from a sternotomy or thoracoscopy scar.

Pneumomediastinum can occur with the rupture of the oesophagus or airways at any level, or air tracking from the neck or peritoneal cavity.

Physical examination
Check whether the person is **systemically unwell**: pulse, blood pressure, temperature, and oxygen saturation. In the post-procedure setting, there may be signs of local infection with tenderness, erythema, warmth, and a discharge. If mediastinitis affects the middle one-third of the oesophagus, there may be a 'click' sound with each heartbeat.

In the presence of a pneumomediastinum, there may be SC emphysema that generally tracks to the base of the neck.

Investigations and management
Prognosis measured in hours to days prior to the onset of this problem (symptom control)
Pain is still the major problem with mediastinitis. Use of opioid analgesia is necessary to provide adequate analgesia. Fever may predominate.

Prognosis measured in weeks prior to the onset of this problem (in addition to symptom control)
On **CXR** there may be evidence of the widening of the mediastinum and evidence of free gas. The definitive examination for mediastinal pathology

is **CT**. With the working diagnosis of a ruptured oesophagus, a **contrast swallowing study** may be helpful.

Check **FBC** for neutrophilia and take **blood cultures**.

For post-surgical mediastinitis, drain any collection and debride any tissue with marginal viability. Use aggressive doses of parenteral antibiotics with broad-spectrum coverage including anaerobic cover (p.48). Monitor carefully until the person is stable.

Prognosis measured in months to years prior to the onset of this problem (in addition to the above)

In the palliative or supportive care setting, a **video-assisted mediastinoscopy** is rarely required. Surgical repair of an oesophageal perforation is rarely an option for people with a life-limiting illness. An attempt at stenting and treating mediastinitis with antibiotics will be the definitive approach for most people. Post-surgical mediastinitis is a serious complication, with a mortality rate still approaching 20%.

Further reading

Chapman SJ, Robinson GV (2021). Mediastinal abnormalities (Chapter 33). In: *Oxford Handbook of Respiratory Medicine*, 4th ed. Oxford: Oxford University Press. Available at: https://doi.org/10.1093/med/9780198837114.003.0033

Large-airway obstruction :O:

Obstruction from growth within the bronchial tree or external compression can narrow the lumen of large airways (Table 5.4).

Table 5.4 Causes of compromise to large airways

	More frequently encountered causes	Less frequently encountered causes
Cancer	Primary or secondary lung cancers, especially bronchoalveolar carcinoma (with potential for transbronchial spread)	Extrinsic compression by malignant mediastinal lymph nodes
Intercurrent illnesses		Bronchial adenomas, sarcoidosis (only 80% have bilateral hilar lymphadenopathy)

History

Symptoms of large-airway obstruction include **cough**, which in the case of adenomas may be present for many years. **Haemoptysis** can frequently occur. **Wheeze**, **stridor**, and **progressive breathlessness** may be dominant findings. (**Inspiratory stridor tends to suggest supraglottic pathology and expiratory stridor subglottic problems.**)

Recurrent or refractory pneumonia (distal to partial or total obstruction) is frequently encountered.

Tracheal obstruction is most commonly from enlarged mediastinal nodes that may cause varying degrees of oesophageal obstruction, recurrent laryngeal nerve paralysis (hoarse voice), or phrenic nerve involvement (sudden worsening in breathlessness as a hemidiaphragm fails to contribute to respiratory effort).

With a life-limiting illness, it is rare that large-airway obstruction will be new pathology. Rather, it is more likely to be progression of documented disease.

Physical examination

Physical findings should reflect the level at which the airway is compromised. Horner's syndrome (small pupil, partial ptosis, ipsilateral loss of sweating, and enophthalmos (loss of the tarsal muscles)) will occur with damage to the cervical sympathetic chain.

Do the lungs expand symmetrically (a relatively small airway may be affected) or is expansion largely absent on one side (a main bronchus is obstructed)? Percussion and careful auscultation may help localization. With loss of a hemidiaphragm in phrenic nerve lesions, the spleen or liver may appear unusually high.

Investigations and management

Prognosis measured in hours to days prior to the onset of this problem (symptom control)

Ensure **adequate oxygenation** and use supplemental oxygen if there is hypoxaemia. Most symptoms are related to **cough** or **breathlessness**. Cough can be particularly problematic. A combination of regular, low-dose morphine and anxiolytics may help with these symptoms.

Prognosis measured in weeks prior to the onset of this problem (in addition to symptom control)

CXR will demonstrate any collapse or consolidation. It may also demonstrate any lymphadenopathy. A chest CT will further define pathology.

Bronchoscopy will define the pathology. Bronchoscopic stenting may help with extrinsic compression of airways and be of use if there is no post-obstruction collapse/consolidation. (If consolidation is already evident, stenting will not produce re-expansion of the lung.) Laser ablation of endobronchial tumours or their removal can be offered at endoscopy.

Bronchomalacia can occur after lung transplantation. Because the blood supply to the bronchi is not directly restored at surgery, the anastomosis relies on retrograde blood flow. Anastamotic leaks or later stenosis are frequently encountered. Bronchoscopic stenting may help with some anastomotic problems. A bronchial fistula can occur if the anastomosis breaks down.

Further reading

Chapman SJ et al. (2021). Bronchoscopy (Chapter 63). In: *Oxford Handbook of Respiratory Medicine*, 4th ed. Oxford: Oxford University Press. Available at: https://doi.org/10.1093/med/978019 8837114.003.0063

Haemoptysis ☠️

Haemoptysis is a feared complication of many end of life respiratory illnesses. Malignancy, infection, and valvular heart disease need to be considered as causes (Table 5.5).

Table 5.5 Causes of haemoptysis

	More frequently encountered causes	Less frequently encountered causes
Cancer	Primary lung cancer Cancers of the upper aero-digestive tract	
Intercurrent illnesses	Bronchiectasis Pulmonary infarction Vigorous coughing rupturing mucosal blood vessels	TB Fungus ball Lung abscess Mitral stenosis Acute left ventricular failure Primary pulmonary hypertension

History
Bleeding can occur at any time in people with lung cancer.
With large bleeds, there is rarely a sentinel bleed. Volume of bleeding is difficult to estimate, but in extensive bleeding, the blood appears bright red and at times frothy. **Bleeding that causes any difficulty in breathing is significant**.

Define likely mechanisms of bleeding. For example, haemoptysis that arises from pulmonary embolism is an important diagnosis even with a life-limiting illness.

Other bleeding that may mimic haemoptysis includes upper GIT bleeding, when both coughing and vomiting are present, and bleeding from the naso-pharynx. Secondary malignancies in the lungs rarely generate haemoptysis.

Physical examination
Establish the **person's haemodynamic status**: blood pressure, pulse, and oxygen saturation. Look for other evidence of bleeding or bruising. Look for the cause of haemoptysis: pneumonia, pulmonary infarction from pulmonary embolus, underlying mitral stenosis, or evidence of left ventricular failure.

Investigations and management
Prognosis measured in hours to days prior to the onset of this problem (symptom control)
With significant haemoptysis, **stop any medications that may exacerbate bleeding**: anticoagulants, NSAIDs, and clopidogrel. **Consider**

vitamin K for people who have been on warfarin, or, if there are no contraindications, **oral tranexamic acid** 1 g orally four times daily.

Haemoptysis is frightening.

Everyone around the bed is likely to be frightened. In someone for whom this is the terminal event and where active measures are not appropriate, provide adequate analgesia and sedation with a combination of crisis medications (opioids and benzodiazepines (IV if necessary; p.54)) as death from bleeding is mostly from obliteration of airways with irritative blood. Red or green linen may reduce the visual impact of bleeding.

Prognosis measured in weeks prior to the onset of this problem (in addition to symptom control)

If seeking a distinction between bleeding from lung and stomach, check **pH** as respiratory bleeding will be slightly alkaline.

Check **coagulation studies**, looking for coagulopathies including DIC (low platelets, APTT, red cell fragments which may be present on a blood film, and raised fibrinogen degradation products; p.196).

A **CXR** may show evidence of lobar pneumonia, lobar collapse (because of a more proximal intraluminal lesion obstructing that lobe), or a wedge-shaped peripheral lesion of pulmonary infarct.

In people with more than streaks of blood in sputum, a **bronchoscopy** should be carried out on a semi-urgent basis if there is no explanation for the bleeding. This may also be therapeutic as there is the ability to use a laser in diathermy of a bleeding vessel.

Prognosis measured in months to years prior to the onset of this problem (in addition to the above)

Most bleeding from the lungs stops spontaneously. Larger volume bleeds (>500 mL in 24 h) are likely to require intervention. If the bleeding is from primary lung cancer, explore local treatment options: laser coagulation, external beam radiotherapy, or brachytherapy.

Rarely, selective intubation to isolate a lobe where there is bleeding may preserve the rest of the lung's function while a definitive plan is put in place. Bronchial artery catheterization and selective embolization is an option for ongoing low-level bleeding. Open surgery is very rarely indicated.

Further reading

Chapman SJ, Robinson GV (2021). Haemoptysis (Chapter 7). In: *Oxford Handbook of Respiratory Medicine*, 4th ed. Oxford: Oxford University Press. Available at: https://doi.org/10.1093/med/9780198837114.003.0007

Pneumonitis ①

Pneumonitis occurs most commonly as an iatrogenic complication of radiotherapy or chemotherapy, infection, or connective tissue diseases (Table 5.6).

Table 5.6 Causes of pneumonitis

	More frequently encountered causes	Less frequently encountered causes
Cancer	Chemotherapy (acutely) Radiotherapy (2–3 months after treatment)	
Intercurrent illnesses	Rheumatoid arthritis Occupational lung disease including asbestosis	SLE

History

People with pneumonitis present with **cough** and **breathlessness**, and are often systemically unwell with **fever and malaise**.

The syndrome may mimic an atypical pneumonia in time course, presentation, and physical findings. An acute clinical course may follow exposure to a number of chemotherapeutic agents including cyclophosphamide, methotrexate, gemcitabine, bleomycin, busulphan, chlorambucil, taxanes, and temozolomide.

Lung signs and symptoms are delayed until some months after treatment with radiotherapy. Unlike other complications of radiotherapy, the respiratory findings can be more widespread than the irradiated area. Mucous plugs with fibrous tissue (bronchiolitis obliterans with organizing pneumonia (BOOP)) may be seen.

Rheumatoid arthritis can be associated with fibrosing alveolitis and interstitial fibrosis. Along with SLE and drug-induced pneumonitis, these changes predominate in the lower lobes.

Physical examination

Physical examination may be **normal throughout the clinical course**. Look for central cyanosis on lips or ear lobes. Clubbing suggests that there is long-standing pathology. Look for evidence of respiratory distress including tachypnoea at rest or on minimal exertion. Fine, late inspiratory crackles may be heard in the affected area.

Right-sided heart strain may manifest as overt failure or evidence of increased pressures on the right side of the heart with a loud pulmonary component of the second heart sound.

Investigations and management

Prognosis measured in hours to days prior to the onset of this problem (symptom control)

The breathlessness caused is often progressive and associated with significant fear as function worsens and breathlessness intensifies. Adequate psychological support and relaxation techniques are an important adjunct to pharmacological interventions. Energy conservation techniques are an integral part of management.

Check oxygenation.

Exclude an atypical pneumonia that may mimic the presentation. Discontinue the offending agent if pneumonitis is medication related.

Prognosis measured in weeks prior to the onset of this problem (in addition to symptom control)

The **CXR** may show little change early in the course of the clinical presentation. The pattern of interstitial changes will confirm clinical suspicions.

Mild hypoxaemia with normal or low partial pressure of carbon dioxide is seen on **arterial blood gases**.

Chest CT may delineate the extent of lung changes.

In long-standing changes, a restrictive pattern may be seen on **pulmonary function tests** and secondary polycythaemia may be present on **FBC**.

Glucocorticoids may play a role in reducing local inflammation and reducing the intensity of symptoms early in its course.

Prognosis measured in months to years prior to the onset of this problem (in addition to the above)

Treat any underlying connective tissue disorder.

Further reading

Chapman SJ, Robinson GV (2021). Drug and toxin induced lung disease (Chapter 25). In: *Oxford Handbook of Respiratory Medicine*, 4th ed. Oxford: Oxford University Press. Available at: https://doi.org/10.1093/med/9780198837114.003.0025

Lymphangitis carcinomatosis ①

The blockage of lung lymphatics by tumour creates the clinical presentation of lymphangitis carcinomatosis. Some malignancies are more likely to cause this (Table 5.7).

Table 5.7 Malignancies associated with lymphangitis carcinomatosis

	More frequently encountered causes	Less frequently encountered causes
Cancer	Adenocarcinoma of the lung or breast	Other malignancies

History

Lymphangitis presents with breathlessness, mimicking pulmonary oedema, atypical pneumonia, or pulmonary emboli. Progressive severe breathlessness is seen with rapidly developing hypoxaemia.

Physical examination

Early in the clinical course, physical examination may be normal. Look for central cyanosis of the lips or ear lobes. Look for respiratory distress including tachypnoea at rest or on minimal exertion.

Investigations and management

Prognosis measured in hours to days prior to lymphangitis (symptom control)
Exclude an atypical pneumonia that may mimic the presentation.

The major symptomatic intervention is the **relief of breathlessness**. Oxygen may be of limited benefit until hypoxaemia develops. **Regular, low-dose morphine and anxiolytics** may reduce symptoms.

Prognosis measured in weeks prior to the onset of this problem (in addition to symptom control)
CXR may be normal early in its course but progress to hilar enlargement with fan-shaped opacities, reflecting tumour spread through lymphatic channels. Kerley B lines may be visible.

Sputum cytology may be positive for malignant cells.

Check pulse oximetry.

Unless the underlying malignancy is responsive to chemotherapy, little is likely to reverse this problem. Case reports suggest glucocorticoids may offer some early symptomatic benefit.

Prognosis measured in months to years prior to the onset of this problem (in addition to the above)
Transthoracic or transbronchial biopsy may confirm the diagnosis.

People with a primary breast cancer with submaximal systemic treatment should be offered hormone therapy for oestrogen- or progesterone-positive tumours or systemic cytotoxic chemotherapy to which the cancer has not been previously exposed. The presence of lymphangitis carcinomatosis is a very poor prognostic sign, with median survival measured in weeks.

Further reading

Chapman SJ, Robinson GV (2021). Lung cancer (Chapter 32). In: *Oxford Handbook of Respiratory Medicine*, 4th ed. Oxford: Oxford University Press. Available at: https://doi.org/10.1093/med/9780198837114.003.0032

Chapter 6

Gastrointestinal disorders

Oral mucositis *148*
Gastrointestinal mucositis *150*
Colitis *153*
Acute abdomen *156*
Upper gastrointestinal tract bleeding *158*
Lower gastrointestinal tract bleeding *161*
Bowel obstruction *163*
Ascites *166*
Sudden onset of jaundice *169*
Biliary sepsis *172*
Acute pancreatitis *174*
Acute hepatocellular failure *177*
Fistula formation *180*

Oral mucositis ☼

- Mucositis may be a complication of radiotherapy to the head and neck, chemotherapy, or bone marrow transplants (Table 6.1) (p. 151).
- Mucositis may affect the mucosa of any part of the GIT (p. 151).
- Oral mucositis may cause pain, decreased oral intake, and increased incidence of infections (p. 151).
- Mucositis of the pharynx and oesophagus may cause dysphagia, odynophagia, ulceration, or perforation (p. 151).
- Mucositis of the larynx may cause a hoarse voice, painful earache, cough, breathlessness, or stridor (p. 151).

The World Health Organization (WHO) grades of oral mucositis are:
- Grade 0: none.
- Grade 1: mild erythema, mild pain.
- Grade 2: oral erythema, mouth ulcers but a solid diet is tolerated.
- Grade 3: mouth ulcers; only a liquid diet is tolerated.
- Grade 4: oral alimentation is not possible.

Reproduced with permission from the World Health Organization.

Table 6.1 Causes of oral mucositis

	More frequently encountered causes	Less frequently encountered causes
Cancer	Radiotherapy to the mouth, oropharynx, or oesophagus	Chemotherapy containing 5-fluorouracil, cisplatin, or melphalan
	Chemotherapy for haematological malignancy aimed at severe bone marrow suppression	
Intercurrent illness		Aphthous ulcers, widespread oral herpes simplex

History

- People with oral mucositis will complain of a **sore mouth**.
- The most important issue is to distinguish between inflammation due to therapy and other additional pathology such as **herpes simplex**.
- A history of cold sores in someone with widespread oral ulceration signals the need for **viral swabs**.

Physical examination

- Check **hydration** (tissue turgor, pulse rate, blood pressure, and moisture of mucous membranes) and nutritional status if mucositis is severe (grade 3 or 4) or has been prolonged.
- Exclude other skin and oral lesions, specifically simplex lesions of the lips, oral candida, or evidence of more widespread mucosal/

skin damage (Stevens–Johnson syndrome (p.84) or toxic epidermal necrolysis (p.84)).
- If a primary herpetic infection is suspected, exclude central signs of encephalitis.

Investigations and management

Prognosis measured in hours to days prior to the onset of this problem (symptom control)

Further investigations are not indicated. However, these people all require **good mouth care**, with the frequency with which the care is attended seeming to be the most important issue. Agents that have been used include 0.9% NaCl, sodium bicarbonate, and 0.2% chlorhexidine. Care must be exercised if chlorhexidine is commenced as it can worsen pain because of the alcohol content.

Ensure that there are no colonies of oral candida.

People with oral mucositis, regardless of the severity, must have access to **analgesia**. This includes topical agents (benzydamine gel) and systemic opioids with morphine the best choice. In this poor-prognosis group, morphine is most easily administered as SC injections. While grade 1–2 oral mucositis may be managed with opioids as requested, people with grade 3 or 4 require regular morphine. The starting dose depends upon prior exposure and the overall condition of the person.

Prognosis measured in weeks prior to the onset of this problem (in addition to symptom control)
- Check FBC, EUC, and albumin.
- Hydration must be assessed and supplemental fluids administered parenterally (IV or SC) if necessary.
- Pain management requires a combination of local and systemic interventions. Morphine is best administered as PCA if patients are well enough.

Prognosis measured in months to years prior to the onset of this problem (in addition to the above)

Additional considerations include the management of superimposed infections and early consideration of **supplemental feeding** (total parenteral nutrition) while waiting for severe mucositis to settle.

Further reading

Davies AN (2021). Oral care (Chapter 10.4). In: *Oxford Textbook of Palliative Medicine*, 6th ed. Oxford: Oxford University Press. Available at: https://doi.org/10.1093/med/9780198821328.003.0063

Watson M et al. (eds) (2019). Gastrointestinal symptoms (Chapter 9). In: *Oxford Handbook of Palliative Care*, 3rd ed. Oxford: Oxford University Press. Available at: https://doi.org/10.1093/med/9780198745655.003.0009

Gastrointestinal mucositis ☼

GIT mucositis causes abdominal pain and diarrhoea and is usually iatrogenic (Table 6.2). Other symptoms depend upon the level of the GIT involved and may include:
- upper GIT: anorexia, nausea, vomiting, melaena, haematemesis, ileus, perforation.
- lower GIT (including rectum): change in bowel habits, rectal blood or mucus, tenesmus, ileus, perforation, fistula formation.

Table 6.2 Causes of GI mucositis

	More frequently encountered causes	Less frequently encountered causes
Cancer	Radiotherapy to abdomen or pelvis	Chemotherapy containing 5-fluorouracil, cisplatin, irinotecan, docetaxel
	Chemotherapy for haematological malignancy aimed at severe bone marrow suppression	

History

People will complain of **abdominal pain and altered bowel habits**. Other problems will depend upon the level of the GIT involved and its severity (Table 6.3). Symptoms may include nausea and vomiting, melaena, tenesmus, and the passage of mucus through the rectum.

Physical examination

- Check **hydration** and **nutritional status** (people can rapidly lose large amounts of fluid and protein).
- Inspect the **mouth and oropharynx**.
- Check **pulse, temperature, and blood pressure**.
- Palpate the abdomen for pain and exclude an acute abdomen (p.156).
- Auscultate for bowel sounds.

Investigations and management

Prognosis measured in hours to days prior to the onset of this problem (symptom control)

In this group of people, further investigations are not indicated. Despite the poor prognosis, people who have diarrhoea or vomiting may benefit from parenteral fluids, either SC or IV.

Nausea and vomiting must be addressed regardless of prognosis. In the absence of an ileus or perforation, metoclopramide 10 mg SC three or four times daily may be used. Haloperidol 0.5–2.5 mg SC daily or cyclizine 12.5–25 mg SC four times daily may provide additional relief. If mucositis is a complication of chemotherapy or radiotherapy, consider the addition of a 5-HT$_3$ antiemetic (ondansetron 4 mg SL/SC/IV or tropisetron 5 mg SC/IV).

Pain and diarrhoea will require SC morphine.

If diarrhoea fails to settle with regular opioids, SC octreotide (100 micrograms three times daily as a starting dose) may be of benefit.

Table 6.3 Radiation Therapy Oncology Group (RTOG) grading of gastrointestinal mucositis

Organ	Grade 0	Grade 1	Grade 2	Grade 3	Grade 4
Pharynx and oesophagus	No change	Moderate dysphagia or odynophagia	Moderate dysphagia requiring opioids	Severe pain and weight loss Parenteral feeding needed	Complete obstruction, ulceration, perforation
Larynx	No change	Mild hoarseness	Hoarse but able to speak, sore ear and throat, cough	Whispering voice, ear and throat pain requiring opioids	Breathlessness, stridor, tracheotomy needed
Upper GIT	No change	Weight loss <15% from baseline Nausea and pain not requiring treatment	Weight loss <5% from baseline Opioids for pain	Anorexia with weight loss >15% from baseline Severe pain despite treatment	Ileus, obstruction, may require surgery Blood transfusions needed
Lower GIT and pelvis	No change	Increasing frequency of bowel actions Pain not requiring treatment	Diarrhoea requiring medications Pain requiring opioids	Diarrhoea requiring parenteral support Must wear pads	Acute or subacute obstruction, pain, and tenesmus requiring surgery Blood transfusions needed

Reprinted from *International Journal of Radiation Oncology, Biology, Physics*, 31, 5, JD Cox et al., Toxicity criteria of the Radiation Therapy Oncology Group (RTOG) and the European organization for research and treatment of cancer (EORTC), pp. 1341–1346. Copyright 1995, with permission from Elsevier.

Prognosis measured in weeks prior to the onset of this problem (in addition to symptom control)

- Check **FBC**, **EUC**, and **albumin**.
- Collect **stool cultures** for *Clostridium difficile*.
- If **pain** is a problem, parenteral opioids (morphine, hydromorphone) must be prescribed.
- People should receive either **ranitidine** (150 mg orally twice daily or 50 mg IV three times daily) or **omeprazole** (20 mg orally daily or 40 mg IV daily) for epigastric pain with the route of administration dependent upon associated nausea and vomiting.
- **Oral sulfasalazine** 500 mg twice daily may help with **diarrhoea**.
- In people with **rectal mucositis**, sucralfate enemas (20 mL of 10% sucralfate solution twice daily) may provide relief from pain, tenesmus, and rectal bleeds.

Prognosis measured in months to years prior to the onset of this problem (in addition to the above)
- Consider endoscopy if symptoms persist for more than a week.
- If severe or prolonged, supplemental feeding (total parenteral nutrition) must be considered.

Further reading

Cassidy J et al. (eds) (2015). Principles of symptom control in palliative care (Chapter 6). In: *Oxford Handbook of Oncology*, 4th ed. Oxford: Oxford University Press. Available at: https://doi.org/10.1093/med/9780199689842.003.0006

Colitis ☼

Colitis is commonly seen in people who are unwell. It is often a major stressor on already compromised body systems at the end of life. Manage reversible causes even late in life (Table 6.4).

Table 6.4 Causes of colitis

	More frequently encountered causes	Less frequently encountered causes
Cancer	Radiation colitis	External pressure on two or more branches of mesenteric blood supply, neutropenia
End-stage organ failure		Hypotension, hypokalaemia, cardiac arrhythmias, atherosclerosis, pancreatitis, vasculitis
Intercurrent illnesses	Recent use of antibiotics Crohn's disease Ulcerative colitis	Medications (opioids, anticholinergics)

History

- *Clostridium difficile* accounts for about 20% of all antibiotic-associated diarrhoea. Watery diarrhoea with abdominal pain, fever, and leukocytosis suggests pseudomembranous colitis.
- **Diarrhoea may be bloody with colitis**.
- An **ileus** may develop late and proceed to a toxic megacolon, mimicking an acute abdomen (p.156).
- Check for bleeding from the gut. Crohn's disease may have local, high-volume bleeding when surgery or embolization should be considered in people well enough to tolerate the procedure.
- **Shoulder-tip pain and well-localized or diffuse abdominal pain associated with shock alerts to the possibility of gut perforation** (p.156).
- The severity of signs of colitis may be **masked by immunosuppressants or advanced disease**.

Ischaemic colitis may occur with:
- vascular occlusion (thrombus, embolus, long-term radiation damage, or vasculitis)
- hypoperfusion (hypotension, hypovolaemia)
- vasoconstriction or venous compromise (pancreatitis, malignancy).

The gut may initially be hypermotile with poorly localized pain progressing to the intense abdominal pain of an acute abdomen (especially in uncontrolled atrial fibrillation; p.156).

In people with known inflammatory bowel disease, inability to take anti-inflammatories or immunosuppressants, hypokalaemia, opioids, or other anticholinergics can precipitate toxic colitis.

Physical examination

Fever, dehydration, and tachycardia may be seen in all forms of colitis. Examine for atrial fibrillation and cardiac failure (ischaemic colitis). Seek bruising or bleeding suggesting coagulopathy. Look for cutaneous vasculitis (p.92). Localize any site of abdominal pain to indicate the level of gut involved.

Abdominal examination may **not** have specific signs early in ischaemic colitis.

Investigations and management

Prognosis measured in hours to days prior to the onset of this problem (symptom control)

Regardless of the cause of colitis, address pain and diarrhoea. Give opioid **analgesia** SC or IV which may also help to reduce diarrhoea. If diarrhoea persists, consider **octreotide 100 micrograms SC three times daily. Discontinue prokinetic medications (metoclopramide, senna, domperidone)**.

Even late in life, if **C. difficile** is considered the cause of diarrhoea, causative antibiotics should be stopped and treatment with IV metronidazole or vancomycin commenced.

People with **ischaemic colitis** may be very unwell and this is likely to be a terminal event (p.153). In addition to opioid analgesia, these people may benefit from SC hyoscine butylbromide (20 mg four times daily) or octreotide to reduce any cramping pain.

Prognosis measured in weeks prior to the onset of this problem (in addition to symptom control)

Check **FBC**, **EUC**, and a **stool specimen**.

A **plain abdominal X-ray** with colon diameter of >7cm suggests toxic megacolon which has a high perforation risk. This carries a very poor prognosis and crisis medications (p.53) must be available.

In the presence of clinical or biochemical evidence of **dehydration**, gently hydrate for comfort.

Managing **diarrhoea** can also employ loperamide (two tablets now followed by two tablets after each loose bowel action) or atropine sulphate/diphenoxylate (two tablets three times daily).

Treat the diarrhoea of **C. difficile** with oral or parenteral metronidazole or oral vancomycin. Oral cholestyramine (1 g three times daily) may be useful.

In **ischaemic colitis**, partial-thickness damage with no systemic manifestations of sepsis or haemodynamic compromise can be treated with gut rest and hydration. With full-thickness damage, surgery needs to be considered if comorbidities and prognosis allow. If inoperable, prognosis is poor.

Prognosis measured in months to years prior to the onset of this problem (in addition to the above)

Investigate and manage simultaneously.
- **Blood cultures** if febrile.
- Ensure **IV access and commence hydration**.

- In the absence of perforation, further investigations include **abdominal CT**.
- Sigmoidoscopy will show raised 2–10 mm yellow plaques in pseudomembranous colitis.
- If subdiaphragmatic free air, seek an **urgent surgical consultation**. Commence IV antibiotics.
- In people with **ischaemic gut**, seek an **urgent surgical consultation** to consider excision.
- In inflammatory bowel disease, continue or reintroduce long-term immunosuppressive therapy.

Further reading

Gimson A (2020). Miscellaneous disorders of the bowel (Chapter 15.19). In: *Oxford Textbook of Medicine*, 6th ed. Oxford: Oxford University Press. Available at: https://doi.org/10.1093/med/9780198746690.003.0314

Acute abdomen ☼

The clinical presentation of an acute abdomen can range from the very classic presentation seen as acute appendicitis develops through to a much more subtle presentation where the person becomes progressively unwell with subtle signs that need to be interpreted carefully in the light of their clinical history and their overall condition (Table 6.5).

Table 6.5 Causes of an acute abdomen

	More frequently encountered causes	Less frequently encountered causes
Cancer		Tumour eroding through gut wall
		Perforation secondary to radiation colitis
		Fistula formation
		Peritonitis secondary to infected ascites
End-stage organ failure		Atrial fibrillation causing perforation secondary to gut ischaemia
		Ischaemia due to prolonged hypotension or hypovolaemia
Intercurrent illnesses	Acute cholecystitis	Ruptured gastric ulcer
	Acute appendicitis	Ischaemic colitis
	Flare of Crohn's disease or ulcerative colitis	
	Diverticulitis	
	Acute pancreatitis	

History

- A classical presentation of poorly localized pain becoming well defined and localized, together with an ileus can occur.
- In people late in life, the signs may be far more subtle, with the person appearing unwell with little or no obvious localizing symptoms. In ischaemic colitis, early signs may be quite non-specific.
- If there has been previous abdominal surgery or radiotherapy where bowel may have been within the field, consider whether any gut perforation was localized due to previous adhesions.
- The severity of signs of an acute abdomen can be **masked by immunosuppressants or advanced disease**. Background analgesia is unlikely to mask an acute abdomen, but consider why a person has suddenly increased their use of 'as-needed' doses.
- If ascites is present, have a low threshold for considering the presence of spontaneous infection, or infection following previous instrumentation.

Physical examination

Fever, dehydration, and tachycardia may be seen with any cause of an acute abdomen. Check for atrial fibrillation and cardiac failure (ischaemic colitis).

Carefully seek to localize the site of pain. Listen carefully for any bowel sounds.

Abdominal examination may *not* have specific signs especially in the presence of previous surgery with adhesions.

Investigations and management

Prognosis measured in hours to days prior to the onset of this problem (symptom control)

Regardless of the cause of an acute abdomen, address pain. Give regular opioid **analgesia** SC or IV. Consider how best to maintain (or gently improve) hydration. This may range from ice chips to slow SC hydration.

Prognosis measured in weeks prior to the onset of this problem (in addition to symptom control)

Check **FBC** and **EUC**.

A plain abdominal X-ray may demonstrate free gas under the diaphragm (or rostrally in lateral films if supine). If there is a perforation, consideration needs to be given to imaging to show the source and an urgent laparotomy after fluid resuscitation and adequate broad spectrum antibiotic cover.

An **abdominal CT** may help to identify the pathology that has led to an acute abdomen if it is not clinically obvious.

If there is ascites, consider cultures of blood and ascites.

Seek an **immediate surgical consultation**. Carefully weigh whether surgical intervention will be tolerated by the person or whether the catabolic insult of surgery will be too much for the person (and hasten their death).

If cholecystitis or pancreatitis is due to a gallstone, consider the role of ERCP with the hope of removing any ductal calculi.

Diverticulitis can cause distressing symptoms, but if there is no perforation, it can be managed conservatively.

Prognosis measured in months to years prior to the onset of this problem (in addition to the above)

Manage actively while investigating the cause. Seek an urgent surgical consultation.

- **Blood cultures** if febrile.
- Ensure **IV access and commence hydration**.
- In the absence of perforation, further investigations include **abdominal CT**.
- If subdiaphragmatic free air, seek an **urgent surgical consultation**. Commence IV antibiotics. Given the procedures that can now be done safely laparoscopically, the threshold for intervention is lower than it used to be because it is better tolerated.
- In inflammatory bowel disease, ensure continuation/reintroduction of long-term immunosuppressive therapy while evaluating other options.

Further reading

Woodward J (2020). Symptoms of gastrointestinal disease (Chapter 15.2). In: *Oxford Textbook of Medicine*, 6th ed. Oxford: Oxford University Press. Available at: https://doi.org/10.1093/med/9780198746690.003.0285

Upper gastrointestinal tract bleeding ☠️

- There are many potential causes of upper GIT bleeding in life-limiting illnesses (Table 6.6).
- This is initially a clinical diagnosis for which there needs to be a high index of suspicion. It may mimic other causes of systemic decompensation.
- Upper GIT bleeding is an emergency. Prompt treatment minimizes premature mortality.

History

Table 6.6 Causes of upper GIT bleeding

	More frequently encountered causes	Less frequently encountered causes
Cancer	Abnormal platelet function (cytotoxic agents, renal failure, NSAIDs, myelodysplasia, paraproteinaemias, acute leukaemias)	Gastric tumours Small bowel tumours
	Thrombocytopaenia (increased consumption, splenic pooling, decreased production)	
	Mucosal bleeding	
End-stage organ failure	Portal hypertension (oesophageal varices, splenomegaly, gastropathy)	
Intercurrent illnesses	Peptic ulceration Oesophagitis Gastritis Sepsis (DIC)	Mallory–Weiss tear Angiodysplasia Haemangiomas

People often describe **nausea and vomiting** ('coffee-grounds' or haematemesis). **Melaena** may be reported but its absence does not exclude upper GIT bleeding. Postural symptoms may predominate in association with hypotension and hypovolaemia.

Check if the person is currently or has previously received NSAIDs (including COX-2 inhibitors) alone or with corticosteroids, or anticoagulants. Many over-the-counter products contain NSAIDs, and must be specifically asked about.

Check a history of long-term alcohol use, previous chronic liver disease, or previous GIT bleeding.

Physical examination

- Check conjunctiva and palmar creases for anaemia.
- Examine for **shock** (cold peripheries, a thready tachycardia, hypotension).

- Exclude an **acute abdomen** (suggesting perforation; p.156). Do a digital rectal examination looking for melaena.
- Look for any **bruising or bleeding** suggesting a coagulopathy. A high index of suspicion is needed, as physical findings may be relatively normal in people even with significant bleeding.

Investigations and management

Prognosis measured in hours to days prior to the onset of this problem (symptom control)

Whatever the cause of bleeding, ensure adequate parenteral analgesia. If the person is shocked, IV opioids may be more effective than SC, given impaired absorption.

Ongoing bleeding may cause **anxiety**. Benzodiazepines (clonazepam 0.5–1.0 mg SL/SC twice daily, midazolam 2.5–5.0 mg as needed or a starting dose of 10 mg SC over 24 h) may be needed.

GIT tract bleeding can cause **nausea and vomiting**, and regular antiemetics are indicated: monitor response to metoclopramide (10 mg SC four times daily). Alternative agents include haloperidol or cyclizine. Usually a combination of agents is required. Intractable nausea may need chlorpromazine (25–50 mg SC) or levomepromazine (6.25 mg SC at night or via syringe driver).

Stop heparin, warfarin and review the need for NSAIDs or clopidogrel.

If **torrential bleeding** occurs as a life-threatening event, crisis medications (p.53) must be available. Torrential bleeding is very distressing for family and carers. In this situation, red or green sheets may reduce the visible evidence of bleeding.

Prognosis measured in weeks prior to the onset of this problem (in addition to symptom control)

- Define the likely cause of bleeding. Catastrophic bleeding is likely to be a terminal event.
- In this group, it is important to assess fluid status and hydrate if necessary.
- **Cross-match for a packed cell transfusion** at the same time as taking baseline bloods (Hb, renal function, coagulation studies, LFTs).
- Low-flow **oxygen** may be useful if shocked.
- Correct any coagulopathy with vitamin K 10 mg orally or IV, FFP, and platelets.
- In bleeding with an adequate platelet count, **tranexamic acid 500 mg** four times daily may stabilize clots. Use cautiously with simultaneous urological bleeding to avoid clot retention.
- If there is **upper GIT bleeding**, an IV PPI (omeprazole 40 mg IV daily) or H$_2$ blocker (ranitidine 50 mg IV three times daily) and oral sucralfate (1 g four times daily) may be useful.
- Consider **endoscopy** for localized therapies (diathermy, fibrin, banding of varices). Surgery is rarely indicated in this patient population. If surgery is not an option for uncontrolled bleeding, embolization through visceral angiography is an option in a selected subgroup.

Prognosis measured in months to years prior to the onset of this problem (in addition to the above)

This is a medical emergency. **Contact surgical teams urgently for an urgent endoscopy**.

- Examine the person for **shock**. If shocked, immediately insert two large-bore cannulae.
- **Cross-match** 6 U of packed cells. **Rapidly correct fluid loss** with colloids and packed cells.
- **Correct clotting abnormalities** with vitamin K, FFP, and platelets.
- If **bleeding varices** are suspected, commence octreotide 50 micrograms/h IV.
- All people should **receive IV omeprazole** (or locally available IV PPI).

Further reading

Brown V, Rockall TA (2020). Gastrointestinal bleeding (Chapter 15.4.2). In: *Oxford Textbook of Medicine*, 6th ed. Oxford: Oxford University Press. Available at: https://doi.org/10.1093/med/9780198746690.003.0291

Lower gastrointestinal tract bleeding :☻:

Approximately two-thirds of episodes of GIT bleeding originate from the lower tract (Table 6.7).

History

Table 6.7 Causes of lower GIT bleeding

	More frequently encountered causes	Less frequently encountered causes
Cancer	Malignancy (primary or secondary with direct invasion of the bowel wall)	
	GIT mucositis	
End-stage organ failure	Bleeding haemorrhoids (portal hypertension)	
Intercurrent illnesses	Diverticulosis	Inflammatory bowel disease
		Benign anorectal disease

- Rather than the altered blood of upper GIT bleeding, most people will describe **bright blood**. **Melaena** may still be present with bleeding of the terminal ileum.
- The larger the volume of bleeding in the proximal gut, the more likely that unchanged blood will be seen in stools.
- A history of previous episodes of lower GIT bleeding is important, as is any tendency to bleeding.
- Localized pain or tenderness suggests **diverticulitis**.

Physical examination

- Look for any evidence of a **coagulopathy** (peripheral bruising or bleeding).
- **Blood pressure drop** of >10 mmHg or a rise in pulse of >10 beats/ min when standing from sitting suggests significant (>10%) blood loss.
- Abdominal examination should seek any rebound, guarding, or tenderness suggesting an acute abdomen (p.156).

Investigations and management

Prognosis measured in hours to days prior to the onset of this problem (symptom control)

- Manage pain, nausea, and anxiety.
- Crisis interventions must be available (p.53).
- Unnecessary medications must be discontinued. Stop medications such as aspirin, clopidogrel, or anticoagulants that may worsen bleeding.

Prognosis measured in weeks prior to the onset of this problem (in addition to symptom control)

- Examine for an **acute abdomen** (p.156). This may indicate **perforation**.
- A **plain X-ray** may show free gas under the diaphragm. This group is unlikely to tolerate major surgery for perforation. Focus on comfort care and discuss with the patient and their family.
- Check FBC, EUC, and coagulation studies.
- **If Hb <10 g/dL**, transfuse packed cells if breathlessness or anxiety are prominent.
- **Sigmoidoscopy** will assess anorectal sources of bleeding. **Colonoscopy** may be performed if the sigmoidoscopy is negative. Colonoscopy should not be performed if there is a concern about ischaemic gut or with suspected severe mucosal inflammation. Colonoscopy can definitively treat most bleeding polyps, bleeding cancers, telangiectasia, and arteriovenous malformations with either diathermy or laser. With no other known gut pathology, a labelled red cell scan or selective mesenteric angiography may localize bleeding and allow selective embolization.

Prognosis measured in months to years prior to the onset of this problem (in addition to the above)

Consult the surgical team immediately.

- A large-bore cannula must be inserted and fluid resuscitation administered if shocked or haemodynamically unstable.
- Correct any bleeding diathesis with FFP and vitamin K.
- Discontinue medications likely to be contributing to bleeding.
- If febrile, take blood cultures and commence broad antibiotic cover.

Further reading

Brown V, Rockall TA (2020). Gastrointestinal bleeding (Chapter 15.4.2). In: *Oxford Textbook of Medicine*, 6th ed. Oxford: Oxford University Press. Available at: https://doi.org/10.1093/med/9780198746690.003.0291

Bowel obstruction :☼:

- Obstruction of the small bowel due to advanced cancer is more common than large bowel.
- 20% of malignant bowel obstructions are multilevel.
- Up to 50% of obstructions in advanced cancer are due to causes other than cancer (Table 6.8).
- Bowel perforation or strangulation complicating malignant bowel obstructions is rare.

Table 6.8 Causes of bowel obstruction

	More frequently encountered causes	Less frequently encountered causes
Cancer	Primary or metastatic cancers within the lumen of the gut, within the wall of the gut, or compressing the gut	Radiation strictures
		Infiltration of the myenteric plexus
	Primary or metastatic peritoneal disease reducing motility	Severe constipation
Intercurrent illnesses	Adhesions	Intestinal hernias
	Inflammatory bowel disease	Sigmoid volvulus
		Constipation

History

- People with bowel obstruction most often present with insidious onset of **cramping abdominal pain**, **distension**, and **nausea** and vomiting.
- In small bowel obstruction, **nausea** is an early symptom with copious vomiting, often of undigested food.
- Obstruction at any level can cause **feculent vomiting** due to bacterial overgrowth with stasis.
- **Abdominal pain** can be a constant dull ache and cramping. Pain is typically periumbilical for small bowel obstruction perceived more laterally with less severity for large bowel obstruction.
- Incomplete bowel obstruction may present with severe cramping pain, followed by the passage of stools or flatus. In complete obstruction, the person passes no stools or flatus.

Physical examination

- Abdominal distension and visible peristalsis may be present but not needed for the diagnosis.
- Localized or generalized abdominal tenderness may be present, but pain may be mild.
- A palpable mass may be present.
- Bowel sounds may be hyperactive and high pitched, or absent. High obstruction may yield a gastric splash.

- Rectal examination may be unremarkable or reveal an empty and dilated rectum.

Investigations and management

Prognosis measured in hours to days prior to the onset of this problem (symptom control)

Investigations are not indicated.

Assess abdominal distension, and bowel sounds. Perform a rectal examination. If the rectum is full, a glycerine suppository followed by a bisacodyl (Dulcolax®) suppository may be administered.

Analgesia with parenteral opioids must be available. In people with moderate to severe pain or an acute abdomen, give regularly, not 'as needed'. Co-prescribe antispasmodic agents with cramping pain or vomiting (hyoscine butylbromide 20 mg SC four times daily up to 120 mg via SC infusion).

Ranitidine reduces volume of upper GIT secretions by 50% and can be given 50 mg SC four times daily.

Nausea is prominent. Vomiting is associated with complete proximal obstruction or high oral or parenteral intake. For nausea, choices include haloperidol (0.5–3.0 mg SC daily) with cyclizine (12.5–25 mg SC twice to four times daily). Intractable nausea may require ondansetron 10 mg wafers or SC injection twice daily, or levomepromazine 6.25–12.0 mg using a SC infusion.

Despite oral intake often exacerbating vomiting, allow people to take in what they want. Occasionally, severe vomiting should be managed initially with an NG tube to decompress the gut.

Initiate a mouth care regimen.

Prognosis measured in weeks prior to the onset of this problem (in addition to symptom control)

If this is the first presentation of a malignant bowel obstruction, management includes:
- Gentle **hydration** with either IV or SC fluids.
- Temporary **NG tube placement** may occasionally be necessary to decompress the upper gut.
- **Abdominal X-ray** (diagnostic of bowel obstruction with dilated loops of small bowel, more than three air–fluid levels, and no air in the rectum). X-rays may be normal in people with low tumour volume, or distal obstruction.
- **Gastrografin® contrast studies** may be used to define partial or single-level obstructions.
- **Abdominal CT** scan may best define the cause of obstruction.

Procedures can include bypass, defunctioning, or stenting. If surgical or stenting procedures are inappropriate, management should revert to good symptom control.

Prognosis measured in months to years prior to the onset of this problem (in addition to the above)

The site and completeness of the obstruction help to dictate the management. People require:

- **abdominal CT scan**
- IV hydration and correction of electrolyte abnormalities
- a grossly dilated large bowel, volvulus, perforation, or strangulated hernia requires **urgent surgical intervention**.

Further reading

Boland JW, Boland EG (2021). Malignant bowel obstruction (Chapter 14.10). In: *Oxford Textbook of Palliative Medicine*, 6th ed. Oxford: Oxford University Press. Available at: https://doi.org/10.1093/med/9780198821328.003.0085

Watson M et al. (eds) (2019). Gastrointestinal symptoms (Chapter 9). In: *Oxford Handbook of Palliative Care*, 3rd ed. Oxford: Oxford University Press. Available at: https://doi.org/10.1093/med/9780198745655.003.0009

Ascites ⓘ

- Ascites is defined as the pathological accumulation of fluid in the peritoneal cavity.
- The pathogenesis is poorly understood, differing according to underlying causes (Table 6.9).

Table 6.9 Causes of ascites

	More frequently encountered causes	Less frequently encountered causes
Malignancy	Primary peritoneal cancers or secondary cancer (bowel, pancreas, breast, ovary, lung cancer)	Hepatocellular carcinoma
End-stage organ failure	Cirrhosis (alcoholic, viral hepatitis, autoimmune)	Cardiac failure including constrictive pericarditis
Intercurrent illnesses	Pancreatitis Nephrotic syndrome	Protein-losing enteropathy Malnutrition Budd–Chiari syndrome (hepatic vein thrombosis) Hypothyroidism

History

People describe **increasing abdominal girth**, at times associated with shortness of breath, early satiety, nausea and vomiting, and abdominal discomfort. It is often multifactorial.

Fevers or an influenza-like illness raise the question of **spontaneous bacterial peritonitis**.

Previous episodes of ascites and risk factors for first presentations need to be explored. Associated portal hypertension with oesophageal varices (melaena, haematemesis) point to a hepatic cause. A sudden onset of ascites makes malignancy or Budd–Chiari syndrome more likely.

Physical examination

Ascites is graded on its volume:
- **Grade 1** (1–4 L) is detectable only by ultrasound.
- **Grade 2** (4–8 L) is detected clinically with evidence of shifting dullness.
- **Grade 3** (>8 L) is associated with tense swelling and a fluid thrill.

Check for anaemia, jaundice, stigmata of chronic liver disease (Dupuytren's contractures, parotid enlargement, spider naevi in SVC's distribution) and, in males, gynaecomastia and testicular atrophy. Check for hepatomegaly and splenomegaly, and scrotal or labial oedema.

Investigations and management

Prognosis measured in hours to days prior to the onset of this problem (symptom control)

It is **not appropriate to investigate** the causes or to drain ascites in people this close to death.

It is very appropriate to ensure that any **discomfort** or **breathlessness** that is associated with gross ascites is managed with opioids. Ensure any SC needle is not placed in an oedematous area.

Nausea may be due to squashed stomach, hypomotile gut, or a combination of factors. Antiemetics may include metoclopramide 10 mg SC four times daily, haloperidol 0.5–3.0 mg SC daily.

Prognosis measured in weeks prior to the onset of this problem (in addition to symptom control)

The only definitive treatment of ascites is to **control the underlying cause**. If there is tense ascites associated with breathlessness, pain, or nausea, paracentesis is indicated.

Prior to an ascitic tap, **check coagulation** (platelets $>40 \times 10^9$/L, international normalized ratio (INR) <1.4). Cease diuretics 24 h before the procedure. Potentially less rapid drainage may decrease the risk of a peritoneal bleed. While 90% of people get symptom relief, **adverse effects** include hypovolaemia, hypotension, renal dysfunction (less likely with peripheral oedema), perforated viscus, peritonitis, or fistula formation.

In the management of non-malignant ascites, guidelines support the benefit of concentrated albumin replacement when >5 L of fluid is drained (replace 8 g/L of fluid drained).

Prognosis measured in months to years prior to the onset of this problem (in addition to the above)

- Establish a cause for ascites.
- **FBC** looking for anaemia or neutrophilia. Check coagulation studies.
- Check serum protein and albumin, liver and renal function, and serum amylase.
- **Ultrasound** will define hepatic metastases or cirrhosis.
- **Doppler studies** will assess patency of the hepatic and portal veins.
- To help establish a primary cause, **analyse peritoneal fluid** for cell count (<250/dL is normal), microscopy, cytology, protein and albumin, amylase, and culture.
- Serum-to-ascites albumin gradient (SAAG) can help differentiate the cause (>11 g/L probably due to cirrhosis, fulminant hepatic failure, liver metastases, alcoholic hepatitis, cardiac failure).
- Turbid ascites is seen in pancreatitis or TB.
- White (chylous) fluid suggests lymphatic obstruction.
- People with new malignant ascites should receive an oncology consultation.

In non-malignant ascites, **diuretics** are the initial choice for symptomatic management—spironolactone (100 mg twice daily) and a loop diuretic (furosemide 40–80 mg daily) if tolerated. With adequate doses, a response may be seen in a few days, but postural symptoms, renal impairment, and electrolyte abnormalities may limit the efficacy of the intervention. There is little evidence to support this treatment in malignant ascites.

If repeated paracentesis is needed for **malignant ascites**, consider a permanent peritoneal drain.

In people with a shorter prognosis (months), **placement of a tunnelled catheter** (Tenckhoff catheter or modified venous port) with an external portal for drainage may be effective.

In people with a longer prognosis (years), **a peritoneal–venous** shunt may be useful although DIC can complicate this. Completely draining ascites prior to placement may reduce this risk.

Ascites associated with cirrhosis carries a median survival of 2 years. Except for ovarian and breast cancer, the development of malignant ascites carries a median prognosis of 3 months.

Further reading

Fernandex J, Arroyo V (2020). Cirrhosis and ascites (Chapter 15.22.2). In: *Oxford Textbook of Medicine*, 6th ed. Oxford: Oxford University Press. Available at: https://doi.org/10.1093/med/9780198746690.003.0318

Sudden onset of jaundice ☼

- The three main reasons for hyperbilirubinaemia are liver disease, obstruction of bile ducts, or isolated disorders of bilirubin metabolism (Table 6.10).
- Jaundice is classified according to the type of circulating bilirubin (conjugated or unconjugated) or the site of the problem (pre-, intra-, or post-hepatic).

Table 6.10 Causes of a sudden onset of jaundice

	More frequently encountered causes	Less frequently encountered causes
Cancer	Nodes at the porta hepatis Hepatic metastases	Pancreatic carcinoma Cholangiocarcinoma
Intercurrent illnesses	Gallstones Gilbert syndrome Shock Septicaemia Alcohol	Sarcoidosis Sickle cell crisis Haemolysis Resorption of a haematoma
Drugs	Phenothiazines Tricyclic antidepressants Sulphonylureas Penicillins	Haloperidol Cyproheptadine NSAIDs Phenytoin Carbamazepine Phenobarbital Thiazides Allopurinol
Spurious	Carotenaemia (sparing of the sclera)	

History

Check for recent infections, blood transfusions, medications (the list of medications causing cholestasis, or cholestatic hepatitis is almost endless), and any previous episodes of jaundice.

Check for fever and right upper quadrant pain (choledocholithiasis), and for fatigue, myalgia, and malaise (viral illness).

Physical examination

- Check **temperature**, **blood pressure**, and **pulse rate** to assess for fluid status and sepsis.
- **Altered skin colour and scleral icterus** suggest serum bilirubin >35 mmol/L.
- **Scratch marks** reflect severe pruritus.

- Examine for tattoos and needle tracks, and peripheral stigmata of chronic alcohol use (parotid enlargement, Dupuytren's contracture, gynaecomastia in males).
- **Abdominal examination** includes checking Murphy's sign (p.172), liver size and contour, ascites, and bruising.
- Exclude splenomegaly and other evidence of **portal hypertension**.
- Auscultate over the liver for a **venous hum** (alcoholic hepatitis, hepatocellular cancer).
- Examine for **encephalopathy** (p.177).

Investigations and management

Prognosis measured in hours to days prior to the onset of this problem (symptom control)

People with **jaundice** have nausea (p.41) and pruritus. **Pruritus** in incomplete biliary obstruction may respond to cholestyramine. In complete obstruction, use 5-HT$_3$ antagonists (ondansetron 4 mg SL or IV/SC twice daily) or paroxetine (20 mg daily). Antihistamines are only useful in pruritus caused by urticaria and allergy.

Although these people are at the very end of life, dehydration should be treated to reduce itch.

Stop hepatoxic medications if possible.

Prognosis measured in weeks prior to the onset of this problem (in addition to symptom control)

Investigations include the following:

- **LFTs** (cholestatic, isolated elevated bilirubin, or globally impaired).
- **FBC** (anaemia, platelet count, reticulocyte count).
- **Blood film** (to suggest haemolysis).
- **Coagulation studies**.
- **Electrolytes and renal function**.
- Liver ultrasound looking for obstruction of the biliary tree.
- Febrile people should have immediate blood cultures and it may be appropriate to commence IV hydration and antibiotics while awaiting the result (p.48).
- Any hepatoxic medications should be stopped.
- Treat hepatic encephalopathy if it is present (p.177).
- Cholestasis secondary to gallstones or malignant obstruction may be improved with an ERCP or percutaneous drainage of the biliary tree and, for malignant obstruction, stenting.

Prognosis measured in months to years prior to the onset of this problem (in addition to the above)

Investigations are indicated to define the cause of the problem.

- Failure to reach a diagnosis based on preliminary screen indicates further investigations including **conjugated and unconjugated bilirubin estimation**.
- Cholestasis secondary to gallstones requires **endoscopic or surgical intervention**.

- Jaundice secondary to biliary duct compression (cancer, lymphoma) may be suitable for insertion of a **biliary stent**, with subsequent radiotherapy or chemotherapy in responsive cancers.
- **Hypoperfusion** and toxic liver damage require **supportive management** while avoiding further episodes of insult.
- Viral and autoimmune hepatic disease requires **specialist consultations**.

Further reading

Collier J (2020). Investigation and management of jaundice (Chapter 15.22.1). In: *Oxford Textbook of Medicine*, 6th ed. Oxford: Oxford University Press. Available at: https://doi.org/10.1093/med/9780198746690.003.0317

Biliary sepsis ☼

- Acute cholangitis is a life-threatening complication of biliary obstruction.
- Cholangitis occurs when the normally sterile bile is affected by ascending infections.
- This is most commonly due to translocation of bacteria from the portal system or introduction by biliary instrumentation (Table 6.11).
- Early diagnosis is necessary to minimize the high mortality rate associated with biliary sepsis, especially in elderly people or people with significant comorbidities.

Table 6.11 Causes of biliary sepsis

	More frequently encountered causes	Less frequently encountered causes
Cancer	Carcinoma of the pancreas	Duodenal carcinoma
	Cholangiocarcinoma or porta hepatis disease	
End-stage organ failure		Post-liver transplant
Intercurrent illnesses	Biliary stones (choledocholithiasis, hepatolithiasis)	Primary sclerosing cholangitis
	Pancreatitis	Biliary surgery
	Post-ERCP	AIDS (benign stricture)
	Change of biliary stent	Spontaneous or surgical biliary–enteric fistula

History

The classical presentation of **fevers, jaundice, and right upper quadrant pain (Charcot's triad)** is usually a late presentation. If associated with drowsiness, confusion, and shock, **prognosis is poor**.

Most people present with non-specific signs of **fluctuating fever, nausea and vomiting, and abdominal pain** (which may be generalized). **Pain** may mimic angina or radiate to the right shoulder.

When obstruction is present, people describe dark urine and pale stools.

Physical examination

- In acute cholangitis, severe pain on inspiration while palpating the right upper quadrant (**Murphy's sign**) may be positive.
- Additional findings include **fever, jaundice, abdominal distension, and signs of peritonism** and, in malignant biliary obstruction, a painless palpable gall bladder (**Courvoisier's sign**).

Investigations and management

Prognosis measured in hours to days prior to the onset of this problem (symptom control)

- Acute cholangitis is a life-threatening condition with a high mortality.

- Worse prognostic features include old age and acute kidney injury.
- In the very final stages of life, it may not be appropriate to commence regular antibiotics.
- Possible symptoms include **pain**, best managed with SC opioids.
- People may have **pruritus**, and if these people have pain, the opioid of choice is hydromorphone which may cause less itching than other opioids.
- Other symptoms include nausea, vomiting, and fever. The management of fever is both pharmacological (regular paracetamol 1 g three times daily, IV/rectal 500 mg three times daily), and non-pharmacological (tepid sponge, fan, and cool ambient temperatures).
- People with jaundice may develop itch. The **itch of cholestasis** may be relieved by relieving the obstruction, but symptomatic treatments include 5-HT$_3$ antagonists as first-line therapy or an androgen (methyltestosterone 25 mg SL). Non-pharmacological measures to address itch include avoiding very hot baths or showers, and treating anxiety and insomnia. Ensure that the skin is not dry and discourage the use of soap. Ensure that the person's room is not overheated. Maintain hydration.

Prognosis measured in weeks prior to the onset of this problem (in addition to symptom control)

These people may be **shocked**. **Fluid resuscitation, pain relief, antiemetics, and broad-spectrum antibiotics** should be initiated (IV ampicillin 2 g every 6 h and gentamicin 4–6 mg/kg IV daily). Prior to commencing antibiotics, blood should be drawn for blood cultures. Further investigations should include **FBC, LFTs, and coagulation studies**.

LFTs are usually abnormal, with a cholestatic picture (raised gamma-glutamyl transferase, alkaline phosphatase, and bilirubin). Transaminases may also be elevated and suggest a hepatic rather than biliary cause. In elderly or debilitated people, WCC may be normal, reflecting a poor inflammatory response.

If **INR >1.4**, commence vitamin K 10 mg IV or orally daily.

A **biliary ultrasound** may identify the cause of the obstruction.

In someone with no obvious cause, an ERCP may be considered.

Despite the poor prognosis of these people, **endoscopic** or **percutaneous drainage** of a dilated biliary tree may provide good symptom relief.

Prognosis measured in months to years prior to the onset of this problem (in addition to the above)

Once stabilized, **laparoscopic** or **open cholecystectomy** should be performed.

Further reading

Johnson C, Wright M (2020). Diseases of the gallbladder and biliary tree (Chapter 15.25). In: *Oxford Textbook of Medicine*, 6th ed. Oxford: Oxford University Press. Available at: https://doi.org/10.1093/med/9780198746690.003.0334

Acute pancreatitis :☉:

- Pancreatitis is an inflammatory reaction in the pancreas from a variety of insults (Table 6.12).
- It is divided into mild acute pancreatitis, severe acute pancreatitis, and chronic pancreatitis.
- The classification of severe pancreatitis is made when any of the following is present:

    1. Organ failure with one or more of the following:
        - shock (systolic blood pressure <90 mmHg)
        - pulmonary insufficiency (PaO_2 ≤60 mmHg)
        - renal failure (serum creatinine level >180 μmol/L after rehydration)
        - GIT bleeding (>500 mL in 24 h).
    2. Local complications such as necrosis, pseudocyst, or abscess.
    3. At least three of Ranson's criteria (hypoxaemia as above):
        - age >55 years
        - WCC >16 × 10^9/L
        - blood glucose >11 mmol/L
        - serum lactate LDH >400 IU/L
        - serum aspartate transaminase >250 IU/L
        - low calcium (corrected for albumin).

Reprinted from *Surgery Gynaecology & Obstetrics*, 139, 1, Ranson JH et al., 'Prognostic signs and the role of operative management in acute pancreatitis', pp. 69–81, Copyright 1974, with permission from the American College of Surgeons and Elsevier.

Table 6.12 Causes of acute pancreatitis

	More frequently encountered causes	Less frequently encountered causes
Cancer	Pancreatic cancer Metastatic disease to liver or porta hepatis	Cancer of the ampulla of Vater
Intercurrent illnesses	Gallstones Alcohol Idiopathic	Post-ERCP Hypertriglyceridaemia Medications (valproate, steroids, azathioprine, L-asparaginase) Infections (mumps, Coxsackie B, viral hepatitis)

History

- People present with a **sudden onset of pain**, which may be mild to extreme.
- Pain is localized to the **epigastrium** or may **radiate to the back** or lower abdomen.
- The pain is often relieved by sitting upright and bending forward.

- People may also experience **nausea and vomiting, anorexia, and fever**.
- There may be a change in bowel habits, progressing to a **paralytic ileus**.

Physical examination

- People look unwell and may be **agitated**.
- Check **vital signs** and assess **hydration urgently**. They may be **febrile** and **shocked**.
- Abdominal examination may be unremarkable compared with the level of distress or may reveal a generally tender distended abdomen, with reduced or absent bowel sounds.
- Severe necrotizing pancreatitis can lead to tissue catabolism of haem giving **Cullen's sign** (periumbilical blue discoloration) and **Grey–Turner's sign** (flank discoloration).
- **Pleural effusions** may be present.

Investigations and management

Prognosis measured in hours to days prior to the onset of this problem (symptom control)

The **pain of pancreatitis may be extreme**. Morphine is the analgesia of choice (and is unlikely to cause contraction of the sphincter of Oddi). Give at least the first dose IV.

People may have **nausea with vomiting**. Manage with metoclopramide (10 mg oral/SC/IV four times daily) except when there is a paralytic ileus. Other medications include haloperidol (0.5–3.0 mg oral/SC daily) and cyclizine (12.5–25 mg oral/SC three times daily).

Agitation secondary to pain, shock, hypoxaemia, infection, and possibly alcohol withdrawal may be seen. Despite the poor prognosis, consider and gently treat any reversible causes of agitation (hypoxia, urinary retention, pain, fever). Manage agitation with diazepam 2.5–5.0 mg three times daily.

Prognosis measured in weeks prior to the onset of this problem (in addition to symptom control)

- Although this is mostly a self-limiting disease, initially these people may be extremely unwell.
- **Fluid resuscitation, analgesia, antiemetics**, and treatment of **infection** are indicated.
- If **LFTs** and **ultrasound examination** confirm gallstone pancreatitis, urgent **ERCP** is indicated.
- With severe pancreatitis and no gallstones, consider not transferring to a high dependency unit.
- For prognosis, **assess severity** checking amylase, lipase, FBC, EUC, LFTs, calcium, glucose, and LDH.

Prognosis measured in months to years prior to the onset of this problem (in addition to the above)

Seek support from a high dependency unit while checking:

- **serum amylase and lipase** are elevated (amylase >3–4 times the upper limit of normal)
- **renal function** (to help determine hydration status)

- liver function (looking for underlying pathology) with albumin
- **FBC** (anaemia, neutrophilia)
- **serum calcium** (corrected for albumin), **LDH**
- arterial blood gases
- a **plain abdominal and CXR** is seeking evidence of perforation
- **abdominal ultrasound** will identify gallstones, dilatation in the biliary tree, and pseudocysts
- an **abdominal CT** may show loss of peripancreatic tissue planes with acute inflammation.

The initial management includes:
- **urgent fluid resuscitation** (fluid sequestration) and careful monitoring; an indwelling urinary catheter should be inserted with **hourly monitoring** of vital signs and urine output
- **opioid** analgesia is required
- **daily FBC, EUC, LFTs, calcium, amylase, glucose**, and **arterial blood gases**.

Mortality is 7–35%, mostly due to multiorgan failure and later infected necrosis of the pancreas.

Further reading

Carter R et al. (2020). Acute pancreatitis (Chapter 15.26.1). In: *Oxford Textbook of Medicine*, 6th ed. Oxford: Oxford University Press. Available at: https://doi.org/10.1093/med/9780198746 690.003.0335

Acute hepatocellular failure ☠

- Acute liver failure is a syndrome of sudden hepatic dysfunction leading to encephalopathy, coagulopathy, circulatory collapse, renal failure, and infection.
- Acute hepatic failure is divided into hyperacute, acute, and subacute defined by the speed with which encephalopathy develops after the onset of jaundice. In advanced disease, its prognosis is poor whatever the underlying aetiology (Table 6.13).
- Mortality with fulminant or acute hepatic failure is high and with infiltrating metastatic malignancy, mortality is 100%. Poor prognostic factors include rapidly developing jaundice, raised intracranial pressure, hypotension, sepsis, being HIV positive, or being elderly.

Table 6.13 Causes of acute hepatic failure

	More frequently encountered causes	Less frequently encountered causes
Cancer	Lymphoma	Malignant infiltration
Intercurrent illnesses	Acute viral hepatitis	Viruses (cytomegalovirus, Epstein–Barr virus)
	Autoimmune hepatitis	Budd–Chiari syndrome (hepatic vein thrombosis)
		Veno-occlusive disease of the liver
		Haemochromatosis
		Wilson's disease
Drugs	Paracetamol overdose	Halothane, isoniazid, antiretrovirals

History

People present with **non-specific** fatigue, nausea and vomiting, anorexia, and jaundice. The time course for these symptoms is usually very short. Check for risk factors and exposures.

Physical examination

The only finding may be **new jaundice**. Check **fluid status** as people may be severely dehydrated.

Neurological examination must be undertaken to exclude encephalopathy. Specifically test for asterixis, constructional apraxia, and a full mental state evaluation.

These people are at risk of **cerebral oedema**, and should be observed for changes of hypertension, bradycardia, papillary changes, seizures (p.249), and decerebrate posturing.

The physical examination will allow the person to be graded as:
- grade 1: altered mood or behaviour
- grade 2: increasing drowsiness, confusion, slurred speech
- grade 3: stupor, incoherence, restlessness.

Investigations and management

Prognosis measured in hours to days prior to the onset of this problem (symptom control)

- These people will **deteriorate very rapidly**.
- **Nausea and vomiting** will require parenteral medications. Metoclopramide may be used.
- In an agitated person, haloperidol may be preferred.
- Consider cyclizine (12.5–25 mg SC four times daily) in a person with pruritus and jaundice.
- **Seizures** need to be addressed even in the terminal phases of care. Load with phenytoin (10–15 mg/kg by *slow* IV infusion, then continue 100 mg IV three times daily) and ensure a rescue dose of benzodiazepine (diazepam 5 mg IV or midazolam 5 mg SC) is available if seizures occur.
- If seizure activity persists, consider phenobarbital (100 mg SC loading dose, then 30 mg three times daily). Phenobarbital causes cerebral vasoconstriction, is sedative, and is an antiepileptic.
- **Pain** due to inflammation of the hepatic capsule will require opioid analgesia.
- Even late in life, **dehydration** can cause significant symptoms, and gentle parenteral hydration may be of benefit.
- If there is **bleeding**, give vitamin K 10 mg IV daily. Have crisis medications (p.53) available.
- The **jaundice may cause itch**. Parenteral ondansetron 4 mg SL/IV twice daily may help.

Prognosis measured in weeks prior to the onset of this problem (in addition to symptom control)

- Poor prognostic factors include grade III, IV encephalopathy; age >40 years; albumin <30 g/L; metastatic or drug-induced.
- Check **FBC, EUC, LFTs, and albumin**.
- Check serum levels if **paracetamol overdose** is suspected. Treat with acetylcysteine.
- **Gentle hydration** with glucose-containing fluids should be continued. **Avoid constipation**.

Prognosis measured in months to years prior to the onset of this problem (in addition to the above)

Few people with an established life-limiting illness will recover from fulminant hepatic failure. An urgent hepatology consultation should be sought. Transfer to a high dependency unit.

Investigations and management include the following:

- **LFTs** (elevated bilirubin, aspartate transaminase, alanine transaminase); LDH.
- **FBC** (infection, GI bleed)
- **Coagulation studies** (prothrombin time (PT)/INR).
- **Renal function**, **electrolytes**, and blood sugar level (BSL).
- **Viral serology**.
- **Serum paracetamol levels**.

- **Hepatic ultrasound**, looking specifically for Doppler flow in the hepatic and portal vasculature.
- High-resolution **spiral CT scan** may demonstrate miliary spread of malignancy to the liver.
- Cease all **potentially hepatotoxic medications**. Treat paracetamol overdose.
- Nurse people who are becoming **encephalopathic** in a quiet room, with bed-head elevation.
- Initiate oral or rectal **lactulose** to empty bowel and minimize encephalopathy.
- People who are **bleeding** should have vitamin K (10 mg IV daily for 3 days), platelets, and FFP.
- **PPIs** should be commenced for all people.
- Carefully monitor **fluid resuscitation** (40–80% incidence of renal failure).
- There is **high risk of infection** (impaired complement synthesis), with 50% risk of pneumonia and 30% risk for urinary tract infections. Actively treat sepsis (ceftriaxone 1 g IV/IM daily).
- **Hypoglycaemia** should be treated with 50% glucose (glucagon alone will not be effective).

Further reading

Coggle S et al. (2020). Acute medical presentations (Chapter 30.1). In: *Oxford Textbook of Medicine*, 6th ed. Oxford: Oxford University Press. Available at: https://doi.org/10.1093/med/978019 8746690.003.0647

Fistula formation ☼

- A fistula is an abnormal opening connecting two hollow organs or a hollow organ and the skin.
- The most common acquired fistulae originate in the GIT (Table 6.14).
- Fistulae are associated with significant morbidity and mortality.

Table 6.14 Causes of fistula formula

	More frequently encountered causes	Less frequently encountered causes[a]
Cancer	Any intra-abdominal malignancy	Previous radiotherapy
Intercurrent illnesses	Diverticulitis	Pancreatitis
	Inflammatory bowel disease	Cholecystitis
	Previous stenting	Appendicitis
		Trauma
		Previous abdominal surgery
		Ischaemic bowel
		Crohn's disease

[a] See also TOF (p.135).

History

- A fistula between the gut and the biliary system is often subclinical except when **gallstone ileus develops**. These people present with nausea and vomiting mimicking small bowel obstruction.
- **Enterocutaneous fistulae** are typically preceded by an erythematous swelling. Once the fistula has developed, the diagnosis is very clear.
- Internal gut fistulae may cause a change in bowel habits, often with diarrhoea and pain.
- A **fistula between the pelvic organs and the gut** is accompanied by the passage of faecal matter or flatus when voiding or faecal matter through the vagina. This is often associated with incontinence (urinary and faecal), cystitis, and urinary tract infections.
- Rarely, **fistulae may develop between the upper gut and major blood vessels**. **This is rapidly fatal**.

Physical examination

- The physical examination may be unremarkable.
- An already formed enterocutaneous fistula is obvious, with discharge of intestinal contents through the skin, often with surrounding cellulitis and excoriation.
- If the small bowel is involved, there is a significant risk of dehydration.
- Examine the abdomen for any other localized tenderness or palpable mass as the pathology may be multifocal.
- For vaginal fistulae, inspect the perineal region for localized excoriation.

- Check temperature, pulse, and blood pressure (standing and sitting) for fluid status and sepsis.

Investigations and management

Prognosis measured in hours to days prior to the onset of this problem (symptom control)

The **immediate priority** is to **control pain**, **infections**, and **dehydration**. The other therapeutic aim is to decrease output from a fistula: carefully manage any parenteral fluid; use octreotide (100 micrograms SC three times daily titrated up).

People with enterocutaneous fistulae require review by a **specialist stoma therapy/wound care nurse** for the best application of drainage bags and to minimize skin problems, including autodigestion, and secondary bacterial and fungal infections.

There is a risk of **torrential bleeding** from fistulae. Ensure crisis medications (p.53) are at hand.

Prognosis measured in weeks prior to the onset of this problem (in addition to symptom control)

Investigations are dictated by the presumed site of the fistula and the condition of the person. For enterocutaneous fistulae, check **FBC, electrolytes** (there can be significant loss of K^+ and Na^+ in small bowel enterocutaneous fistulae), and renal function, and **assess the output** from the fistula. For internal fistulae, **FBC (Hb, WCC), coagulation studies** (bleeding risk), **electrolytes, renal function, liver function, albumin, blood cultures**, and **urine cultures** (if febrile) are indicated.

Diagnosis of bowel-to-bowel fistulae can be difficult. Plain abdominal X-rays may be of no help, and contrast studies are sometimes difficult to interpret. A **Gastrografin® study** should be done if a bowel-to-bowel fistula is suspected. An **abdominal CT** scan will give information about the site and, potentially, the cause.

Endoscopy may be useful to assess whether stenting is possible especially for rectal lesions.

Surgical closure depends upon the location and the likelihood of cure. Malignant fistulae or fistulae at the site of previous radiotherapy are unlikely to gain good outcomes from surgery.

Fistulae may be amenable to **palliative stenting** if the oesophagus, gastric outlet, duodenum, or rectum are involved.

Enterocutaneous fistulae are usually accompanied by malnutrition, and there needs to be early consideration of parenteral feeding on a case-by-case basis.

Vitamin deficiencies need correction, especially if the distal small bowel is involved.

Regular **octreotide** may reduce outputs from enteric fistulae and assist with spontaneous closure.

Prognosis measured in months to years prior to the onset of this problem (in addition to the above)

Mortality remains high as fistula formation is often evidence of progressive disease.

Further reading

Buchs NC et al. (2020). Colonic diverticular disease (Chapter 15.14). In: *Oxford Textbook of Medicine*, 6th ed. Oxford: Oxford University Press. Available at: https://doi.org/10.1093/med/978019 8746690.003.0309

Watson M et al. (eds) (2019). Gastrointestinal symptoms (Chapter 9). In: *Oxford Handbook of Palliative Care*, 3rd ed. Oxford: Oxford University Press. Available at: https://doi.org/10.1093/med/9780198745655.003.0009

Chapter 7

Haematological disorders

Neutropenic sepsis *184*
Anaemia *187*
Thrombocytopenia *191*
Bone marrow failure *194*
Disseminated intravascular coagulation *196*
Bleeding secondary to disorders of the coagulation cascade *198*
Leukocytosis *200*
Hyperviscosity *203*
Sickle cell crisis *205*

Neutropenic sepsis ☠

- Severe neutropenia is an absolute neutrophil count of $<0.5 \times 10^6/\mu L$ from decreased production or increased destruction (Box 7.1). The risk of infection increases as the neutrophil count decreases to $<1.0 \times 10^6/\mu L$.
- Neutropenic fever is defined as a single oral temperature ≥38.3°C or temperature ≥38.0°C for 1 h in a neutropenic person.
- Acute neutropenia is more often associated with bacterial infections while chronic neutropenia is associated with fungal infections.

Box 7.1 Causes of neutropenia

Impaired production of neutrophils
- Drugs (cytotoxic chemotherapy, immunosuppressive therapy, sulfonamides, antithyroid medications, anticonvulsants).
- Post-infection.
- Primary marrow failure especially with malignant infiltration.
- Congenital (cyclic, congenital).
- Nutritional deficiencies (vitamin B$_{12}$, folate, copper).

Increased destruction of neutrophils
- Infection.
- Immune-mediated destruction (SLE, rheumatoid arthritis with Felty's syndrome).
- Increased sequestration.
- Splenomegaly.

History

- A person with **acute neutropenic** sepsis may fail to develop localizing signs except for fever or general influenza-like symptoms.
- Take a history of **recent cytotoxic chemotherapy** and **other medications**.
- Check for **localizing symptoms of sepsis** with the most common sites of infection in decreasing order being the **GIT, blood, skin, lung, and urinary tract**.
- Chronic neutropenia may cause chronic sinusitis or mouth ulcers as its only evidence.

Physical examination

- Aside from fever, many people do not display typical inflammatory effects of infections.
- Along with vital signs, examine the mouth and ears, check for signs of meningism (photophobia, neck stiffness, and pain on straight leg raising (Kernig's sign)), examine chest and abdomen, palpate lymph nodes, palpate over the facial sinuses, and examine skin (including the perineum, injection sites (SC or IV) and between the toes).

Investigations and management

Prognosis measured in hours to days prior to neutropenia (symptom control)
It is not appropriate to initiate further investigations in this group.

Treat fever and rigors:
- Tepid sponges and control the ambient temperature.
- Regular paracetamol (1 g orally or 500 mg rectally three times daily) or NSAIDs (indomethacin 25 mg orally three times daily or 100 mg rectally twice daily or ketorolac 10 mg SC four times daily).
- Consider a single dose of gentamicin 160 mg and ceftriaxone 1 g IV (or IM) in suspected sepsis.
- Ensure adequate hydration.

Prognosis measured in weeks to months prior to neutropenia (in addition to symptom control)
- Collect a FBC with differential, **two sets of blood cultures (aerobic and anaerobic)**, including one set from each lumen of indwelling devices plus one peripheral set or two cultures from separate venipuncture sites, liver and renal function tests, electrolytes, and lactate.
- Review CXR to exclude pneumonia.
- If diarrhoea is present, ensure stool cultures are collected, microscopy requested, and stools are tested for *Clostridium difficile* toxin.
- Swab any wounds.
- The three most important steps are:
  - suspension of myelosuppressive medications
  - **prompt initiation of antibiotics**
  - **adequate fluid resuscitation**.

The choice of antibiotic is dictated by local pathogens informing local practice. **Prolonged neutropenia** or **prior use of antibiotics** will increase the likelihood of fungal infections. A person **without a spleen** (either surgically or functionally) must be covered for capsulated organisms (*Streptococcus pneumoniae*, *Haemophilus influenzae*, *Neisseria meningitis*). Infectious disease review should be sought in people with fever failing to resolve in 72 h. A person who is haemodynamically stable, who can swallow, and who is expected to have normal absorption may be managed with oral antibiotics. Otherwise, use parenteral therapy.

Growth factors (granulocyte colony-stimulating factor (G-CSF), granulocyte–macrophage colony-stimulating factor (GM-CSF)) are used in cytotoxic-induced neutropenia and in some people with chronic neutropenia (congenital, cyclic autoimmune, or HIV/AIDS). These agents reduce the period of neutropenia, but do not reduce mortality.

Autoimmune neutropenia may require regular corticosteroids and growth factor injections.

Prognosis measured in months to years prior to the onset of neutropenia (in addition to the above)
Further investigations will be necessary if the source of sepsis is not identified. These include a **CT of the facial sinuses, high-resolution CT of the chest** looking for fungal infections, **echocardiogram**, and **bone marrow examination**.

The risk of mortality for people with acute neutropenia is about 7%. Factors predicting poorer outcomes include continuing haemodynamic instability, organ failure, fever lasting >6 days, and gut or IV line infections.

Further reading

Cassidy J et al. (eds) (2015). Spinal cord compression and bone marrow suppression (Chapter 30). In: *Oxford Handbook of Oncology*, 4th ed. Oxford: Oxford University Press. Available at: https://doi.org/10.1093/med/9780199689842.003.0030

Anaemia :✪:

- Anaemia is when haemoglobin concentration is <13.0 g/dL (men) and <11.5 g/dL (women).
- Acute anaemia is caused by blood loss, haemolysis, or lower red cell production (Table 7.1).

Table 7.1 Causes of anaemia

Blood loss	Erosion of a major blood vessel
	Failure of normal haemostasis
	Surgery/trauma
	GIT blood loss
Haemolysis	*Inherited disorders*
	• Hereditary spherocytosis or elliptocytosis
	• Red cell enzyme defects
	Acquired disorders: non-immune
	• Hypersplenism
	• Membrane defects
	• Infections
	• Drug-related
	• Thrombotic microangiopathies
	• Vasculitis
	• Mechanical
	Acquired disorders: immune
	• Autoimmune
	• Transfusion
Ineffective haemopoiesis	Reduced red cell production secondary to bone marrow infiltration
	Chemotherapy-induced marrow suppression
	Nutritional deficiencies (iron, vitamin B_{12}, or folate)
	Reduced erythropoietin
Other	Anaemia of chronic disease

History

- Anaemia may cause **fatigue, increasing breathlessness on exertion, angina, palpitations, headache, impaired concentration, anorexia, and weakness**.
- People may describe **symptoms of heart failure** (orthopnoea, paroxysmal nocturnal dyspnoea, or increasing ankle oedema).
- Check for a **history of bleeding** (rectal, vaginal, urinary tract).
- Check the **drug history** (NSAIDs, aspirin, heparin, warfarin).

Physical examination

- Check for **pallor of the palmar creases** and **pale conjunctiva**. There may be a tachycardia.

- If anaemia is due to blood loss, the **pulse may be thready** and the person **hypotensive**. Alternatively, there may be a **hyperdynamic state** with cardiac enlargement (in chronic anaemia) and flow murmurs leading to cardiac failure.
- Examine for **signs of bleeding**, including a rectal examination.

Investigations and management

Prognosis measured in days to hours prior to the onset of this problem (symptom control)

This is a clinical diagnosis. Contributing medications should be discontinued if possible.

Active bleeding should be addressed by local measures (tranexamic acid mouthwashes, local pressure, or epinephrine-soaked sponges). Consider an infusion of packed cells if breathlessness or clouded cognition are causing distress, and a primary site of bleeding can be identified and controlled. If the person is at risk of, or clinically in heart failure, transfuse slowly with furosemide 20–40 mg IV/SC cover. Dosing depends on previous diuretic use and any history of renal dysfunction.

Ensure that crisis medications (p.53) are available with the presence of active bleeding.

Prognosis measured in weeks prior to the onset of this problem (in addition to symptom control)

The initial investigations include a FBC and **examination of the blood film**. This allows the anaemia to be classified into:
- microcytic (mean corpuscular volume (MCV) <80 fL)
- normocytic (MCV 80–100 fL)
- macrocytic (MCV >100 fL).

A **microcytic anaemia** is most likely to be due to:
- iron deficiency, increased red cell distribution width (RDW), anisocytosis, poikilocytosis, thrombocytosis
- anaemia of chronic disease
- thalassaemia (polychromasia, target cells).

The **ferritin level** will be low in iron deficiency and normal to high in chronic disease or with any inflammatory process. Transfuse packed cells if the person is symptomatic. If tolerated, oral iron may be commenced.

A **normocytic anaemia** may occur in people who have:
- active bleeding
- anaemia associated with chronic disease including renal failure
- haemolysis (spherocytes, schistocytes, bite cells)
- marrow failure (abnormal differential count, blast cells, dimorphic blood cells, Pelger–Huet cells, rouleaux).

People **actively bleeding** require stabilization (local control, fluid resuscitation). Check **coagulation studies** and administer packed cells and, if necessary, FFP and platelets. If bleeding is not controlled, **consider surgical or radiological review** to help to achieve haemostasis. A person with anaemia from chronic disease is best managed supportively.

A screen for active haemolysis includes LDH (raised), **haptoglobins** (raised), **indirect bilirubin** (very high), and **reticulocyte count** (low).

Haemolysis may occur secondary to genetic disorders including:
- red cell membrane disorders (e.g. hereditary spherocytosis)
- haemoglobin disorders (e.g. sickle cell anaemia, thalassaemia)
- enzyme defects (e.g. glucose-6-phosphate dehydrogenase deficiency (G6PD)).

Causes of acquired haemolysis include:
- immune:
  - isoimmune (blood transfusion reaction)
  - autoimmune (warm or cold autoantibodies)
  - drug reaction (penicillin, α-methyldopa, mefenamic acid, or L-dopa)
- non-immune:
  - trauma (prosthetic heart valve, microangiopathic anaemia secondary to haemolytic uraemic syndrome (HUS))
  - septicaemia
  - membrane disorders (paroxysmal nocturnal haemoglobinuria, liver disease)
  - previous episodes or a family history of haemolysis should identify familial causes.

Known precipitants to genetic haemolysis include medications (ciprofloxacin, sulfonamides, primaquine), infections, or dehydration. Management is supportive. Discontinue likely medications, maintain hydration, and provide analgesia.

In people with **warm autoimmune** haemolytic anaemia, a trial of steroids is indicated.

Cold autoimmune haemolytic anaemia typically presents with a symptomatic anaemia and Raynaud's syndrome and is managed by ensuring that the person is nursed in a warm ambient temperature.

A **macrocytic anaemia** with increased RDW may be due to:
- medications (oval macrocytes): zidovudine, hydroxyurea
- nutritional (oval macrocytes): thiamine, folate, or vitamin B_{12} deficiency
- myelodysplasia or marrow infiltration (dimorphic blood cells)
- liver disease (normal RDW, round macrocytes)
- hypothyroidism (normal RDW, round macrocytes)
- bone marrow failure (abnormal differential count, blast cells, dimorphic blood cells, Pelger–Huet cells, rouleaux).

Thiamine deficiency may present with neurological abnormalities (confusion, ataxia, ophthalmoplegia, nystagmus) and cardiac dysfunction (general oedema, biventricular failure). Commence thiamine replacement with 100 mg orally or IV daily.

Vitamin B_{12} deficiency may present with subacute combined degeneration of the spinal cord. This affects the posterior and/or lateral columns. A peripheral neuropathy occurs, with joint position and vibration sense the first to be affected. Later, sensory changes with increasing weakness and stiffness occur. Replace vitamin B_{12} with cyanocobalamin 1000 micrograms/mL IM daily for 3 days and then monthly.

Bone marrow failure may be due to stem cell failure (aplastic anaemia occurring secondary to drugs, viral hepatitis, autoimmune causes, inherited causes, and cytotoxic therapy), malignant infiltration, or myelodysplasia. These people require transfusion support and treatment of infections.

Discontinue medications that may have precipitated this problem (chemotherapy agents, gold).

Further reading

Sankaran VG (2020). Erythropoiesis (Chapter 22.6.1). In: *Oxford Textbook of Medicine*, 6th ed. Oxford: Oxford University Press. Available at: https://doi.org/10.1093/med/9780198746690.003.0531

Zhu N, Wu C (2021). Anaemia, cytopenias, and thrombosis in palliative medicine (Chapter 14.13). In: *Oxford Textbook of Palliative Medicine*, 6th ed. Oxford: Oxford University Press. Available at: https://doi.org/10.1093/med/9780198821328.003.0088

Thrombocytopenia ☠

- Thrombocytopenia is a reduction in platelets to <150 × 10⁹/L.
- Spontaneous bleeding generally does not occur until the platelet count is 10 × 10⁹/L or less, unless platelet function is affected. Suspect with spontaneous bleeding—a medical emergency.
- Bleeding with trauma may occur with counts <40 × 10⁹/L.
- The most common cause of low platelets in people who are hospitalized is a critical illness or medications. In the community, the most common cause is idiopathic thrombocytopenic purpura (ITP) (Table 7.2).
- When considering bleeding disorders, also consider impaired platelet function even in the presence of a normal platelet count (Table 7.3).

Table 7.2 Causes of low platelet counts

	More frequently encountered causes	Less frequently encountered causes
Decreased production	Bone marrow infiltration from malignancy Haematological malignancies	Myelodysplasia Toxic (alcohol) Folate/B₁₂ deficiency Paroxysmal nocturnal haemoglobinuria
Increased destruction	ITP Lymphoproliferative disorders HIV SLE Antiphospholipid antibodies Sepsis Hypersplenism	Drug-induced including heparin-induced Evans syndrome DIC Thrombotic thrombocytopenic purpura (TTP) HUS Malignant hypertension
Increased sequestration	Splenomegaly Cardiopulmonary bypass Haemodilution	Hypothermia

Table 7.3 Causes of impaired platelet function

More frequently encountered causes	Less frequently encountered causes
NSAIDs including aspirin, clopidogrel, ticlopidine	Marrow failure Myelodysplasia Renal failure

History

A **drug history** includes recent use of heparin, antibiotics (rifampicin, trimethoprim, sulfur-containing medications), cardiac medications (amiodarone, quinine, procainamide, thiazide diuretics), immune checkpoint inhibitor (pembrolizumab), rheumatoid arthritis disease-modifying agents, ranitidine, and antiepileptics (phenytoin, carbamazepine).

Check for recent blood transfusions or surgery, fever, arthralgia, a diagnosis of HIV (or risk factors), and heavy alcohol use.

Physical examination

- Check for **fever**, pulse, and **postural blood pressure**.
- Inspection of the skin may reveal **petechiae** and **ecchymoses**. Inspect the mouth for **mucous membrane bleeding** or **haemorrhagic bullae**.
- Check the person's **mental state** (alcohol use, confusion in TTP or HUS, intracranial bleed).
- Examine the abdomen for **splenomegaly** or signs of **chronic liver disease**.
- Check urine analysis for blood and stools for occult blood.

Investigations and management

Prognosis measured in days to hours prior to the onset of this problem (symptom control)

- This is a **clinical diagnosis** based on the appearance of petechiae and ecchymoses.
- If there is active bleeding, a **platelet transfusion** may be indicated despite the short prognosis but **platelet transfusions are contraindicated in TTP and DIC**.
- Cease **medications likely to worsen bleeding** (NSAIDs, heparin, warfarin).
- Administer **vitamin K** (10 mg IV or orally) if the person has liver disease, or a history of alcohol misuse or recent antibiotic use.
- Institute **good mouth care**. Add tranexamic acid mouthwashes (1 g orally four times daily) if there is oral mucosal bleeding.
- For **topical bleeding**, apply local pressure with epinephrine-soaked sponges.
- In the absence of haematuria, coronary artery disease, and DIC, **tranexamic acid** 1 g orally three times daily may be tried even at the end of life.
- **Crisis medications** (p.53) must be available in the event of catastrophic bleeding.

Prognosis measured in weeks prior to the onset of this problem (in addition to symptom control)

- **FBC with a blood film** will establish the degree of thrombocytopenia and may suggest the underlying aetiology: schistocytic red blood cells suggests DIC or TTP; clumping of platelets suggests pseudo-thrombocytopenia.
- Bleeding in the presence of a **platelet count >40 × 10⁹/L** suggests disordered coagulation or non-functioning platelets.

- Further investigation includes **haptoglobins** (raised), **LDH** (raised), **coagulation studies**, D-dimer, **renal and liver function tests**, and **COVID-19 screening**.
- Carry out a **septic screen** for people who are febrile, hypotensive, or hypothermic.
- In the absence of ITP/DIC/TTP and the presence of a major bleed, administer platelets. Measure the effect of platelet transfusion by repeat counts taken 10 min and 24 h later.
- Medication-induced thrombocytopenia may resolve with discontinuation of the medication.
- **Heparin-induced thrombocytopenia** is potentially catastrophic. Discontinue heparin immediately. Confirm by *in vitro* testing to detect heparin-dependent platelet antibodies.
- **TTP** and **HUS** are haematological emergencies presenting with thrombosis. These people are extremely unwell and may require plasma exchange and dialysis. A haematological opinion must be sought urgently. **Platelet transfusion is contraindicated**. Initially treat hypovolaemia or hypertension.
- ITP may respond to steroids or Intragram® within 1–2 days.

Prognosis measured in months to years prior to the onset of this problem (in addition to the above)

- **A specialist haematology consultation is indicated**.
- **TTP, HUS**, and **DIC** all cause elevated **LDH** and **haptoglobins** due to haemolysis resulting in fragmented blood cells. Only DIC will also cause abnormal coagulation studies (p.196).
- Sequestering of platelets due to hypersplenism is best treated with a splenectomy for people with adequate bone marrow reserve.
- **ITP** is a diagnosis of exclusion after checking for connective tissue disease (antinuclear antibodies), lymphoproliferative disorders, and HIV infection (serology). In the short term, the management should be supportive while these diagnoses are clarified.
- Prolonged thrombocytopenia and failure to achieve any increase in the platelet count are independent factors predicting a worse outcome.

Further reading

Curry H, Shapiro S (2020). Thrombocytopenia and disorders of platelet function (Chapter 22.7.3). In: *Oxford Textbook of Medicine*, 6th ed. Oxford: Oxford University Press. Available at: https://doi.org/10.1093/med/9780198746690.003.0545

Zhu N, Wu C (2021). Anaemia, cytopenias, and thrombosis in palliative medicine (Chapter 14.13). In: *Oxford Textbook of Palliative Medicine*, 6th ed. Oxford: Oxford University Press. Available at: https://doi.org/10.1093/med/9780198821328.003.0088

Bone marrow failure :O:

Either genetic or acquired, bone marrow failure presents with pancytopenia or a single cytopenia (erythroid, myeloid, megakaryocytic) (Table 7.4).

Table 7.4 Causes of bone marrow failure

	Congenital	Acquired
Pancytopenia	Fanconi anaemia Dyskeratosis congenita	Idiopathic, toxin, drugs (chloramphenicol), chemicals, radiation, viral infection, malnutrition or vitamin deficiencies including vitamins B_{12} and folate, myelodysplastic syndrome (MDS)
Single haematopoietic lineage	Congenital neutropenia, including Kostmann syndrome Diamond–Blackfan anaemia Shwachman–Diamond syndrome Congenital amegakaryocytic thrombocytopenia (CAMT) Thrombocytopenia absent radii (TAR) syndrome	Aplastic anaemia

History

- People may present with fatigue that develops over an extended time. The most frequent reason that people present is either due to bleeding or infection.
- A family history is important.

Physical examination

- Examine for signs of anaemia including pallor and respiratory distress.
- As a result of thrombocytopenia, people may display ecchymoses, petechiae, bleeding gums, or nose bleeds.
- Check for fever, cellulitis, pneumonia, or sepsis as complications of a low WCC.

Prognosis measured in hours to days prior to the onset of this problem (symptom control)

Although the prognosis is short, ensuring **adequate hydration** may improve comfort.

Prognosis measured in weeks to months prior to the onset of this problem (in addition to symptom control)

- **FBC with a blood film** will identify any anaemia or leukopenia. Bone marrow examination is not indicated. Check **renal function** and **coagulation factors**.
- Ensure adequate hydration.
- **Plasmapheresis** may be necessary to keep the symptoms of hyperviscosity under control in people who are too unwell for definitive treatment.

Prognosis measured in months to years prior to the onset of this problem (in addition to the above)

Seek definitive treatment of the cause. If active disease-modifying measures have been exhausted, symptomatic support is based on optimizing renal function and hydration in myeloma, and in reducing viscosity with plasmapheresis in hyperleukocytosis.

Further reading

Cassidy J et al. (eds) (2015). Spinal cord compression and bone marrow suppression (Chapter 30). In: *Oxford Handbook of Oncology*, 4th ed. Oxford: Oxford University Press. Available at: https://doi.org/10.1093/med/9780199689842.003.0030

Zhu N, Wu C (2021). Anaemia, cytopenias, and thrombosis in palliative medicine (Chapter 14.13). In: *Oxford Textbook of Palliative Medicine*, 6th ed. Oxford: Oxford University Press. Available at: https://doi.org/10.1093/med/9780198821328.003.0088

Disseminated intravascular coagulation

- DIC is a syndrome that occurs due to serious underlying conditions such as sepsis, cancer (solid or haematological), or obstetric emergencies (Table 7.5).
- It is characterized by a systemic activation of coagulation that may lead to thrombosis obstructing small and medium-size vessels which in tun may cause acute organ failure. At the same time, platelets and coagulation proteins are consumed leading to significant haemorrhagic complications.
- DIC doubles the mortality of the underlying condition.

Table 7.5 Causes of DIC

	More frequently encountered causes	Less frequently encountered causes
Cancer	Haematological malignancy Adenocarcinoma	Carcinoid Sarcoma
Intercurrent illnesses	Pancreatitis Sepsis	Fat embolism (bone fracture, crush injury) Aortic aneurysms
End-stage organ failure	Hepatic failure Graft-versus-host disease	

History

People are already **seriously unwell** from the underlying cause. They may develop **bleeding** from any site and **extensive bruising**. At any point, **thrombosis** may cause organ failure or gangrene.

Physical examination

People may have widespread **bruising and bleeding** from mucous membranes, IV catheter sites, wounds, or indwelling catheters. They may have impaired blood supply to the digits, nose, and ear lobes because of fibrin deposition, resulting in ischaemic skin ulcers. They are also at risk of acute respiratory distress and neurological complications.

Investigations and management

Prognosis measured in hours to days prior to the onset of this problem (symptom control)

- **The symptoms and signs of DIC demand good palliation**.
- The most severe consequence of DIC is the occurrence of **organ failure secondary to microthrombi**.
- Symptoms must be considered and managed as necessary. It is likely that people will require:
  - **analgesia** (digital and visceral infarcts, internal bleeding, pulmonary emboli)

- management of **delirium** (organ failure, CNS microthrombi)
- management of other symptoms which may include increasing **shortness of breath** (pulmonary emboli, anaemia), anxiety, and **nausea and vomiting** (organ failure, internal bleeding, gut ischaemia).

- Although the risk of catastrophic bleeding is low, it is necessary to ensure that **crisis medications** (p.53) are available.
- Platelet half-life in DIC is short, and platelet transfusion is unlikely to benefit.
- Mouth care with tranexamic acid solution as a mouthwash (1 g orally four times daily) may reduce oozing from oral mucosa.

Prognosis measured in weeks prior to the onset of this problem (in addition to symptom control)

The definitive diagnosis of DIC requires the person to have an underlying disorder that is known to be associated with DIC. Widespread activation and consumption of the coagulation cascade occurs leading to diagnostic findings of:

- decreased platelet count
- increased fibrin degradation markers (e.g. D-dimer)
- prolonged PT
- reduced fibrinogen levels.

Treatment of the underlying cause is the only definitive treatment of DIC.

Consideration must be given to the cause of the DIC and whether or not this is likely to be reversible in this group of people.

Investigations include:

- **FBC** (low Hb, low platelets)
- **blood film** (fragmented red cells)
- **coagulation studies** (prolonged PT, APPT, decreased fibrinogen)
- increased **D-dimer** (product of fibrin degeneration).

Supportive measures to address DIC include the following:

- Administration of **vitamin K** 10 mg orally or IV.
- Cryoprecipitate should be given only if fibrinogen is low.
- FFP should be given to correct coagulation disorders but it also replaces antithrombin III, protein C, and protein S.
- **Platelets** should only be given to reverse clinically serious bleeding or to cover invasive procedures.
- Although the net benefit of heparin in DIC has yet to be proven in clinical trials, it may be used in clinically significant thrombus. This should be discussed with a haematologist.

Prognosis measured in months to years prior to the onset of this problem (in addition to the above)

Some people, especially with malignancy, may have low-grade DIC with which they coexist over long periods of time.

Further reading

Warkentin TE (2020). Acquired coagulation disorders (Chapter 22.7.5). In: *Oxford Textbook of Medicine*, 6th ed. Oxford: Oxford University Press. Available at: https://doi.org/10.1093/med/9780198746690.003.0547

Zhu N, Wu C (2021). Anaemia, cytopenias, and thrombosis in palliative medicine (Chapter 14.13). In: *Oxford Textbook of Palliative Medicine*, 6th ed. Oxford: Oxford University Press. Available at: https://doi.org/10.1093/med/9780198821328.003.0088

Bleeding secondary to disorders of the coagulation cascade ①

This section briefly summarizes bleeding disorders secondary to abnormalities of the coagulant cascade which may be inherited or acquired (Table 7.6).

Table 7.6 Inherited and acquired coagulopathies

Inherited	Acquired
Haemophilia A (factor VIII deficiency)	Acquired haemophilia A
Haemophilia B (factor IX deficiency)	Acquired von Willebrand disease
Von Willebrand disease	Acute traumatic coagulopathy
	Severe liver disease
	Vitamin K antagonists (warfarin)
	Parenteral and oral factor Xa Inhibitors

History

The history of the bleeding episode is imperative including the onset, and whether this is new or a recurrent problem. Explore the type of bleeding (bruising versus active blood loss) and the bleeding site.

Check for a childhood or family history of bleeding or bruising and recent exposure to any new medications. Although very rare, consider the diagnosis of acquired haemophilia when unexplained bleeding affects a person.

Physical examination

- Examine the skin and joints for sites of bleeding including the oral mucosa.
- Examine the skin for bruising and joints for swelling.
- Active bleeding is a critical event and examination needs to include assessments of haemodynamic stability (pulse, blood pressure, respiratory rate).

Investigations and management

Prognosis measured in hours to days prior to the onset of this problem (symptom control)

Active bleeding at the end of life is an emergency. People will require the following:

- A staff member or relative to stay with the dying person at all times.
- Manage any pain, anxiety, or shortness of breath.
- Provide green or red towels to help disguise any blood.
- Protective equipment including googles, gloves, aprons, and waste bags.
- Mouth care with tranexamic acid solution as a mouthwash (1 g orally four times daily) may reduce oozing from oral mucosa.

Prognosis measured in weeks prior to the onset of this problem (in addition to symptom control)

Additionally, if there is an active bleeding site, attempt to stop this with local pressure using epinephrine-soaked gauze.

Investigations include:

- FBC (including platelet function)
- coagulation studies (prolonged PT, APPT)
- cross-match (ABO typing is required to administer FFP).

Depending upon the differential diagnosis, cease any contributing medication(s).

Consider the administration of FFP or prothrombin complex concentrate, depending on the specific disorder and the severity of bleeding (Table 7.7).

Table 7.7 Differentiating the choice between prothrombin complex concentrate and fresh frozen plasma

Prothrombin complex concentrate	FFP (ABO typing required)
Acquired coagulation inhibitors	Liver disease
Acquired haemophilia	Vitamin K deficiency
Liver disease	Inherited bleeding disorders
Factor Xa inhibitors	

In comparison, the management of acute traumatic coagulopathy requires the concurrent administration of tranexamic acid and blood products including platelets and packed red blood cells.

Prognosis measured in months to years prior to the onset of this problem (in addition to the above)

These people all require referral to haematology for consideration of whether there is a need for ongoing factor replacement or just as required.

Further reading

Warkentin TE (2020). Acquired coagulation disorders (Chapter 22.7.5). In: *Oxford Textbook of Medicine*, 6th ed. Oxford: Oxford University Press. Available at: https://doi.org/10.1093/med/9780198746690.003.0547

Leukocytosis ⓘ

Elevated white blood cells are diagnosed on a peripheral blood film.

The WCC value represents the sum total of white blood cell subtypes: neutrophils, eosinophils, lymphocytes, and monocytes. It may also include cells not normally present on blood films including lymphoblasts.

Leukocytosis is classified by defining the main white blood cell subtype contributing to the increase (Table 7.8).

Table 7.8 Important causes of leukocytosis

Cell type	Acute elevation of WCC	Chronic elevation of WCC
Neutrophils (40–60%)	Reactive: recent physical or emotional stress, infection, medications, trauma, and smoking Clonal: as an autonomous response to dysregulation of the bone marrow such as leukaemia	Reactive: chronic inflammation (long-term use of corticosteroids, rheumatoid arthritis) Bone marrow stimulation (haemolytic anaemia, ITP) Hereditary: Down syndrome, hereditary idiopathic neutrophilia
Lymphocytes (20–40%)	Reactive: acute viral infections (cytomegalovirus, hepatitis, Epstein–Barr), *Bordetella pertussis*, toxoplasmosis Hypersensitivity reactions Clonal: lymphoma, leukaemia	Reactive: chronic infections (TB) Clonal: lymphoma, leukaemia
Eosinophils (1–4%)	Reactive: malignancy Allergy and drug hypersensitivity Infections: parasitic infections, scarlet fever (recovery phase), viral infections (recovery phase), and chlamydial infections Skin disorders including dermatitis herpetiformis, pemphigus, and erythema multiforme cause eosinophilia	Clonal: hypereosinophilia syndrome
Monocytes (2–8%)	Reactive: bone marrow recovery Infections, exercise Post-splenectomy, stress Medications, acute coronary syndrome Solid tumours Clonal: leukaemia	Reactive: chronic infection Medications Rheumatoid conditions granulomatous conditions (sarcoid) Solid tumours Clonal: leukaemia
Basophils (0.5–1%)	Inflammatory conditions: allergic reactions to food or medications, viral infections, endocrinopathies, myeloproliferative disorders, other malignancies	Reactive: solid tumours, myeloproliferative disease

History

Review previous blood tests to understand any trend. Key questions on history by subtype of leukocytes include:

- **Neutrophilia:** smoking, recent travel, surgery, current medications, contact with other people who have been unwell.
- **Lymphocytosis:** contact with other people who have been unwell, recent flu-like illnesses, medications, recent and past immunization history, recent travel.
- **Monocytosis:** family history, surgical history (splenectomy), travel history.
- **Eosinophilia:** allergic reaction, parasitic infection, dermatological conditions, current medications, reaction/hypersensitivity, eosinophilic oesophagitis.
- **Basophilia:** signs and symptoms of malignancy or allergic reactions.

Most isolated elevations of white blood cells do not require further investigation. There are two key exceptions:

1. Persistent elevations of basophils, eosinophils, and monocytes should prompt a symptom review for problems such as shortness of breath, pallor, unusual bleeding, petechiae, frequent infections, and fatigue that might accompany a diagnosis of malignancy including leukaemia.
2. Significant elevations such as a leukocytosis close to 100×10^9/L, should always prompt immediate evaluation for leukaemia or myeloproliferative disorders. Even if the person is asymptomatic, this is a medical emergency. For those people who present with symptoms they may include vision changes, bleeding, stroke or neurological changes, infarction, ischaemia, and/or multiorgan failure due to hyperviscosity syndrome (p.203).

Physical examination

Physical examination is directed by the history, the degree to which blood counts are elevated, and the main white cell type elevated.

Investigations and management

Prognosis measured in hours to days prior to the onset of this problem (symptom control)

Management needs to focus on the symptoms that a person is experiencing, especially any pain or shortness of breath.

Prognosis measured in weeks to months prior to the onset of this problem (in addition to symptom control)

The main approach to care is to identify the cause of the leukocytosis and, depending upon this, manage the underlying cause.

In the case that this is a hyperleukocytosis, management should focus on addressing symptoms associated with this very poor prognostic problem.

Prognosis measured in months to years prior to the onset of this problem (in addition to the above)

Hyperleukocytosis is a medical emergency. This can be associated with severe complications including a hyperviscosity syndrome and is likely to accompany a diagnosis of leukaemia, lymphoma, or a myeloproliferative disorder.

Appropriate recognition and prompt treatment, including rehydration, phlebotomy, and plasmapheresis, can prevent death and reduce long-term complications.

An urgent referral to a haematologist is required in order to initiate optimal management which includes leukapheresis, hydration, urine alkalinization, and administration of allopurinol or rasburicase (uric acid oxidase) to reduce serum uric acid with the aim of minimizing the effect of tumour lysis syndrome (p. 223). Treatment of the underlying cause is indicated.

Further reading

Sinning J, Berliner N (2020). Granulocytes in health and disease (Chapter 22.3.1). In: *Oxford Textbook of Medicine*, 6th ed. Oxford: Oxford University Press. Available at: https://doi.org/10.1093/med/9780198746690.003.0513

Hyperviscosity ⚠

- Blood viscosity is a function of the concentration of the plasma and the components of blood. Clinical manifestations are mostly due to the effect of the volume of abnormal cells or immunoglobulins (Table 7.9).
- Its clinical manifestations are due to impaired microcirculation.

Table 7.9 Causes of hyperviscosity syndrome

	More frequently encountered causes	Less frequently encountered causes
Cancer	Myeloma	Chronic myelocytic leukaemia (CML), chronic lymphocytic leukaemia (CLL), AML
Intercurrent illnesses	Polycythaemia secondary to COPD	Primary polycythaemia Waldenström's macroglobulinaemia

History

A history of **headaches**, **blurred vision**, and **increasing confusion** may be present. In severe cases, **cerebral ischaemia** may present with vertigo, ataxia, and diplopia. People may describe **increasing shortness of breath** and **chest pain**. Check for haematuria, rectal bleeding, or melaena.

Physical examination

- There may be **digital infarcts**.
- Examine for **nystagmus**, **gait disorder**, and confusion. Examination should also include **fundoscopy** for retinal vein engorgement or flame-shaped haemorrhages.
- Check for signs of **left ventricular failure** or **tender hepatosplenomegaly**.

Investigations and management

Prognosis measured in hours to days prior to the onset of this problem (symptom control)

Although the prognosis is short, ensuring **adequate hydration** may improve comfort.

Prognosis measured in weeks to months prior to the onset of this problem (in addition to symptom control)

- **FBC with a blood film** will identify polycythaemia or leukocytosis. Bone marrow examination is not indicated. Check **renal function and coagulation factors**.
- Ensure adequate hydration.

- **Plasmapheresis** may be necessary to keep the symptoms of hyperviscosity under control in people who are too unwell for definitive treatment.

Prognosis measured in months to years prior to the onset of this problem (in addition to the above)

Seek definitive treatment of the cause. If active, disease-modifying measures have been exhausted, symptomatic support is based on optimizing renal function and hydration in myeloma, and in reducing viscosity with plasmapheresis in hyperleukocytosis.

Sickle cell crisis :❂:

- The inherited haemoglobin variants responsible for sickling crises are HbSS, HbSC, HbS/beta thalassaemia, and HbSD.
- HbS forms polymers when deoxygenated, which cause the normally pliable red blood cells to become stiff and crescent shaped, clogging capillaries and leading to veno-occlusion and tissue hypoxia necrosis. A number of other insults may precipitate a sickle cell crisis (Box 7.2).

Box 7.2 Precipitants of a sickle cell crisis

- Hypoxaemia.
- Infection.
- Dehydration.
- Temperature extremes.
- Physical stress.
- Psychological stress.

History

Serious complications in sickle cell disease include:

- Acute pain is the hallmark symptom. It may be localized or diffuse as the result of vascular occlusion, hypoxaemia, or ischaemia. This is often associated with **fever**, and **nausea and vomiting**.
- Infections as a result of splenic dysfunction, inflammation, and ischaemia with more common problems including systemic sepsis, osteomyelitis, or pneumonia.
- Anaemia as the result of sickling and hypersplenism leading to profound fatigue, shortness of breath, weakness, and chest pain.
- Organ dysfunction as the result of ischaemia, infarction, or haemorrhage resulting in the clinical problems of stroke, acute coronary syndrome, renal failure, or splenic infarcts.

Physical examination

- Check **temperature** and other **vital signs** including **oxygen saturations**.
- Perform a peripheral examination for stigmata of **anaemia**, **digital infarcts**, or **leg ulcers**.
- Perform a **neurological examination** to seek evidence of cerebral ischaemia.
- Check for **hepatosplenomegaly** and ensure that **priapism** is not present.

Investigations and management

Prognosis measured in hours to days prior to the onset of this problem (symptom control)

Management includes **adequate hydration and analgesia**. This should be opioids (either continuous by PCA or IV). Sickle cell crisis may require significant doses of opioid even in the opioid-naïve person along with NSAIDs and paracetamol. **Oxygen** is only indicated with hypoxaemia.

Maintain an **even temperature** and do not allow the person to become cold.

Prognosis measured in weeks prior to the onset of this problem (in addition to symptom control)

Check FBC (anaemia, increased WCC, platelet count may be either increased or decreased, increased reticulocyte count). Check **renal and liver function**, especially for bilirubin levels. Check **pulse oximetry** and **arterial blood gases** looking for hypoxaemia. Regardless of whether or not the person is febrile, a **septic screen** is indicated, including a **CXR** and **blood cultures**. An **ECG** is indicated if there is chest pain.

A broad-spectrum antibiotic should be added, even without the results of a septic screen because of the risk of functional hyposplenism. Maintain an even temperature and do not allow the person to become cold. Exchange transfusion may be necessary in the presence of priapism, cerebral ischaemia, or cardiac ischaemia.

Further reading

Hay D, Weatherall DJ (2020). Disorders of the synthesis or function of haemoglobin (Chapter 22.6.7). In: *Oxford Textbook of Medicine*, 6th ed. Oxford: Oxford University Press. Available at: https://doi.org/10.1093/med/9780198746690.003.0537

Chapter 8

Renal and metabolic disorders

Acute kidney injury 208
Hyperkalaemia 212
Hypokalaemia 214
Hypercalcaemia 215
Hypernatraemia 217
Hyponatraemia 219
Acute gout 221
Tumour lysis syndrome 223

Acute kidney injury :☢:

- Acute kidney injury refers to an acute (hours to days) deterioration in the GFR leading to an accumulation of nitrogenous waste products (creatinine and urea).
- This is commonly (although not universally) associated with decreasing urine output, sometimes anuria, while fluid balance, electrolyte balance, and acid–base balance are impaired.
- The causes of acute kidney injury are grouped according to aetiology as:
  - pre-renal failure (under-perfused kidneys)
  - post-renal failure (compression of the collecting system)
  - intrinsic renal failure
  - decompensated (or acute-on-chronic) chronic renal failure (Table 8.1).

Table 8.1 Causes of acute kidney injury

	Frequently encountered causes	Less frequently encountered causes
Pre-renal failure	Hypoperfusion (haemorrhage, volume depletion)	
	Inadequate effective vascular volumes (heart failure, hypoalbuminaemia, ascites)	
	Acute disruption to renal artery blood flow	
	Drugs that interfere with GFR and renal blood flow (ACE inhibitors, angiotensin II inhibitors, NSAIDs)	
Post-renal failure	Obstruction of the collecting system (bladder outlet obstruction, ureteric obstruction)	
Intrinsic renal failure	Acute tubular necrosis (ischaemic, gentamicin, radio-contrast, cisplatin, uric acid, myoglobinuria, haemoglobinuria, HUS, TTP)	Vasculitis
		Acute interstitial nephritis
		Glomerular nephritis
		Malignant hypertension
		Hepatorenal syndrome
Decompensated chronic renal failure	Glomerular nephritis	Myeloma
	Pyelonephritis	Amyloidosis
	Interstitial nephritis	SLE
	Diabetic nephropathy	Scleroderma
	Hypertensive nephropathy	Gout
	Polycystic kidney disease	Vasculitis
	Analgesic nephropathy	HUS
	Renovascular disease	Renal tumours
	Nephrolithiasis	

History

Pre-renal failure may present with symptoms associated with diminished fluid reserve. These people may have **thirst**, **symptoms of postural hypotension**, **dry mouth**, and **sensation of anxiousness and un-ease**, which is often associated with bleeding.

A recent **change in medications** (ACE inhibitors, angiotensin II inhibitors, NSAIDs), recent radiology studies, or recent chemotherapy should be sought.

A history of acute deterioration and rapid changes in blood pressure should be sought (ischaemic acute tubular necrosis, pre-renal failure).

Difficulties passing urine, **nocturia**, **haematuria**, and **flank pain** radiating **to the groin suggest an obstructive cause**.

A past history of chronic renal failure and recent changes that may account for this acute deterioration should be sought. Check for any recent changes to medications (NSAIDs, ACE inhibitors, angiotensin II inhibitors, diuretics, lithium, ciclosporin). Check also for symptoms that suggest obstruction (difficulty voiding, haematuria), infection (fever, sweats, dysuria), hypercalcaemia, or hyperglycaemia.

As people become more unwell with **uraemia**, they may become drowsy, nauseated, and confused. Eventually, they may develop myoclonic jerking and seizures.

Physical examination

- Check **pulse**, **blood pressure** (include postural blood pressure), **pulse oximetry**, and **temperature**. Check for visible signs of bleeding, bruising, and anaemia.
- Check for a **flap** and skin for **scratch marks** (uraemic itch) and **palpable purpura** (vasculitis).
- **Cardiovascular** and **respiratory examination** includes an assessment of fluid status (JVP tissue turgor, pulmonary oedema, peripheral and sacral oedema, pleural effusions). Auscultate the heart for a **pericardial rub**.
- Palpate the abdomen for **ascites**. Check for **ballotable renal masses** and percuss for a bladder.
- There may be **muscle weakness** or **muscle paralysis** in the presence of severe **hyperkalaemia**.
- Assess **mental state**.

Investigations and management

Prognosis measured in hours to days prior to the onset of this problem (symptom control)

- Despite the poor prognosis of this group, assess **fluid status**. Cease **nephrotoxic medications** and reduce doses of medications that are renally excreted.
- People who are **fluid overloaded** and in pulmonary oedema require oxygen, diuretics (furosemide 40–80 mg IV/SC) (if not anuric). If in **respiratory distress** or **breathless**, consider low-dose, SC morphine 2.5mg every 6–8 h and titrate to response.
- In people who are **fluid depleted**, rehydration with either SC or IV fluids is indicated (0.9% NaCl 1 L in 8–10 h). This must be reviewed

frequently as eventually the ability to tolerate the fluid load will become impaired.
- Other problems of increasing uraemia that need palliation include the following:
  - **Nausea:** haloperidol 0.5–2.5mg SC daily. Alternatives include cyclizine 12.5–25 mg SC twice to four times daily and ondansetron 4–8 mg SL once or twice daily.
  - **Itch:** ondansetron 4–8 mg SL twice daily. Keep skin moist with regular moisturizers (sorbolene cream).
  - **Myoclonic jerks:** clonazepam 0.5 mg SC/SL twice daily.
  - **Dry mouth** with halitosis from uraemic saliva: institute regular mouth care.

Prognosis measured in weeks prior to the onset of this problem (in addition to symptom control)

Check **FBC** and **coagulation studies** (including bleeding time), **EUC**, **LFT**, **albumin**, **BSL**, and **calcium**. The aim is both to assess the severity of renal impairment and to identify factors that can easily be reversed. It is unlikely that this group would be considered for dialysis.

Immediate life-threatening problems that need to be considered and addressed include the following:

- **Pulmonary oedema:** management of this problem includes sitting the person upright. Administer oxygen, diuretics (if not anuric), and morphine, and apply a glyceryl trinitrate patch (25–50 mg depending on the blood pressure). People who are very frightened by this breathlessness may require an anxiolytic (lorazepam 0.5–1.0 mg SL).
- **Hyperkalaemia** (p.212): organize an ECG. Changes of hyperkalaemia include tenting of the T wave, reduced height of the P wave, widening of the QRS, and increased PR interval. If the potassium is elevated biochemically but the ECG is normal, the first step should be IV administration of 50 mL of 50% glucose and rapidly acting insulin (Actrapid® 10 U) over 10 min. This should be followed by either oral or rectal sodium or calcium polystyrene sulphonate (Resonium® 15 g orally or 15–30 g rectally). If there are ECG changes, the initial step should be 10 mL of IV 10% calcium carbonate to stabilize the cardiac membranes.
- **Bleeding:** acute bleeding may be the precipitating problem that may be exacerbated by the uraemic state. These people require fluid resuscitation and administration of packed cells and platelets. Desmopressin 0.3 U/kg IV will help prolong bleeding time.

Once these acute issues have been addressed, attention will need to be paid to:
- maintenance of fluid balance
- avoidance of nephrotoxic medications
- dose modifications of renally excreted medications
- treatment of underlying problems such as hyperglycaemia and hypercalcaemia
- correcting or preventing urinary tract obstruction.

Prognosis measured in months to years prior to the onset of this problem (in addition to the above)

The investigations and management of these people is best approached in a stepwise fashion. First, complications should be treated:

- Treat **hyperkalaemia** as above.
- **Pulmonary oedema:** organize a CXR, EUC, FBC, and ECG. Treat with diuretics (if not anuric), morphine, and nitrates. Administer oxygen. Consult high dependency services for transfer to coronary care if not settling.
- **Bleeding:** check FBC, coagulation studies including bleeding time. Insert a large-bore cannula and commence fluid resuscitation if dehydrated. Administer packed cells, platelets, and desmopressin. Seek a surgical consultation.
- Once these acute problems have been stabilized, the precipitating factor should be sought and addressed if possible:
  - sepsis
  - cardiac failure
  - urinary obstruction.

A renal consultation should be sought to ascertain whether or not dialysis is indicated in this person. Indications for dialysis include:

- persistent hyperkalaemia or disordered acid–base balance
- uraemic encephalopathy
- pericarditis
- refractory pulmonary oedema.

Oliguric renal failure carries a better prognosis than anuric renal failure.

Further reading

Cassidy J et al. (eds) (2015). Biochemical crises (Chapter 36). In: *Oxford Handbook of Oncology*, 4th ed. Oxford: Oxford University Press. Available at: https://doi.org/10.1093/med/9780199689 842.003.0036

Fielding RE, Farrington K (2020). Clinical presentation of renal disease (Chapter 21.3). In: *Oxford Textbook of Medicine*, 6th ed. Oxford: Oxford University Press. Available at: https://doi.org/10.1093/med/9780198746690.003.0475

Hyperkalaemia ☠

- A low-level increase in serum potassium will be asymptomatic.
- Higher levels are an emergency which can cause premature mortality.

History

For most people, hyperkalaemia is an **incidental finding** associated with mild uraemia. Review their medications and recent fluid intake (Table 8.2). **Muscle weakness** presenting as fatigue should prompt review of serum potassium. The most serious complication is **cardiac arrhythmia**.

Table 8.2 Causes of hyperkalaemia

	Frequently encountered causes	Less frequently encountered causes
Cancer		Tumour lysis syndrome
Intercurrent illnesses	Renal failure	Rhabdomyolysis
	Potassium-sparing diuretics (spironolactone, triamterene, amiloride)	Digoxin toxicity
	Hypoaldosteronism	Beta-blockers (redistribute K^+ to the extracellular space)
	Addison's disease	Any cause of acidosis
	ACE inhibitors, angiotensin II receptor blockade, NSAIDs, tacrolimus, excessive potassium intake	

Physical examination
Physical examination will most often be normal.
Check **hydration status** to exclude hypovolaemia as a pre-renal cause of kidney impairment. Exclude **muscle injury** due to prolonged immobility following a fall or cerebrovascular accident.

Investigations and management
Prognosis measured in hours to days prior to the onset of this problem (symptom control)
No change to comfort care should be initiated unless the person is symptomatically dehydrated.

Prognosis measured in weeks prior to the onset of this problem (in addition to symptom control)
Establish the underlying cause.
Stop contributing medications. Hydrate in renal failure secondary to decreased oral intake. Consider using cation exchange resins which act within 1–2 h (oral or rectal Resonium® 15–30 g 2–3/day). Ensure a **baseline ECG** is done. 'Sine wave' ECG is a late manifestation and is life-threatening.

Prognosis measured in months to years prior to the onset of this problem (in addition to the above)

In this population, consider an insulin–glucose infusion (50 U of Actrapid® in 50 mL 50% dextrose run IV at 5 mL/h initially) which will start to lower potassium within 30 min. In critically high levels, consider immediate dialysis.

Further reading

Firth JD (2020). Disorders of potassium homeostasis (Chapter 21.2.2). In: *Oxford Textbook of Medicine*, 6th ed. Oxford: Oxford University Press. Available at: https://doi.org/10.1093/med/9780198746690.003.0474

Hypokalaemia ⓘ

History

Usually an incidental laboratory finding. Take a thorough medication history (Table 8.3).

Weakness and fatigue should raise the question of **hypokalaemia**. New-onset polyuria or polydipsia can be a symptom of renal tubular dysfunction. GIT symptoms can include the first presentation of an ileus, and hypokalaemia needs to be in the differential consideration of recently developed constipation. In severe hypokalaemia, rhabdomyolysis may occur.

Table 8.3 Causes of hypokalaemia

	Frequently encountered causes	Less frequently encountered causes
Intercurrent illnesses	Vomiting and/or diarrhoea, diuretics (except those that cause K^+ retention), diabetic ketoacidosis	Renal tubular acidosis
		Causes of acute metabolic or respiratory alkalosis
		Primary hyperaldosteronism
		Fludrocortisone excess
		β_2 adrenergic excess
		Cushing's syndrome or disease

Physical examination

Physical examination will most often be normal.

Check **hydration status** if vomiting or diarrhoea are the likely cause of low potassium. Check cardiac function. Check for muscle tenderness.

Investigations and management

Prognosis measured in hours to days prior to the onset of this problem (symptom control)

Continue to focus on comfort measures. Hypokalaemia will be mostly asymptomatic in this population.

Prognosis measured in weeks or more prior to the onset of this problem (in addition to symptom control)

Establish the underlying cause. Obtain a **baseline ECG**. **Replace potassium orally** unless the person is unable to tolerate oral administration or oral replacement is unsuccessful. Refractory cases without obvious precipitant should prompt investigation for Cushing's syndrome, particularly in small cell lung cancer or prostate cancer.

Further reading

Firth JD (2020). Disorders of potassium homeostasis (Chapter 21.2.2). In: *Oxford Textbook of Medicine*, 6th ed. Oxford: Oxford University Press. Available at: https://doi.org/10.1093/med/9780198746690.003.0474

Hypercalcaemia ⚠

- The rate of rise of blood calcium levels dictates the symptomatic presentation. A rapid rise in calcium may lead to a wide spectrum of problems. In contrast, a slow rise may be an incidental diagnosis.
- In malignancy, raised serum calcium may be related to:
  - lytic bone lesions
  - production of parathyroid hormone-related peptide (PTHrP)
  - deregulated conversion of 25-vitamin D to $1,25(OH)_2$-vitamin D (Table 8.4).
- Correction of serum calcium for albumin levels can be calculated in a number of ways. A simple way is corrected calcium = serum calcium + [(40 − albumin g/L) × 0.02].

Table 8.4 Causes of hypercalcaemia

	More frequently encountered causes	Less frequently encountered causes
Cancer	Cancers (most commonly breast, lung, myeloma, lymphoma, renal)	
Intercurrent illnesses		Hyperparathyroidism
		Sarcoid
		Vitamin D intoxication
		Immobility
		Pancreatitis

History

- **Altered mentation is prominent** in rapidly rising calcium, with irritability, drowsiness, lethargy, seizures, or even coma.
- **Anorexia, nausea,** and **vomiting** are frequently encountered. People may have **polyuria** and **polydipsia**.
- **Constipation, abdominal pain,** and **muscle weakness** may also be present.

Physical examination

- Assess the **degree of dehydration** (tissue turgor, blood pressure, pulse, urine output).
- Cardiovascular assessment needs to include pulse (exclude sinus bradycardia, or second-degree heart block).
- Assess level of consciousness and formally test cognition.
- **Severe constipation** is often present with a distended uncomfortable abdomen. Auscultate for bowel sounds as a paralytic ileus may be present.

Investigations and management

Prognosis measured in hours to days prior to the onset of this problem (symptom control)

- In very unwell people entering the final hours of life, no interventions to reduce calcium are necessary.
- No investigations should be performed.
- Those with a prognosis of days may feel more comfortable with **gentle hydration** (NaCl 1 L via SC infusion over 24 h) combined with SC calcitonin (50–100 IU daily or twice daily). This may allow correction of the hypercalcaemia more rapidly than IV bisphosphonates which may take up to 48 h or longer to have an effect in the frail elderly.

Prognosis measured in weeks prior to the onset of this problem (in addition to symptom control)

- **Check serum electrolytes and renal function** (pre-renal impairment from nausea and vomiting, polyuria, inability to drink due to somnolence).
- Pancreatitis may be associated with hypercalcaemia; **check amylase**.
- If there is an unlikely association between the life-limiting illness and hypercalcaemia (e.g. prostatic cancer), check parathyroid hormone levels.
- **Commence hydration** with 0.9% NaCl 1 L IV. The aim is to administer 2 L in 24 h. This will depend upon the fragility of the person.
- **Forced diuresis is not necessary**. Carefully monitor fluid status to avoid precipitating cardiac failure. It is necessary to repeat EUC daily.
- **Administer an IV bisphosphonate** (disodium pamidronate 30–90 mg over 1–2 h, or clodronate 1.5 g over 4 h, or zoledronic acid 4 mg over 15 min).
- **In people with haematological malignancies, commence dexamethasone 4–8 mg SC in the morning**.
- Approximately 20% of people fail to respond to hydration and bisphosphonates. This is a poor prognostic group, with life expectancy measured now in days to weeks.

Prognosis measured in months to years prior to the onset of this problem (in addition to the above)

- If this was the first episode of hypercalcaemia, the cause needs to be ascertained.
- The best long-term management of hypercalcaemia is management of the underlying disorder.

Further reading

Ryan R, Casey R (2021). Endocrine and metabolic complications of advanced cancer (Chapter 14.9). In: *Oxford Textbook of Palliative Medicine*, 6th ed. Oxford: Oxford University Press. Available at: https://doi.org/10.1093/med/9780198821328.003.0084

Thakker RV (2020). Parathyroid disorders and diseases altering calcium metabolism (Chapter 13.4). In: *Oxford Textbook of Medicine*, 6th ed. Oxford: Oxford University Press. Available at: https://doi.org/10.1093/med/9780198746690.003.0248

Hypernatraemia ⓘ

Symptomatic hypernatraemia can occur with serum sodium levels >150 mmol/L from a range of causes (Table 8.5).

Table 8.5 Causes of hypernatraemia

	More frequently encountered causes	Less frequently encountered causes
Cancer	Use of exogenous glucocorticoids causing Cushing's syndrome[a]	Cushing's syndrome[a] (adrenocorticotropic hormone (ACTH)-producing tumours (small cell lung carcinoma with hypokalaemia as the only clue) or corticotropin-releasing hormone-producing tumours such as bronchial carcinoid, pancreatic tumours, thymus tumours). Malignant infiltration of the pituitary fossa
Other life-limiting illnesses		Cystic fibrosis[b]
Intercurrent illnesses	Diuretics[b] Any person unable to drink normally[c] (especially with decreased level of consciousness)	Lactulose[b] (osmotic purgative) Renal failure[b] Cushing's syndrome[a] Primary hyperaldosteronism[a] Central diabetes insipidus[b] (antidiuretic hormone not synthesized or not secreted)

[a] Salt retention greater than water retention.

[b] Water loss greater than salt loss.

[c] Normal total body water content.

History

Clues to hypernatraemia include **new onset of fits** with no known cerebral disease, **decreasing level of consciousness**, or **an acute confusional state from cerebral oedema** (p.29). Review all medications carefully.

Physical examination

Physical examination will often be normal with mild hypernatraemia; carefully assess hydration including tissue turgor and mucous membranes. Examine for tachycardia and hypotension. Signs of significant hypernatraemia include increasing hyper-reflexia, increasing ataxia, and spontaneous muscle twitching. Clues to causes include Cushingoid appearance: fat deposition (face, upper thoracic spine, supraclavicular region, and abdomen) and skin changes (plethora, striae).

Investigations and management

Prognosis measured in hours to days prior to the onset of this problem (symptom control)

Hypernatraemia becomes an incidental finding in the last few hours or days of life. With neurological deficit, it may be reasonable to hydrate gently if hypernatraemia is due to diuretics, lactulose, or renal failure.

Prognosis measured in weeks prior to the onset of this problem (in addition to symptom control)

Establish the underlying cause. Stop or wean any medications that may be contributing to the problem. Hydrate to euvolaemia in people with total body water deficit. If the cause is dexamethasone or prednisolone, ensure that the person is experiencing the proposed benefit.

Prognosis measured in months to years prior to the onset of this problem (in addition to the above)

If hypernatraemia is due to ectopic ACTH, successfully treating the underlying malignancy will treat high sodium levels.

Further reading

Moritz ML, Ayus JC (2020). Disorders of water and sodium homeostasis (Chapter 21.2.1). In: *Oxford Textbook of Medicine*, 6th ed. Oxford: Oxford University Press. Available at: https://doi.org/10.1093/med/9780198746690.003.0473

Hyponatraemia ☠️

- Symptomatic hyponatraemia can occur with serum sodium levels <125 mmol/L.
- The speed of onset of the hyponatraemia will dictate the speed of the response. Acute reductions in sodium need to be treated actively in appropriate people because ensuing acute cerebral oedema will be fatal. Causes vary widely (Table 8.6).

Table 8.6 Causes of hyponatraemia

	More frequently encountered causes	Less frequently encountered causes
Cancer		Ascites or pleural effusions[a]
Other life-limiting illnesses	End-stage cardiac failure[b] Cirrhosis[b] Renal failure[b]	
Intercurrent illnesses	Diuretics[a] Vomiting or diarrhoea[a] Pancreatitis Peritonitis[a]	Syndrome of inappropriate antidiuretic hormone (SIADH)[c] Addison's disease[c] Hypothyroidism[c] Nephrotic syndrome[b] Hyperglycaemia[a]

[a] Salt loss greater than water loss.

[b] Water retention greater than salt retention.

[c] Normal total body water content.

History

Hyponatraemia needs to be considered in people with a change in level of consciousness or impaired mentation.

Lethargy may be a prominent symptom for some people. It is a frequently encountered cause of an **acute confusional state** (p.29). Check serum sodium in anyone presenting with seizure activity (for the first time or with **seizure activity** that has become unstable).

Physical examination

Careful assessment of **hydration** is the key to categorizing hyponatraemia. Assess for **oedema** (cardiac in origin or nephrotic syndrome), but also ensure that there is no dehydration from vomiting or diarrhoea. Establish cognition and record the baseline mental state. Examine for evidence of cardiac failure or third-space relocation (pleural effusions or ascites). Seek signs of hypothyroidism.

Investigations and management

Prognosis measured in hours to days prior to the onset of this problem (symptom control)

In the last few hours of life, **treat symptoms directly**. If fluid overloaded and symptomatic, consider a loop diuretic. If hyponatraemia is severe, consider clonazepam 0.5–1 mg daily as an antiepileptic.

Prognosis measured in weeks prior to the onset of this problem (in addition to symptom control)

Establish the likely causes of hyponatraemia and treat accordingly:

- **Hypervolemic hyponatraemia**—fluid restriction and diuretics.
- **Hypovolaemic hyponatraemia**—normal saline rehydration.
- **Euvolemic hyponatraemia**—treat the underlying cause if possible and fluid restrict. Investigate for hyponatraemia and Addison's disease. Cease medications that could be causing SIADH (Table 8.7). If refractory to fluid restriction, salt tablets with demeclocycline 300–600 mg twice daily may help.

Table 8.7 Causes of SIADH

	More frequently encountered causes	Less frequently encountered causes
Cancer	Small cell lung carcinoma Pancreatic carcinomas Any CNS tumour	Mesothelioma Cyclophosphamide Vincristine Vinblastine
Intercurrent illnesses	Pneumonia (or any chest infection) Tricyclic antidepressants Haloperidol Thiazide diuretics	Meningitis Intracranial bleed Hypothyroidism Chlorpropamide MAOIs

Prognosis measured in months to years prior to the onset of this problem (in addition to the above)

As above, plus:

- Careful evaluation of the underlying causes which need to be explored and treated.

Further reading

Moritz ML, Ayus JC (2020). Disorders of water and sodium homeostasis (Chapter 21.2.1). In: *Oxford Textbook of Medicine*, 6th ed. Oxford: Oxford University Press. Available at: https://doi.org/10.1093/med/9780198746690.003.0473

Acute gout ①

- Gout may manifest as acute joint swelling and pain or as renal disease (calculi or interstitial damage from crystal deposition).
- Consider underlying causes in first presentations (Table 8.8).

Table 8.8 Causes of gout

	More frequently encountered causes	Less frequently encountered causes
Cancer		Following therapy for sensitive tumours
		Myeloproliferative diseases
Intercurrent illnesses	Following alcohol intake	Psoriasis
	Post-surgery	Hypertension
	Prolonged fasting	Sarcoidosis
	Major medical illness	Hypothyroidism
	Primary gout (mostly under-excretion)	Haemolytic anaemia of any cause
	Medications reducing excretion (diuretics, salicylates, ciclosporin)	Secondary polycythaemia

History

For most people with a life-limiting illness, the diagnosis of the first episode of gout will be clear from the **acute painful joint swelling that is time limited to 12–24 h. However, for some people, this will progress to a chronic issue characterized by multiple painful episodes with evidence of joint destruction and uric acid tophi**.

Physical examination

Examine the joints affected. Check the renal angles for pain (consider renal calculi).

Investigations and management

Prognosis measured in hours to days prior to the onset of this problem (symptom control)
Pain relief relies on NSAIDs either orally or parenterally (e.g. ketorolac 10 mg SC three times daily). Corticosteroid SC or locally are alternative options.

Prognosis measured in weeks prior to the onset of this problem (in addition to symptom control)
For acute gout, a short course of colchicine is preferable (1 mg stat orally, 500 micrograms 1 h later).

Prognosis measured in months to years prior to the onset of this problem (in addition to the above)

Having treated an acute episode, it will be important to avoid future episodes especially if there is a precipitant such as tumour lysis. If a person has a risk of tumour lysis, actively hydrate before therapy and use allopurinol prophylactically.

In people with two or more episodes of gout without an obvious precipitant, use allopurinol in the long term.

Further reading

Marinaki AM et al. (2020). Disorders of purine and pyrimidine metabolism (Chapter 12.4). In: *Oxford Textbook of Medicine*, 6th ed. Oxford: Oxford University Press. Available at: https://doi.org/10.1093/med/9780198746690.003.0230

Tumour lysis syndrome ⚙

- Tumour lysis is characterized by a rapid rise in serum urate levels (>900 µmol/L) as tumour cells in highly sensitive tumours are lysed soon after chemotherapy or sometimes when radiotherapy is initiated. Occasionally, it may be seen in untreated acute haematological malignancies because of excessive cell turnover.
- Associated biochemical abnormalities include hyperphosphataemia, raised LDH, and sometimes hypocalcaemia.
- Circulating urate can be deposited widely, including in the distal renal tubules, causing local obstruction and invoking an intense inflammatory reaction.
- Cancers most frequently associated with tumour lysis syndrome are:
  - acute leukaemias
  - high-grade lymphomas
  - small cell lung cancer (less frequently).

Prevention includes aggressive hydration and regular allopurinol (300 mg orally daily) in people with cancers likely to cause the syndrome as chemotherapy is initiated.

Once the syndrome is established, maximally tolerated hydration with normal saline and close monitoring is initiated if the person is not anuric. Renal function should gradually return to normal as uric acid and phosphate levels fall.

Treatment in established renal failure relies on haemodialysis as the renal tubular system becomes clogged with urate crystals or, less commonly, calcium/phosphate compounds.

Further reading

Cassidy J et al. (eds) (2015). Biochemical crises (Chapter 36). In: *Oxford Handbook of Oncology*, 4th ed. Oxford: Oxford University Press. Available at: https://doi.org/10.1093/med/9780199689842.003.0036

Russell N, Burnett A (2020). Acute myeloid leukaemia (Chapter 22.3.3). In: *Oxford Textbook of Medicine*, 6th ed. Oxford: Oxford University Press. Available at: https://doi.org/10.1093/med/9780198746690.003.0515

Endocrine problems

Hypoglycaemia 226
Hyperglycaemia 228
Hypoadrenal crisis 232
Thyroid storm 235
Myxoedema coma 237

Hypoglycaemia ☠

- Hypoglycaemia is the most common metabolic disorder.
- It is defined as a plasma glucose concentration <2.5 mmol/L.
- The symptom threshold varies widely.
- Hypoglycaemia needs to be considered in a range of end-stage diseases other than just diabetics being treated with insulin or oral hypoglycaemics (Table 9.1).
- **The most common cause of hypoglycaemia in known diabetics is insulin or oral hypoglycaemics**.

Table 9.1 Causes of hypoglycaemia

	More frequently encountered causes	Less frequently encountered causes
Cancer	Cancer cachexia	Insulinoma
	Reduced food intake	Paraneoplastic disease
	Liver tumours (primary or metastatic)	Immune hypoglycaemia (Hodgkin's disease)
	Continued use of hypoglycaemic agents with poor or absent food intake	Retroperitoneal fibrosarcomas
End-stage organ failure	Liver failure	Septic shock
		Panhypopituitarism
		Addison's disease

History

There are two main classes of symptoms of hypoglycaemia:
- **Autonomic:** tremor, sweating, palpitations, hunger.
- **Neuroglycopenic:** confusion, altered behaviour, slurred speech, drowsiness, seizures, coma.

These problems may all be blunted in elderly people, people receiving beta-blocking medications, or individuals receiving sedative medications.

Physical examination

In the setting of any **unexplained neurological deterioration** (drowsy, confused, sweating, agitated, aggressive), check blood glucose levels.

Investigations and management

Prognosis measured in hours to days prior to the onset of this problem (symptom control)
- In a known diabetic who is still receiving glucose-lowering treatment, a finger-prick BSL should be checked.
- If well enough and able to protect their airway, these people should receive oral glucose or dextrose. If they are not able to take oral medications, consider 25 mL of 50% dextrose IV.
- Hypoglycaemia in people with cachexia, extensive liver dysfunction, or replacement of liver with tumour are unlikely to respond to glycogen.

- In the last stages of life, oral hypoglycaemic medications should be discontinued.
- If insulin dependent, stop long-acting agents. Rapid-onset insulin (e.g. Actrapid®) should be substituted and blood sugar monitoring should continue. BSL should be kept in a broad range that is less likely to be associated with symptoms (>8 mmol/L to <14 mmol/L).

Prognosis measured in weeks prior to the onset of this problem (in addition to symptom control)

Check **finger-prick BSL and formal BSL**. Do not wait for the results of the formal BSL. Immediate interventions include the following:

- If unconscious, protect airway.
- If the person can safely swallow, give glucose by mouth.
- If not, administer 50% glucose IV into a large-bore vein with a saline flush. If there is any question of previous long-term alcohol intake, give with thiamine 100 mg to avoid inducing Wernicke's encephalopathy.
- Follow the oral sugar with a carbohydrate load (e.g. bread).
- If the person is a known type 1 diabetic, glucagon 1 mg may be administered IM or IV (avoid SC in an emergency because of unreliable absorption). **(In type 2 diabetes mellitus, glucagon will stimulate insulin secretion as well as glycogenolysis and so should not be used.)**

Once the individual has recovered from this acute episode, review glycaemic control.

Renegotiating the aims of glycaemic control can be difficult. Liberalize diet. Reduce or withdraw oral hypoglycaemics in type 2 diabetes and reduce or cease doses of long-acting insulin in type 1 diabetics.

Prognosis measured in months to years prior to the onset of this problem (in addition to the above)

It is reasonable to expect that individuals should recover quickly. However, if recovery is prolonged, recheck the BSL and consider the addition of dexamethasone 4 mg IV four times daily. This is to reduce associated cerebral oedema that may accompany a prolonged and severe episode of hypoglycaemia. Once they have recovered, repeat BSL and perform a septic work-up.

If a person is taking a sulphonylurea, check that renal function has not deteriorated. Renal impairment may prolong their hypoglycaemic effects.

In non-diabetics who are hypoglycaemic, check:

- C-peptide (insulinoma)
- insulin levels (insulinoma, exogenous insulin, sulphonylurea administration)
- thyroid function (thyrotoxicosis)
- random cortisol levels (pituitary and adrenal failure)
- hepatic function (liver failure, excess alcohol).

Further reading

Evans M, Challis B (2020). Hypoglycaemia (Chapter 13.9.2). In: *Oxford Textbook of Medicine*, 6th ed. Oxford: Oxford University Press. Available at: https://doi.org/10.1093/med/9780198746690.003.0260

Watson M et al. (eds) (2019). Endocrine and metabolic complications of advanced cancer (Chapter 15). In: *Oxford Handbook of Palliative Care*, 3rd ed. Oxford: Oxford University Press. Available at: https://doi.org/10.1093/med/9780198745655.003.0015

Hyperglycaemia ☠☺

- The most serious hyperglycaemic complications of diabetes are diabetic ketoacidosis (type 1 diabetes) and hyperosmolar hyperglycaemia (type 2 diabetes).
- Hyperglycaemia in non-diabetic people occurs in extremely unwell individuals (Table 9.2) and may worsen an already poor prognosis because of the risk of impaired fluid balance, impaired immune function and increased inflammation, and increased risk of thrombosis.

Table 9.2 Causes of hyperglycaemia in non-diabetics

	More frequently encountered causes	Less frequently encountered causes
Cancer	Insulin resistance in pancreatic cancer	
End-stage organ failure		High-glucose peritoneal dialysis fluids
Intercurrent illnesses	Infection Inflammation Excessive intake (TPN, 5% dextrose) Corticosteroids	Medications (thiazide diuretics, sympathomimetics, tacrolimus, ciclosporin)

History

In type 1 diabetes, the onset of hyperglycaemia complicated by ketoacidosis is usually short (<24 h) with precipitants including:
- infection
- AMI
- pancreatitis
- medications (glucocorticoids, thiazide diuretics, sympathomimetics, tacrolimus, ciclosporin)
- alcohol binge.

People present with polyuria, polydipsia and polyphagia, nausea and vomiting, abdominal pain, increasing fatigue, and altered consciousness.

In type 2 diabetes, the onset of hyperglycaemia complicated by a hyperosmolar state is often very subtle over a period of days.

Confusion or drowsiness suggests significant CNS impairment.

In non-diabetics, the person who is hyperglycaemic may be thirsty and polyuric. It may be an incidental finding on routine biochemical testing.

Physical examination

- **Assess hydration** (tissue turgor, blood pressure, pulse, urine output).
- A **full neurological assessment** is indicated (level of consciousness, cognition).

- **Deep sighing respirations (Kussmaul breathing)** may be present. The person may be either hypothermic or febrile if an infection is the presenting precipitant.

Investigations and management

Prognosis measured in hours to days prior to the onset of this problem (symptom control)

- It is appropriate to **investigate BSL by finger-prick** testing.
- More invasive blood tests are not indicated.
- A **urine specimen may be collected for ketones**.

Despite the limited prognosis of these people, it is still necessary to **reduce the BSL to <14 mmol/L** to minimize the symptoms of polyuria, thirst, nausea and vomiting, and drowsiness. This is best done by using a **gentle sliding-scale insulin regimen with short-acting insulin** (human Actrapid®, Humulin S®) (Table 9.3).

Hydration should be considered and fluid gently replaced if necessary 0.9% NaCl either SC or IV at a rate of 1 l/24 h. Medications that may elevate BSL should be ceased if possible.

Table 9.3 Sliding scale of insulin to treat symptomatic hyperglycaemia at the end of life.

BSL (mmol/L)	Insulin dose (Actrapid®)
<10	No insulin
10.1–15.0	4 U
15.1–20.0	6 U
>20	8 U

Prognosis measured in weeks prior to the onset of this problem (in addition to symptom control)

- The aim for people with diabetic ketoacidosis or hyperosmolar hyperglycaemia is to reduce symptoms. They are very unwell.
- Assess formal **blood glucose level**. Check **serum electrolytes (especially K+ and Na+** which may be artificially high, and **renal function** which may be grossly impaired), **serum osmolality**, **arterial blood gases** to assess acid–base status, and **urine for ketones**. Check for any source of **sepsis** (urine analysis, CXR, blood cultures).
- Insulin needs to be administered. Initially, it may be appropriate to do this using a sliding-scale regimen with BSL, checked every 2 h. Long-acting insulin (Mixtard®) should be commenced later.
- Restore adequate hydration and correct electrolyte abnormalities.
- It is reasonable to repeat the serum electrolytes and renal function tests daily.
- People need to be observed for cognitive decline that may suggest cerebral oedema or increasing shortness of breath due to (non-cardiac) pulmonary oedema.

Prognosis measured in months to years prior to the onset of this problem (in addition to the above)

Hyperglycaemia presenting in known diabetics requires prompt attention.

In type 1 diabetes, ketoacidosis must be considered in people who present with high blood glucose who are systemically unwell. This is a medical emergency and the following investigations and treatments must be initiated while a high dependency consultation is urgently sought:

- **Serum electrolytes, renal function, HCO_3, amylase, serum osmolality,** Mg^{2+}, PO_4.
- **FBC**.
- **Urinalysis for ketones**.
- **Septic screen** (blood cultures, urinalysis, CXR).
- **Arterial blood gases**.
- **Start IV insulin** 10 U (Actrapid®) and **commence hydration** (1 L 0.9% NaCl immediately then 1 L over the next hour, then 1 L over 2 h, and continue in this manner based on the individual fluid balance).
- **Commence an IV insulin infusion** (50 U Actrapid® in 50 mL 0.9% NaCl), with the infusion rate based on the hourly BSL; check serum electrolytes after 24 h.
- **Check vital signs hourly**.
- **Insert an indwelling catheter** and monitor urine output hourly.
- **Commence DVT prophylaxis**.
- Ensure that the decline in BSL is **not** precipitous as this increases the risk of cerebral oedema.
- Treat suspected infection with IV antibiotics; do not wait for septic screen results.

Hyperosmolar hyperglycaemia occurs in older people with type 2 diabetics. These individuals may present with **dehydration** and a **BSL >35 mmol/L**. This is a medical emergency. Investigate and treatment while a high dependency consultation is urgently sought.

- Serum electrolytes and renal function, serum osmolality.
- FBC.
- Septic screen.
- Rehydrate with 0.9% NaCl.
- **Repeat BSL every hour** while rehydration is occurring; it may not be necessary to use an insulin infusion; it is imperative to avoid rapid changes in electrolytes or BSL.
- **Commence DVT** prophylaxis.

Hyperglycaemia in hospitalized people who are not diabetics requires attention when BSL >12 mmol/L.

In the medically unstable, the most appropriate management is with regular insulin (e.g. Mixtard® 30/70) rather than sliding-scale insulin. It is important to seek specialist endocrine input. These people and any individual who is found to have a random BSL of >6.9 mmol/L in hospital should be tested for diabetes within a month of hospital discharge.

Further reading

Dayan C, Platts J (2020). Diabetes (Chapter 13.9.1). In: *Oxford Textbook of Medicine*, 6th ed. Oxford: Oxford University Press. Available at: https://doi.org/10.1093/med/9780198746690.003.0259

Watson M et al. (eds) (2019). Endocrine and metabolic complications of advanced cancer (Chapter 15). In: *Oxford Handbook of Palliative Care*, 3rd ed. Oxford: Oxford University Press. Available at: https://doi.org/10.1093/med/9780198745655.003.0015

Hypoadrenal crisis :☠:

- Addisonian or hypoadrenal crisis is a rare event but requires a high index of suspicion when underlying causes are present (Table 9.4).
- The symptoms and signs are non-specific and may be mistaken for other serious medical problems (e.g. sepsis, haemorrhage, acute abdomen).
- If missed, it may be a fatal event, and so a high index of suspicion is needed in people who are otherwise unwell and have a sudden deterioration in condition.

Table 9.4 Causes of hypoadrenal crisis

	More frequently encountered causes	Less frequently encountered causes
Cancer		Bilateral adrenal metastases
		Aminoglutethimide
Intercurrent illnesses	Sudden withdrawal of long-term glucocorticoids	Autoimmune adrenal disease
	Superimposed stressors (e.g. septicaemia) on a background of glucocorticoid use	Bilateral adrenal haemorrhage (especially people on anticoagulants)
		Bilateral adrenal infarcts
		Pituitary apoplexy
		Meningococcal sepsis
		TB
AIDS		Ketoconazole
		AIDS (opportunistic infections)

History

In a typical **hypoadrenal crisis, people present with hypotensive shock**. This occurs because of sodium loss with consequent fluid loss, low renin and prostacyclin levels, and decreased response to catecholamines.

More non-specific symptoms include **unexplained fever**, abdominal pain mimicking an acute abdomen, **nausea and vomiting, lethargy, dizziness, confusion, myalgia, arthralgia, and ultimately coma.**

Physical examination

- **Tachycardia**, **fever**, and **shock** (check tissue turgor, blood pressure including postural drop, pulse, urine output).
- Assess level of consciousness (Glasgow Coma Score (Appendix 3) and higher centres (Mini-Mental State Examination)).
- Pigmentation and vitiligo only occur in people with chronic adrenal insufficiency.

Investigations and management

Prognosis measured in hours to days prior to the onset of this problem (symptom control)

- People with suspected hypoadrenal crisis who have a previous history of corticosteroid use should receive corticosteroids (hydrocortisone 100 mg IV or dexamethasone 4–8 mg SC) immediately.
- Treat other symptoms of pain, nausea and vomiting, and increasing confusion as necessary.

Prognosis measured in weeks prior to the onset of this problem (in addition to symptom control)

- Check **serum electrolytes** (decreased K^+, increased Na^+), **renal function**, and **urinary sodium** levels (abnormal urinary sodium loss, altered renal function secondary to fluid loss).
- If there is a decreased level of consciousness, **check BSL** for hypo- or hyperglycaemia.
- **A full septic work-up** is indicated (FBC, mid-stream urine, blood cultures, CXR).
- If the person does not have a past history of corticosteroid use, an **abdominal CT** to image the adrenals is indicated.
- Management of the problem includes:
  - **rehydration** with IV fluids
  - **commence hydrocortisone 100 mg IV infusion** every 6 h
  - **commence IV broad-spectrum antibiotics** (aminoglycoside, third-generation cephalosporin)
  - **monitor for hypoglycaemia**.
- When more stable, the hydrocortisone may be reduced to 50 mg daily and tapered down to 5–10 mg daily. Fludrocortisone (starting dose of 0.05 mg daily) is not indicated acutely. It may be necessary if postural hypotension continues.
- It will be necessary to ensure that steroids are continued for the rest of this individual's life.

Prognosis measured in months to years prior to the onset of this problem (in addition to the above)

In people in whom an adrenal crisis is suspected, management and early investigations must be performed simultaneously. An **endocrine consultation should be sought**.

- Take blood for **random cortisol** and **ACTH, BSL, EUC, TFTs, and septic screen**.
- **Commence rehydration**. Initially a plasma expander may be necessary; then replace with 0.9% NaCl.
- Monitor **blood glucose and administer IV 50% glucose if necessary**.
- Once the person is stabilized, the cause of the hypoadrenal episode will need to be investigated further in people who were not previously taking steroids.
- Investigations include an **abdominal CT scan** and Synacthen test.

Further reading

Coggle S et al. (2020). Acute medical presentations (Chapter 30.1). In: *Oxford Textbook of Medicine*, 6th ed. Oxford: Oxford University Press. Available at: https://doi.org/10.1093/med/978019 8746690.003.0647

Ryan R, Casey R (2021). Endocrine and metabolic complications of advanced cancer (Chapter 14.9). In: *Oxford Textbook of Palliative Medicine*, 6th ed. Oxford: Oxford University Press. Available at: https://doi.org/10.1093/med/9780198821328.003.0084

Thyroid storm ☠

- An acute presentation of hyperthyroidism is characterized as a 'thyroid storm'. A number of underlying aetiologies may cause this (Table 9.5).
- This is a presentation with a spectrum of non-specific signs and symptoms where the diagnosis will only be made with a high index of suspicion.

Table 9.5 Causes of a hyperthyroid crisis

	More frequently encountered causes	Less frequently encountered causes
Cancer		Thyroid cancer
End-stage organ failure		Acute myocardial infarct
Intercurrent illnesses	Exposure to an iodine load (radiographic dyes)	Amiodarone
		Sepsis
	Any pre-existing thyroid disease (painful subacute thyroiditis may proceed to thyroid storm after a viral illness)	Omission of thyroid-suppressing medications
		Overmedication on thyroid replacement therapy

History

- People present systemically unwell with **fever and tachycardia**. The tachycardia may be associated with arrhythmias including atrial fibrillation and other supraventricular tachycardias.
- Additionally, people may be **confused, agitated, or even moribund**.
- They may also have GIT symptoms including nausea and vomiting, **diarrhoea, and abdominal pain that may mimic an acute abdomen**.

Physical examination

- Physical examination may reveal **tachycardia, warm skin, tremor**, and **hyper-reflexia**.
- Other physical signs may be largely absent.
- Evidence of lid-lag, proptosis, and goitre should be sought but are rarely found.

Investigations and management

Prognosis measured in hours to days prior to the onset of this problem (symptom control)

- This is a **clinical diagnosis that should be based on past history and the current clinical situation**.
- Agitation, if present, will need to be addressed with antipsychotic medications (chlorpromazine 50 mg IM or orally twice or three times daily, levomepromazine 25–50 mg via SC infusion).

- **Treat tachycardia** with propranolol (40 mg orally three times daily if able to tolerate oral medications or IV 1 mg over 1 min and repeat up to eight times if necessary).
- **Treat fever** with tepid sponging and paracetamol 1 g orally or IV/ rectally 500 mg three times daily.
- **Control vomiting and abdominal pain**. Vomiting may be profuse from high gastric output.

Prognosis measured in weeks prior to the onset of this problem (in addition to symptom control)

- Despite the limited prognosis of this group, **an endocrine consultation is indicated** as the mortality from this problem is high.
- Thyrotoxicosis may be associated with a significant symptom burden and so directed management is indicated. However, given the overall limited prognosis, transfer to a high dependency unit is not indicated.
- **Check TFTs**.
- **Blood glucose and corrected serum calcium levels** may be raised.
- **Mild renal impairment** may be present.
- A cholestatic picture may be seen with **LFTs**.
- Leukocytosis is frequently seen on FBC.
- If the person is able to swallow, **commence oral carbimazole 15– 25 mg** four times daily. Administer via NG tube if necessary.
- **Rehydrate** with 0.9% NaCl.
- Consider antibiotics if there is focal evidence of infection.

Prognosis measured in months to years prior to the onset of this problem (in addition to the above)

This is a medical emergency. An urgent endocrine and high dependency consultation must be sought immediately.

While this is occurring, the following investigations and management should be implemented:

- Take blood for tri-iodothyronine **(T_3), thyroxine (T_4), EUC, LFTS, FBC, random cortisol, and blood cultures**.
- **Hydrate** with 0.9% NaCl.
- Sedate if very agitated.
- Administer propranolol 1 mg IV over 1 min and repeat as necessary.
- Insert an **NG tube if vomiting** and administer IV antiemetics (prochlorperazine 12.5 mg IV/IM or haloperidol 0.5 mg SC).
- Transfer to a high dependency unit as soon as possible. The acute presentation of thyroid storm carries a mortality rate of 30%.

Further reading

Ryan R, Casey R (2021). Endocrine and metabolic complications of advanced cancer (Chapter 14.9). In: *Oxford Textbook of Palliative Medicine*, 6th ed. Oxford: Oxford University Press. Available at: https://doi.org/10.1093/med/9780198821328.003.0084

Weetman AP, Boelaert K (2020). The thyroid gland and disorders of thyroid function (Chapter 13.3.1). In: *Oxford Textbook of Medicine*, 6th ed. Oxford: Oxford University Press. Available at: https://doi.org/10.1093/med/9780198746690.003.0246

Myxoedema coma :⚙:

This is mostly a diagnosis in people with known hypothyroidism (Table 9.6).

Table 9.6 Causes of hypothyroid crisis

	More frequently encountered causes	Less frequently encountered causes
Intercurrent illnesses	Non-compliance with thyroid medications Sepsis	Amiodarone Trauma Exposure to cold Opioids Sedatives

History

- This occurs in people who are known to be hypothyroid (surgery, radioactive iodine).
- Precipitants which may lead to acute deterioration that may be sought on history include non-compliance with medications, infection, trauma, or new onset of an additional acute medical problem which may cause physical stress or render the individual unable to take medications.

Physical examination

- The **signs of hypothyroidism may be present** to give a clue: thin hair, dry coarse skin, enlarged tongue, delayed deep tendon reflexes, and pre-tibial oedema.
- Systemically, **bradycardia and hypotension** are likely to be present.
- **Hypothermia and lethargy** are prominent.
- **Slow mentation** which has gradually deteriorated is an important clue.
- Abdominal examination may reveal a **distended abdomen** secondary to decreased gut motility and megacolon.

Investigations and management

Prognosis measured in hours to days prior to the onset of this problem (symptom control)

The most likely scenario at this stage of life is the development of this problem when individuals can no longer swallow their thyroid replacement.

Prognosis is very poor in this clinical setting and the therapeutic aim is good symptom control. People may be hypoxaemic, and low-flow oxygen using nasal prongs is indicated. They may be hypothermic and so warm ambient temperatures and blankets are indicated. Despite the short prognosis, ensure that these people are not dehydrated.

Prognosis measured in weeks prior to the onset of this problem (in addition to symptom control)

- **Myxoedema coma carries a poor prognosis even with treatment**.

- If there has been an acute deterioration due to an acute and easily reversible cause (sepsis, AMI), further interventions may be appropriate.
- This situation needs to be managed with caution. **Despite the poor prognosis, consult an endocrinologist**.
- Take bloods for **TFTs** (thyroid-stimulating hormone, T_4, T_3), **EUC**, **BSL**, **FBC**, and **blood cultures**.
- Thyroid function will show a high thyroid-stimulating hormone and low T_4. Hypoglycaemia and hyponatraemia are frequently seen.
- **Check for any source of sepsis** (urine analysis, CXR, blood cultures, WCC with differential).
- High **serum creatinine kinase levels** and a high mean cell volume on red cell morphology are consistent with the diagnosis.
- Check **oxygen saturation** and commence oxygen if hypoxaemic.
- Treat **hypoglycaemia** if present.
- Commence **hydrocortisone 100 mg IV three times daily or dexamethasone 4 mg SC twice daily**.
- **An IV line should be inserted and T_3 5–20 micrograms administered over 12 h**. This must be in discussion with an endocrinologist. This dose should be repeated for 3 days. If well enough, oral T_4 may be given.
- **Rehydrate very cautiously** as there is a chance of precipitating cardiac failure.
- Ensure that these people are **kept warm**.

Prognosis measured in months to years prior to the onset of this problem (in addition to the above)

These people require urgent endocrine and high dependency consultation. The following investigations and interventions should be initiated:
- **Check arterial blood gases**.
- **Ensure IV access**.
- **Carefully observe for any signs of cardiac failure**.

A mortality rate of 20% is associated with hypothyroid coma. This situation requires transfer to a high dependency unit with thyroid hormone replacement supervised by an endocrinologist.

Further reading

Ryan R, Casey R (2021). Endocrine and metabolic complications of advanced cancer (Chapter 14.9). In: *Oxford Textbook of Palliative Medicine*, 6th ed. Oxford: Oxford University Press. Available at: https://doi.org/10.1093/med/9780198821328.003.0084

Weetman AP, Boelaert K (2020). The thyroid gland and disorders of thyroid function (Chapter 13.3.1). In: *Oxford Textbook of Medicine*, 6th ed. Oxford: Oxford University Press. Available at: https://doi.org/10.1093/med/9780198746690.003.0246

Chapter 10

Neurology

Acute stroke 240
Spinal cord compromise 242
Delirium: acute confusional states 246
Seizures 249
Meningitis 252
Intracranial bleeding 256
Raised intracranial pressure 259

Acute stroke :☠:

- Acute stroke is now a medical emergency.
- Consider in people with any sudden change in neurological status (not limited to weakness).
- Thrombotic strokes are increasingly treatable, and treatment should be considered even late in the course of a life-limiting illness.
- Other than neurological changes (which at times may be vague), there may be few symptoms of a stroke.

History

- People may notice motor or sensory changes or both. Other presentations can include any discrete function of the CNS. For example, speech deficits, such as word finding difficulties, may be the only manifestation.
- Is there a history of strokes or transient ischaemic attacks (TIAs)?
- Has there been any previous imaging of the brain?
- Review any long-term risk factors including hypertension, hypercholesterolaemia, tobacco smoking, and diabetes mellitus (Table 10.1).
- Check whether there is a history of arrhythmias, especially if uncontrolled or with new onset.
- Check on other vascular events including acute coronary syndrome, peripheral vascular disease, or abdominal aortic aneurysms.
- Review medications including the use of anticoagulants (including over-the-counter non-steroidal anti-inflammatory medication) or whether anticoagulation was recently ceased.

Table 10.1 Underlying causes of acute strokes

	More frequently encountered causes	Less frequently encountered causes
Cancer	Bleed into a cerebral primary or metastatic lesion	New presentation of metastatic cancer
Intercurrent illness	Atrial fibrillation Carotid artery disease Hypertension Hypercholesterolaemia Diabetes mellitus	Arteriovenous malformation Patent foramen ovale Cerebral abscess

Physical examination

Careful physical examination looking for any:
- difficulty protecting the person's airway
- motor or sensory asymmetry
- the cranial nerves and seek any evidence of papilloedema (suggesting raised intracranial pressure)
- upper motor neuron signs.

Signs may progress over minutes or hours from worsening bleeding or worsening cerebral oedema.

Physical examination findings may be subtle, depending on the size and position of the compromised circulation. Changes such as a different personality may take time to recognize.

Investigation and management

Prognosis measured in hours to days prior to the onset of this problem (symptom control)

This is a clinical diagnosis in this group. Further investigations are not indicated.

Maximize comfort. Assess the person's gag reflex.

Treat any headache. Depending on the symptoms, having a stroke may be very distressing and an anxiolytic may be necessary.

Sensory inattention or motor weakness can mean that the person may injure themselves inadvertently. Nurse carefully to minimize these risks.

Prognosis measured in weeks prior to the onset of this problem (in addition to symptom control)

Have a very low threshold for imaging the person's brain in order to determine whether there was a stroke and, if so, whether it was a thrombotic or haemorrhagic event.

Thrombotic strokes need urgent consideration for thrombolysis, giving the best possible chance of a positive outcome. Contact your local stroke service. Ideally this should be within 3 h of the initial signs or symptoms. (Some units will treat up to 4.5 h after the onset of symptoms.) Consider how best to treat any underlying factors that may have contributed including atrial fibrillation.

Haemorrhagic strokes have a high risk of extending with further bleeding in the hours after the initial presentation. Cease medications that may increase the risk of bleeding. Check coagulation status including platelet count. Look for other evidence of bleeding.

For all people, carefully manage any hypertension (either long term or acute changes related to raised intracranial pressure).

Prognosis measured in months to years prior to the onset of this problem (in addition to the above)

Management is very similar to people with a prognosis measured in weeks.

Consider whether there are risk factors that need to be treated to lessen the likelihood of another event. This includes imaging the carotid arteries and considering stenting or endarterectomy if there are high-risk lesions.

Further reading

van Gijn J, Rothwell PM (2020). Stroke: cerebrovascular disease (Chapter 24.10.1). In: *Oxford Textbook of Medicine*, 6th ed. Oxford: Oxford University Press. Available at: https://doi.org/10.1093/med/9780198746690.003.0590

Voltz R, Lorenzl S (2021). Neurological disorders other than dementia (Chapter 15.5). In: *Oxford Textbook of Palliative Medicine*, 6th ed. Oxford: Oxford University Press. Available at: https://doi.org/10.1093/med/9780198821328.003.0093

Spinal cord compromise ☠

- Spinal cord compression is a medical emergency.
- Consider the diagnosis in people with cancer and back pain. Investigations and treatment must be initiated urgently to preserve as much function as possible.
- Cord compromise occurs in 3–5% of people with cancer: 70% in the thoracic spine, 20% in the lumbosacral spine, and 10% in the cervical spine.
- Back pain **without neurological changes** is the early presenting symptom for most people.

History

The most frequent cause of spinal cord compromise is due to **malignancy** (Table 10.2). The need to consider this diagnosis and initiate prompt treatment cannot be overemphasized.

People with spinal cord compression typically present with **back pain**. This pain often pre-dates neurological changes by weeks and months. It may be worse on lying flat and may be exacerbated by coughing, bending, or sneezing. The pain may be localized to the back, or people may describe a heavy band-like sensation that radiates anteriorly.

Limb weakness and sensory changes are late changes.

The distribution of changes will depend upon the level of the cord that is compromised.

Bladder and bowel disturbance (urinary retention and incontinence, constipation, and faecal incontinence) occur late.

Table 10.2 Causes of cord compromise

	More frequently encountered causes	Less frequently encountered causes
Cancer	Direct extension of vertebral body metastasis	Vertebral body collapse
		Intradural or leptomeningeal disease
		Tumour extending through the intervertebral foramina
		Vasogenic oedema
		Invasion of the anterior spinal artery by tumour
Intercurrent illness	Cervical disc prolapse	Infection (epidural abscess)
	Transverse myelitis	Haematoma (anticoagulated people)
	Multiple sclerosis	Cord infarct
	Guillain–Barré syndrome	Anterior spinal artery occlusion (atrial fibrillation)
		Vasculitis
		Dissecting aortic aneurysm

Lesions of the cauda equina present with back pain that may radiate down both legs. There may be difficulty in walking because of gluteal muscle weakness. There is loss of perineal sensation. These people will develop urinary problems (incontinence and retention) and may have faecal incontinence (loss of anal tone).

Ongoing intrathecal analgesia or a past history of intrathecal analgesia (epidural injections, epidural catheters, intrathecal catheters) raises the possibility of an **epidural** or **intrathecal abscess**. These people will have fever and complain of severe back pain. Depending upon the level of the problem, they may have other sensory or motor changes.

Physical examination

Physical examination may be unremarkable or reflect the level of the cord lesion.

There may be tenderness along the bony spine, and a sensory level with pin-prick should be sought. (Light touch, if normal, is not sufficient to exclude a sensory level as it is carried in posterior columns and the spinothalamic tract. Pin-prick is only carried in posterior columns, the area often affected earliest in cord impingement.) Lesions occurring above L1 may initially present with a flaccid paralysis but an upgoing plantar reflex. Later, this will become a spastic paralysis (increased tone, clonus, and increased reflexes) reflecting an upper motor neuron lesion at the lesion's level and below.

Physical examination must include an assessment of bladder and bowel function (percuss for a bladder with urinary retention; on rectal examination, check anal tone).

A cauda equina lesion will produce lower motor neuron signs. The leg weakness is flaccid and the reflexes are diminished or absent. Examine for a loss of saddle sensation and decreased anal tone. Percuss for a bladder level.

Malignant cord compressions may be multilevel, giving mixed signs on physical examination.

If an intrathecal catheter is *in situ*, check the skin around the injection site for redness, temperature change, or discharge. Palpate for tenderness and check the temperature. Check for signs of meningism.

Investigation and management

Prognosis measured in hours to days prior to the onset of this problem (symptom control)

This is a clinical diagnosis in this group. Further investigations are not indicated.

To maximize comfort, it may still be reasonable to administer **dexamethasone 8 mg SC daily**. This may improve pain control, although other agents (opioids and paracetamol) must be available. An **indwelling urinary catheter** should be inserted and a **bowel regimen implemented**. At this stage of life, there may be minimal oral intake. Therefore, daily enemas or suppositories may be sufficient (Microlax® enema or Dulcolax® suppository).

In the case of an epidural abscess or infected intrathecal injection site, removal of the catheter depends upon the ongoing effectiveness of the analgesia. Often these devices have been inserted for very difficult pain problems. Despite the local infection, if analgesia is adequate, the device may be best left *in situ*. Antibiotics should be administered to help manage the local painful infection. If analgesia has deteriorated, remove the device and commence alternative analgesia.

Prognosis measured in weeks prior to the onset of this problem (in addition to symptom control)

Decide if the person is well enough to tolerate investigations and treatment.

Although the definitive imaging for suspected cord compression is MRI, in this group **plain X-rays** may be sufficient. Plain X-rays will be positive for vertebral damage in 80% of cases. This is not the case for infection, where more definitive scans will be required (MRI, CT).

Commence **dexamethasone 8 mg** oral/SC twice daily (morning and midday).

A **radiation oncology consultation** should be sought.

A **bowel regimen** should be implemented and bowel actions charted daily. Seek advice from a continence nurse. An **indwelling urinary catheter** may be required.

There may be associated **difficult pain syndromes** due to both somatic and neuropathic pain.

Individuals in whom an infective cause is suspected should undergo imaging if they are well enough. The decision to remove an intrathecal infusion depends upon the adequacy of analgesia. Regardless of whether or not the device is removed, antibiotics should be commenced and drainage of abscesses, if present, under CT guidance should be considered.

Prognosis measured in months to years prior to the onset of this problem (in addition to the above)

The definitive treatment for malignant extradural lesions compressing the cord is usually **radiotherapy** unless the pathology is exquisitely sensitive to chemotherapy (small cell cancer, lymphoma).

An infective cause requires urgent neurosurgical consultation for consideration of drainage.

Where there is vertebral body collapse with bone impingement on the cord, unstable fractures, or areas that have previously had supra-maximal doses of radiotherapy, consideration should be given to **urgent surgical decompression**. For most epidural extension of vertebral disease, the lesion is anterior and therefore surgery requires an anterior approach. This is reserved for people who can tolerate the significant catabolic load associated with surgery. Surgery is not well tolerated late in the course of a life-limiting illness.

Cervical lesions may impair diaphragmatic function.

C3–5 lesions may cause fatal respiratory compromise. This will need to be discussed with the person and their family as soon as it is recognized.

Pain may be prominent at the site of bony collapse and radiating from damaged nerves. Adequate paracetamol, opioids, and medications for neuropathic pain such as amitriptyline should be used early.

Early recognition of reversible cord pathology is crucial. The better the level of neurological function at the time of diagnosis, the more likely it is that neurological function can be maintained.

Further reading

Hoskin P (2021). Radiotherapy for symptom management (Chapter 14.3). In: *Oxford Textbook of Palliative Medicine*, 6th ed. Oxford: Oxford University Press. Available at: https://doi.org/10.1093/med/9780198821328.003.0078

Watson M et al. (eds) (2019). Emergencies in palliative care (Chapter 29). In: *Oxford Handbook of Palliative Care*, 3rd ed. Oxford: Oxford University Press. Available at: https://doi.org/10.1093/med/9780198745655.003.0029

Delirium: acute confusional states :☺:

- Delirium is frequently encountered whatever a person's life-limiting illness.
- Unlike other clinical settings, a reversible cause for the delirium is found in only 50% of people at the end of life (Table 10.3).
- Early recognition is the key to minimizing morbidity:
  - **Hyperactive delirium** is typified by drug withdrawal. Unceasing movement and inability to settle are seen late in delirium.
  - **Hypoactive delirium** is typified by encephalopathy, metabolic disorders, or intoxication. Still ask about perceptual disturbances and test concentration, distractibility, and memory.

Table 10.3 Causes of delirium

	More frequently encountered causes	Less frequently encountered causes
Metabolic causes	Dehydration Hypercalcaemia	Hyponatraemia Hypernatraemia (mostly due to dehydration) Hypoglycaemia
Medications	Anticholinergic load (cumulative—many medications add to anticholinergic load p.68) Opioids NSAIDs	Serotonergic syndromes Withdrawal (alcohol, benzodiazepines, nicotine) Glucocorticoids (psychotropic: depression to hypomania) Digoxin
Sepsis	Pneumonia Urinary tract infection Biliary sepsis	Spontaneous bacterial peritonitis (with ascites)
Cerebral pathology	Intracerebral metastases (including miliary and leptomeningeal disease)	Encephalitis (primary herpes simplex) Subdural haematoma (anticoagulants) Post-ictal
End-stage organ failure	Renal or hepatic failure (exclude upper GIT bleeding)	Urinary retention Constipation

History

Delirium requires four key features for diagnosis:

- Fluctuating disturbance of consciousness.
- Change in cognition not explained by pre-existing, established, or evolving dementia.
- Evolution over a short period of time.

- Evidence that the disturbance is caused by physiological consequences of an underlying medical condition.

The most accurate history will often be obtained from families and nursing staff. They will often give clear account of the time frame for the onset of change and its extent.

Physical examination

- These people may be **quiet and withdrawn** or **agitated and anxious.** Their **speech and train of thought is disordered**. They may be **paranoid** or **hallucinating**.
- Examine to ascertain the cause of delirium. Check **temperature, blood pressure, pulse**, and **pulse oximetry. Assess hydration**.
- Look for a **source of sepsis** including the chest (pneumonia, bronchitis), skin (cellulitis), spontaneous bacterial peritonitis (if there is ascites), or meningism (photophobia, neck stiffness) (p.48). Look for asterixis.
- Use a **delirium rating scale** which includes current orientation and ability to concentrate.
- Ensure that the physical examination includes an assessment of **urinary output** (percuss for a bladder with retention) and **constipation**.

Investigations and management

Prognosis measured in hours to days prior to the onset of this problem (symptom control)

- **Delirium at the end of life requires assessment and management**.
- Review current medications.
- Treatment should be administered while assessment is underway.
- When people are very agitated a dose of a **benzodiazepine** may be offered (lorazepam 1 mg SL or midazolam 2.5–5.0 mg SC). Avoid antipsychotics—they have not been shown to reduce the length of delirium nor to reduce the intensity.
- **Easily reversible aspects of the delirium should be addressed** (e.g. gentle rehydration, treat fever with paracetamol, address pain appropriately, consider inserting an indwelling urinary catheter, low-flow oxygen if hypoxaemic).
- If agitated individuals do not settle with benzodiazepines, consider levomepromazine (start with 12.5–25 mg via SC infusion); or chlorpromazine 25–50 mg IM immediately and repeat twice or three times daily. Titrate carefully to response.

Prognosis measured in weeks prior to the onset of this problem (in addition to symptom control)

- Investigations should be directed to excluding easily treatable causes.
- Check **urea**, **creatinine** (calculate **creatinine clearance**), and electrolytes (**hyponatraemia** and **hypercalcaemia** (corrected for albumin)).
- Check **urea-to-creatinine ratio** (high in upper GIT bleeding, dehydration, use of dexamethasone).
- With evidence of cerebral irritation, do a **cerebral CT**.

- If there is any evidence of sepsis, collect **blood cultures** and **mid-stream urine** and organize a **CXR**.
- Check **FBC** for neutrophilia or lymphopenia.
- **At the same time as investigations are being attended to, management should be commenced**.
- Ensure that the person is not able to harm themselves or others. Move to a quiet, well-lit environment with aids to assist orientation (clock, calendar, light in the daytime, darkness at night).
- Observe closely and reassess every hour until the person is settled and then every 2 h while the person is awake.
- If there is a risk that alcohol withdrawal is contributing, ensure that thiamine 100 mg IM is administered immediately. These people are best managed with diazepam 2–5 mg three times daily and adequate hydration. They should be commenced on an alcohol withdrawal chart, and specialist drug and alcohol support should be sought.

Prognosis measured in months to years prior to the onset of this problem (in addition to the above)

- Delirium may take several days longer to clear than the process of normalizing the underlying cause(s).
- Delirium in the elderly is an independent risk factor for poorer prognosis.
- Many people can recall being delirious. It is often the most frightening experience and helping people to understand what has happened and to talk about it may be helpful.

Further reading

Agar M et al. (2021). Delirium (Chapter 13.4). In: *Oxford Textbook of Palliative Medicine*, 6th ed. Oxford: Oxford University Press. Available at: https://doi.org/10.1093/med/9780198821 328.003.0074

Sheehan B (2020). Delirium (Chapter 26.5.1). In: *Oxford Textbook of Medicine*, 6th ed. Oxford: Oxford University Press. Available at: https://doi.org/10.1093/med/9780198746690.003.0627

Seizures ☠

Seizures are feared by people at the end of life because they are associated with the potential of loss of control, loss of dignity; and unpredictability. They can indicate other pathology with the seizure as a secondary manifestation (Table 10.4).

Table 10.4 Causes of seizures

	More frequently encountered causes	Less frequently encountered causes
Cancer	Primary or secondary lesions (small cell lung, melanoma, and breast) of the CNS More frequent in frontal lobe tumours	Secondary bleed into a cerebral metastasis
End-stage organ failure	Hepatic encephalopathy	Multiple sclerosis Secondary fitting with prolonged hypoxaemia in cardiac arrhythmias
Intercurrent illnesses	Pre-existing epilepsy (especially with changed medication metabolism) Alcohol use Drug withdrawal (including benzodiazepines)	Hypoglycaemia Meningitis Primary herpes simplex encephalitis

History

History from the person and someone who has observed the episode is very valuable. Sometimes the precipitant may not be identified. The history may help to define the type of seizure.
- Primary generalized seizures are associated with loss of consciousness as they start. Seizures with evidence of signs that cross the midline of the brain are associated with loss of consciousness. Generalized seizures include absences where there is no loss of posture but loss of activity.
- Focal seizures that generalize are rarely associated with early loss of consciousness.
- Partial seizures are focal and may be considered as simple (consciousness maintained) or complex (consciousness impaired). They often have a warning or 'aura'.
- Status epilepticus is a seizure that lasts longer than 30 min or a series of seizures where the person continues to have impaired consciousness from the post-ictal state before the next seizure begins. A differential diagnosis includes vasovagal syncope, which usually has warning with sweating and weakness, and is not associated with post-collapse confusion unless there is secondary fitting. Cardiac arrhythmias including

Stokes–Adams attacks, and ventricular arrhythmias can cause syncope with subsequent fitting, especially if the person cannot fall to a prone position.

Physical examination

- **Physical findings may well be absent**.
- The period of time for which people have a depressed level of consciousness or confusion will vary widely after generalized seizures.
- **Todd's paresis** refers to transient paralysis following seizure activity.

Investigations and management

Prognosis measured in hours to days prior to the onset of this problem (symptom control)

Seizures may be seen in the terminal stages of a life-limiting illness.
The initial intervention is to arrest the seizure. Medications that may be used include:

- diazepam 10 mg IV or rectally (administered using a mixing tube)
- midazolam 5 mg SC/SL/IV.

The person should then be commenced on definitive antiseizure treatment. At the end of life, appropriate medications include:

- clonazepam (0.5–1.0 mg SL/SC twice daily or 2–4 mg using a SC infusion over 24 h)
- midazolam (20 mg using a SC infusion over 24 h).

In difficult-to-control seizures, sedation may require phenobarbital (100 mg SC immediately and then 200 mg via SC infusion daily).

Prognosis measured in weeks prior to the onset of this problem (in addition to symptom control)

Check **EUC** (hyponatraemia, electrolyte disturbance, uraemia), **BSL** (hypoglycaemia), **FBC** (infection), and **LFTs** (liver failure).

If the person has a history of epilepsy, **check anticonvulsant levels**. If these are subtherapeutic, consider medication interactions, malabsorption, or poor compliance as contributors.

A **cerebral CT** with contrast should be performed in the setting of concerns for structural lesions. **MRI** should be limited to people who do not have known cerebral disease or who have an unremarkable CT and continued fitting. An **electroencephalogram** (EEG) may be helpful in a small number of people at the end of life with fits which are difficult to characterize.

Therapy is directed to reducing the risk of further fitting. If people are able to swallow, consider:

- for **focal seizures**, sodium valproate (initially 600 mg daily and titrate to response) or carbamazepine (initially 200 mg daily in divided doses and titrate to response)
- for **generalized seizures**, sodium valproate (initially 600 mg daily and titrate) or phenytoin (initially 4–5 mg/kg/day and titrate up to 300 mg as a starting dose)
- in the presence of **cerebral oedema**, use glucocorticoids initially.

If a person cannot swallow:
- administer phenytoin IV. Administer a loading dose of 15 mg/kg by slow injection and then commence 300 mg at night.

If seizures are difficult to control:
- Phenobarbital may be administered using the SC route. Start with a loading dose of 100 mg immediately and then administer 100–200 mg in divided doses over 24 h.

Status epilepticus is an emergency.

Protect the airway by positioning the person. Consider an oral airway or even intubation. Administer oxygen. Establish an IV line. The first medications are to try and arrest the seizure. Administer diazepam 2–10 mg IV (or lorazepam 1–2 mg or midazolam 2.5–5.0 mg). After this, commence phenytoin (with a loading dose parenterally of 15 mg/kg by slow IV injection). These medications must not be administered using the same IV line as they do not mix.
- Check **FBC, EUC, BSL, electrolytes**.
- Administer **100 mg thiamine IV**.
- Give **50 mL of 50% dextrose if low BSL, but thiamine must always be given first**.

An intensive care consultation should be sought if fitting fails to settle.

Prognosis measured in months to years prior to the onset of this problem (in addition to the above)
New-onset seizures in adults are symptomatic of an underlying problem. Investigations include:
- lumbar puncture if there is concern that there may be cryptococcal meningitis
- cerebral CT scan.

If more than one seizure has occurred, long-term antiseizure medication will be required.

Further reading

Caraceni A et al. (2021). Neurological problems in advanced cancer (Chapter 14.8). In: *Oxford Textbook of Palliative Medicine*, 6th ed. Oxford: Oxford University Press. Available at: https://doi.org/10.1093/med/9780198821328.003.0083

Sen A, Johnson MR (2020). Epilepsy in later childhood and adulthood (Chapter 24.5.1). In: *Oxford Textbook of Medicine*, 6th ed. Oxford: Oxford University Press. Available at: https://doi.org/10.1093/med/9780198746690.003.0575

Meningitis ☾

History

Infectious meningitis may have a **short history of headache, irritability, photophobia, and nausea and vomiting**. The person may not be able to describe these changes and a history from family or caregivers must be sought. There is a need to exclude secondary bacterial meningitis in people with an established focus of sepsis (Table 10.5).

Table 10.5 Causes of meningitis at the end of life

	More frequently encountered causes	Less frequently encountered causes
Cancer	Acute myeloid leukaemia (*Listeria*) Myeloma/lymphoma (*Streptococcus pneumoniae*) Carcinomatous meningitis (breast or lung cancer)	Lymphoma/acute lymphocytic leukaemia (non-infectious lymphocytic) Meningitis associated with devices (especially VP shunts) Chemical meningitis (intrathecal medications, contaminants)
HIV/AIDS	Cryptococcal meningitis Toxoplasmosis	
End-stage organ failure		Alcoholism (*S. pneumoniae*) Multiple sclerosis (non-infectious lymphocytic) Nephrotic syndrome (hypogammaglobulinaemia with *S. pneumoniae*) Connective tissue diseases (sarcoidosis, SLE, Behçet's syndrome)
Intercurrent illnesses	Bacteraemia especially urinary tract sepsis (*Escherichia coli*) Prolonged immuno-suppression from glucocorticoids (*Listeria monocytogenes*)	Previous splenectomy (*S. pneumoniae*) Sentinel bleed of arteriovenous malformation Medications (NSAIDs, trimethoprim) Post-spinal anaesthesia
Community-acquired illnesses	Bacterial meningitis (meningococcal, pneumococcal, cryptococcus, TB) Viral (herpes simplex, herpes zoster, Coxsackie, mumps, measles)	

Early symptoms are vague: malaise, myalgias, and influenza-like changes, followed later by headache and vomiting. Photophobia and drowsiness are late signs.

People with meningeal carcinomatosis may describe severe headaches. These typically occur insidiously over weeks together with neurological deficits that cannot be attributed to a single lesion. These people often have associated intractable nausea or unheralded vomiting (p.44), lethargy and drowsiness, diplopia, seizures, and pain (neck, back, radicular distribution).

Physical examination

- Check for **vital signs** (blood pressure, pulse, and temperature) as evidence of sepsis.
- People with infective meningitis may **be febrile**, **bradycardic**, **hypertensive**, and have **irregular respiration.**
- Check for **Kernig's sign** (pain and resistance with passive knee extension when the hips are flexed) and **Brudzinski's sign** (hips flex when the head is tilted forward).
- The **level of consciousness may be reduced** and the person may be **irritable**.
- A transient petechial rash may be seen in meningococcal meningitis (shins, forearms, conjunctiva).
- **Classic signs of neck stiffness, photophobia, and fever may not be present in chronic meningitis or severely immunocompromised people**.
- People with meningeal carcinomatosis often have cranial nerve lesions (III, IV, VI most often).
- Other physical findings commonly include localized back and neck pain, limb weakness (lower > upper), and dermatomal sensory changes. Neck stiffness is not a routine clinical finding. Raised intracranial pressure is common, and extensor plantar responses are frequently seen.

Investigations and management

Prognosis measured in hours to days prior to the onset of this problem (symptom control)

- **This is a clinical diagnosis**. **Further investigations are not indicated**.
- Treatment symptoms: **treat any fever** (paracetamol, NSAIDs, control of ambient temperature); **manage headaches and other pains** with parenteral analgesia (morphine, hydromorphone). Adjuvant analgesia to address associated neuropathic pain may be indicated.
- These people are often **confused with cerebral irritation**. Manage in a quiet environment. Gentle sedation may be required.
- **Pay attention to continence**. People may be incontinent or have impaired bladder and bowel function. An indwelling catheter and a bowel regimen may be required.

Prognosis measured in weeks prior to the onset of this problem (in addition to symptom control)

Where an infective cause is expected, **urgently examine the cerebrospinal fluid** (CSF). **Lumbar puncture** may show increased opening pressure (>200 mmH$_2$O), reduced glucose, and lymphocytosis (>4 mm^3). Any polymorph in CSF is abnormal. Raised protein is likely (but can also be seen in aseptic multiple sclerosis or Guillain–Barré syndrome). Take bloods for **FBC** and **blood cultures**.

People with infective meningitis in this prognostic group will benefit from antibiotics. Seek the organism's identification and sensitivities. If there is risk of *Staphylococcus aureus*, cover should be with vancomycin titrated to blood levels until cultures are available. If there is a VP shunt, it is unlikely that sepsis will be cleared without removal.

In meningeal carcinomatosis, a gadolinium-enhanced MRI scan will show diffuse meningeal changes, with foci around nerve roots. This carries a poor prognosis with limited interventions available to modify the course of the disease. This group may benefit from a trial of dexamethasone 8–16 mg in the morning. It is unlikely they will achieve any benefit from intrathecal or systemic chemotherapy. Radiotherapy directed to sites of pain may provide some symptom relief.

Regardless of the cause of the meningism, treatment of fever and headache are priorities. In people electing not to have further disease-modifying treatment, the major symptom burden comes from raised intracranial pressure and ensuing unheralded vomiting (p.44).

Prognosis measured in months to years prior to the onset of this problem (in addition to the above)

If infectious meningitis is suspected, this must be treated as a medical emergency and infectious diseases consultation should be obtained immediately.
Simultaneous investigations and treatments must be initiated.

- Ensure **IV access** and treat for shock if systolic blood pressure <80 mmHg.
- Collect blood immediately for **FBC**, **blood glucose**, and **blood cultures**.
- If there is suspicion of meningococcal meningitis, treat immediately with benzylpenicillin 1.2 g.
- If **CT scans** are readily available, organize an urgent head CT and, if there is no evidence of raised intracranial pressure, collect **CSF for urgent assessment**. If CT is not readily available, examine for **papilloedema and, if absent, proceed to lumbar puncture**.
- **Ensure headache and nausea are addressed** symptomatically with appropriate medications.
- Once the blood cultures and CSF are collected, initiate antibiotics. The choice depends upon the clinical scenario and this is best discussed with an infectious diseases specialist. Consider:
  - community-acquired meningitis in adults may be due to meningococcus or pneumococcus
  - consider herpes simplex encephalitis and treat actively to avoid long-term neurological complications for the person

- immunosuppressed people are additionally at risk of cryptococcal meningitis, listeria, TB, Gram-negative organisms, and *Cryptococcus*
- hospital acquired or post-surgical meningitis may be due to *Klebsiella*, *Pseudomonas*, or *S. aureus*.

People with a presumed diagnosis of malignant meningeal infiltration require dexamethasone 8–16 mg daily. Address pain, and nausea and vomiting.

The median survival for people with malignant meningeal infiltration is 2–6 months. However, it is important to consult medical and radiation on-cology teams, as appropriate interventions may arrest the development of further neurological deficits.

Further reading

Caraceni A et al. (2021). Neurological problems in advanced cancer (Chapter 14.8). In: *Oxford Textbook of Palliative Medicine*, 6th ed. Oxford: Oxford University Press. Available at: https://doi.org/10.1093/med/9780198821328.003.0083

McGill F et al. (2020). Viral infections. (Chapter 24.11.2). In: *Oxford Textbook of Medicine*, 6th ed. Oxford: Oxford University Press. Available at: https://doi.org/10.1093/med/9780198746690.003.0596

van de Beek D, Thwaites GE (2020). Bacterial infections (Chapter 15.14). In: *Oxford Textbook of Medicine*, 6th ed. Oxford: Oxford University Press. Available at: https://doi.org/10.1093/med/9780198746690.003.0309

Intracranial bleeding ☠

- This encompasses intracerebral, subdural, and subarachnoid bleeding (Table 10.6).
- Any change in level of cognitive function should raise a question of silent intracranial bleeding.

Table 10.6 Causes of intracranial pathology

	More frequently encountered causes	Less frequently encountered causes
Subdural haematoma	Epilepsy Alcohol misuse Anticoagulant therapy In elderly people	Haemodialysis
Subarachnoid haemorrhage	Acquired aneurysms (age being the major risk factor)	
Intracerebral bleeding	Hypertension Arteriovenous malformations (age <45 years) Amyloid deposits	Haemorrhage into a cerebral metastasis Haemorrhage into a completed CVA Haemorrhage complicating septic emboli (infective endocarditis; p.108)

History

- In **subdural haemorrhage**, only 50% of people can identify head trauma to account for the problem. Fluctuating consciousness occurs late in the clinical course. The majority of people present with headache or vomiting.
- **Subarachnoid haemorrhage leads acutely to cerebral vasospasm** and **systemic hypertension**. Without trauma, these are almost always due to aneurysmal bleeds. Sudden onset of severe headache or loss of consciousness account for most clinical presentations.
- **Intracerebral haemorrhage is characterized by progressive changes** over a short time. **Vomiting and headache are the predominant symptoms. Changes in consciousness are prominent as the bleed progresses**.

Physical examination

- A person with a **subdural haemorrhage** is likely to have non-specific signs of cerebral irritation (personality change, irritability, sleepiness, unsteady gait). There may be fluctuation in cognitive function. In some cases, the physical examination may be normal. In other people, there may be focal neurological signs (unequal pupils, hemiplegia). **The presentation can mimic delirium**.

- For **subarachnoid bleeding**, neck stiffness takes hours to develop and its absence does not exclude subarachnoid blood. Other changes include drowsiness, coma, or focal neurological signs. If focal signs occur soon after the onset of the headache, consider cerebral haematoma. If this occurs later, cerebral ischaemia is likely.
- **Intracerebral bleeds** are usually associated with hypertension.

Investigations and management

Prognosis measured in hours to days prior to the onset of this problem (symptom control)

People require **pain relief with opioids and paracetamol**. If the person is clinically dehydrated, start very gentle hydration (0.9% NaCl 1 L SC over 24 h). Changes which suggest a substantial bleed include hypertension and a stiff neck. **Stop anticoagulation**. **Consider treatment of hypertension** with topical nitrates (glyceryl trinitrate patch 25 mg).

Prognosis measured in weeks prior to the onset of this problem (in addition to symptom control)

- The initial investigation is a **cerebral CT**.
- While awaiting the scan, **ensure IV access** and **check FBC**, **EUC**, and **coagulation studies**.
- If a bleed is suspected, **stop anticoagulation, ensure adequate hydration, and commence symptom control** (analgesia, antiemetics). If the person is very agitated, consider sedation.
- If the underlying aetiology on CT scan is a **subarachnoid haemorrhage**, management includes:
  - **analgesia**
  - **careful hydration** (underhydration may worsen vasospasm)
  - **sedation** if very agitated
  - **cautious control of hypertension** (use calcium channel blockers to prevent vasospasm).

There is a high risk of further bleeding leading to death.

This contrasts with a **subdural haematoma** as surgical burr holes may lead to a complete recovery.

- **A bleed into cerebral metastases requires:**
  - **a trial of dexamethasone** (8–16 mg in the morning)
  - **control of headaches**
  - **control of nausea and vomiting**.

People with bleeding into a metastasis may rapidly deteriorate and die or transiently improve.

Prognosis measured in months to years prior to the onset of this problem (in addition to the above)

Investigations and management must be simultaneously attended to.

- **Seek neurosurgical and neurological opinions promptly**.
- **Ensure IV access**.
- **Elevate the head of the bed to 30°**.
- **Ensure that the person is placed on bed rest with analgesia and antiemetics prescribed**.

- Cautiously **manage hypertension and maintain euvolaemia** (to avoid vasospasm).
- If the **head CT is normal and a subarachnoid haemorrhage is suspected, organize a lumbar puncture** (early after the bleed, the CSF is blood-stained; later, xanthochromia develops).

A neurosurgical opinion should be sought following a subarachnoid haemorrhage as surgery is aimed at preventing rebleeds. If the bleed was due to an atrioventricular malformation, surgery, stereotactic radiotherapy, or 'coiling' are options (10% of people rebleed in hours of their first bleed).

Further reading

Molyneux AJ et al. (2020). Imaging in neurological diseases (Chapter 24.3.3). In: *Oxford Textbook of Medicine*, 6th ed. Oxford: Oxford University Press. Available at: https://doi.org/10.1093/med/9780198746690.003.0571

Raised intracranial pressure ☠

- Any increase in the volume of contents in the fixed space of the cranial vault can lead to intracranial hypertension.
- Raised pressure occurs because of:
  - increased capillary permeability (tumours, trauma, infection, ischaemia)
  - hypoxic cell death, or
  - obstructive hydrocephalus (Table 10.7).
- Signs and symptoms occur when compensatory mechanisms are overwhelmed.
- The ultimate consequence is decreased cerebral perfusion leading to death if unchecked.

Table 10.7 Causes of raised intracranial pressure

	More frequently encountered causes	Less frequently encountered causes
Cancer	Any cerebral tumours	Non-communicating hydrocephalus secondary to tumour or oedema
Intercurrent illnesses	Haemorrhage Intracranial haematomas Ischaemic injury to brain Cerebral abscesses	Medications (tetracycline, oral contraceptive, glucocorticoids, vitamin A, perhexiline) Stage IV hepatic encephalopathy

History

- People with **raised intracranial pressure often complain of headache** although it may not be prominent or even absent. If headache is present, it is likely to be worse on waking from sleep, with coughing, or straining.
- **Altered consciousness can be seen**, ranging from mild irritation to profound obtundation.
- People may complain of **visual disturbances**.
- Additionally, people may describe **nausea and vomiting**, which is often worse in the morning.
- Check for recent head trauma.

Physical examination

Check whether the person has **papilloedema** (although even this is not always apparent in people with raised intracranial pressure). Check for **multiple cranial nerve** lesions. When there is herniation of the temporal lobe, an ipsilateral lesion of cranial nerve III combined with contralateral body weakness may occur. Bradycardia and hypertension may be present. Eventually **Cheyne–Stokes** respiration may be present. Later, there may be **decerebrate posturing**.

Investigations and management

Prognosis measured in hours to days prior to the onset of this problem (symptom control)

- **Headache and impaired consciousness** generate symptoms with raised intracranial pressure.
- Titrate opioids to relieve pain.
- **Unheralded vomiting** can be very troublesome (p.44). Use metoclopramide 10 mg SC every 8 h. Consider the addition of haloperidol 0.5–1.5 mg SC at night if nausea is difficult to settle.
- **Dexamethasone** 4 mg SC may reduce headaches, and the nausea and vomiting if the cerebral oedema is due to tumour.

Prognosis measured in weeks prior to the onset of this problem (in addition to symptom control)

Urgent **cerebral CT** is used to define any underlying pathology. While awaiting the scans:

- insert an **IV cannula**
- collect blood for **FBC, coagulation testing, EUC, LFTs, and BSL**
- elevate the head of the bed to 30°
- ensure that **analgesia** and **antiemetics** are available.

A person with focal neurosurgical signs secondary to a subdural haematoma may benefit from burr holes. Additionally, ensure blood pressure control. Maintain oxygen saturation and gently correct hyponatraemia. Do not overhydrate (no more than 1000 mL intake in 24 h).

In people with cerebral oedema secondary to tumours (primary or secondary) it is probably not appropriate to consider radiotherapy given their overall prognosis and lack of benefit in that time.

Prognosis measured in months to years prior to the onset of this problem (in addition to the above)

Seek neurosurgical and neurological opinions early. The initial interventions are to ensure that the person can **protect their airway** and **ensure IV access**.

Cerebral CT is used to define any underlying pathology and may demonstrate compression of the lateral ventricles.

Lumbar puncture is contraindicated if there is significant oedema on CT scanning as transtentorial herniation can occur.

Given that changes of intracranial hypertension, a small reduction in intracranial pressure can lead to marked improvements in function. Measures that may assist include:

- **correction of low serum sodium**
- **maintaining normal blood oxygen and carbon dioxide levels**
- **consider 200 mL of 20% mannitol over 15–30 min.**

Urgent neurosurgical consultation is required if there is tumour, haematoma, or non-communicating hydrocephalus causing the raised intracranial pressure. If a tumour is present, commence the person on regular dexamethasone 16 mg in the morning. Carefully monitor Glasgow Coma Scores (Appendix 3).

If left untreated, raised intracranial pressure carries a very poor prognosis.

Further reading

Caraceni A et al. (2021). Neurological problems in advanced cancer (Chapter 14.8). In: *Oxford Textbook of Palliative Medicine*, 6th ed. Oxford: Oxford University Press. Available at: https://doi.org/10.1093/med/9780198821328.003.0083

Menon DK (2020). Management of raised intracranial pressure (Chapter 17.7). In: *Oxford Textbook of Medicine*, 6th ed. Oxford: Oxford University Press. Available at: https://doi.org/10.1093/med/9780198746690.003.0390

Further reading

[faded, illegible text]

Mental health

Suicide assessment 264
Depression 266
Acute psychosis/hypomania 268
Anxiety 270
Prolonged grief disorder 271

Suicide assessment ☠

Assessment of risk for suicide is the responsibility of every health professional in contact with people who may be perceived to be considering ending their life. It includes the assessment of people with a life-limiting illness and their carers. Urgently seek early psychiatric assessment in someone who is suicidal. Suicide risk assessment is complex, and even with excellent risk assessment and mitigation plans, people may still end their lives (Table 11.1).

Table 11.1 Assessing key risk factors for suicide

Factors of greater relevance in people with life-limiting illnesses	Other risk factors
• A fear of being a burden to others • Social isolation • Advancing disease • Uncontrolled symptoms • Physical illness • Feelings of helplessness, hopelessness	• Male (16–25, 55–70 years) • Depression (or other psychiatric disorders) • Low self-esteem • Feelings of excessive guilt • Alcohol and drug use • Prior suicide attempts • Acute confusional state (delusions, hallucinations; p.29) • Recent bereavement • Family history of suicide

History

Consider the degree of intent where a person has:
• thoughts about suicide
• identified the means for suicide
• acted to make those means ready for suicide, or
• attempted to end their life.

To manage the threat of suicide, identify:
• whether this person can be managed in an outpatient setting, an inpatient setting on a palliative care ward, or in a specialist psychiatric unit
• the suicidal person's support network. Ensure that, with permission, this network is mobilized to provide real support to the person considering suicide
• any precipitating factors that may have focused thoughts on suicide at this time (especially if there is a reversible component to this)
• any reversible cognitive or psychiatric aspects to the current thoughts about suicide including clinical depression (p.266) or an acute confusional state (p.246). (In this case, has the person lost the ability to make informed decisions and are they therefore a greater threat to themselves? Anyone who is acutely suicidal and cognitively impaired should be considered for urgent inpatient psychiatric assessment even, at times, without the suicidal person's consent.)

If a person is to remain in the community and does not appear to be at imminent risks of suicide, contract with the person that they will not seek to kill themselves without initially making contact with someone such as their general practitioner, community nurse, or a trusted relative.

Further reading

Kissane D (2021). Depression, demoralization, and suicidality (Chapter 13.2). In: *Oxford Textbook of Palliative Medicine*, 6th ed. Oxford: Oxford University Press. Available at: https://doi.org/10.1093/med/9780198821328.003.0072

Depression ☯

- The prevalence of depression in people with a life-limiting illness is no different from its prevalence in the population presenting to general practitioners.
- Depression needs to be distinguished from sadness. Reversible causes need to be considered (Table 11.2).
- Depression is underdiagnosed and undertreated in people with a life-limiting illness.

Table 11.2 Causes of depression

	More frequently encountered causes	Less frequently encountered causes
Cancer		Frontal lobe tumours
		Higher rates in people with carcinoma of the pancreas, lung, or kidney
Intercurrent illnesses	Stroke, especially left anterior frontal lobe	Glucocorticoids (as one of their psychotropic effects)
	Higher rates in people with diabetes mellitus, multiple sclerosis, coronary artery disease	Amphetamine withdrawal
		Antihypertensives (beta-blockers, clonidine, reserpine, methyldopa)
		Levodopa

History

- **Assessment includes previous episodes of depression and current medications**.
- **Assess specifically for suicidality** (p.264).
- **Do not rely on somatic symptoms** (anorexia, fatigue, psychomotor retardation, or weight loss) as these physical changes overlap with cachexia in life-limiting illnesses.
- Depressed affect, sleep patterns with early morning insomnia, and loss of pleasure in any aspect of life (anhedonia) are important pointers to depression in this population.

Physical examination

- Physical examination will often be normal.
- Consider signs consistent with frontal lobe spread of malignancy in people with cancers likely to spread to the CNS.
- Check for concrete thinking and primitive reflexes.

Investigation and management

Prognosis measured in hours to days prior to the onset of this problem (symptom control)

Support is the key in people in the terminal phases of their life-limiting illness. Acknowledge that depression is there. There may be a role for intermittent, low-dose ketamine for severe depression given its rapid onset of action.

Prognosis measured in weeks prior to the onset of this problem (in addition to symptom control)

Counselling (stress management, problem-solving) or supportive psychotherapy (e.g. cognitive behavioural therapy) is the first aspect in treating mild or moderate depression.

Adjustment disorder with depressed mood is also best treated with supportive interventions rather than antidepressants as first-line therapy.

Major depression needs early identification and treatment with antidepressants. Choice is largely determined by intercurrent illness (SSRIs have less cardiac toxicity) and interactions with existing medications (see Chapter 2). Although the onset of action may be as long as 2 months, many people will start to notice benefit within 2 weeks, including improved sleep patterns and lighter affect. Seek discussion with a psychiatrist.

Prognosis measured in months to years prior to the onset of this problem (in addition to the above)

In people not responding to an adequate trial (dose and duration) of first-line antidepressants, consider consultation with a psychiatrist.

Further reading

Sherman KA, Kilby CJ (2021). Fear, anxiety, and adjustment disorder in palliative care (Chapter 13.3). In: *Oxford Textbook of Palliative Medicine*, 6th ed. Oxford: Oxford University Press. Available at: https://doi.org/10.1093/med/9780198821328.003.0073

Watson M et al. (eds) (2019). Psychiatric symptoms in palliative care (Chapter 22). In: *Oxford Handbook of Palliative Care*, 3rd ed. Oxford: Oxford University Press. Available at: https://doi.org/10.1093/med/9780198745655.003.0022

Acute psychosis/hypomania ☼

Population-wide, 1–2% have evidence of bipolar disorder. Iatrogenic causes of hypomania are the most frequently encountered when caring for people at the end of life (Table 11.3).

Table 11.3 Causes of hypomania

	More frequently encountered causes	Less frequently encountered causes
Intercurrent illnesses	Glucocorticoids	Levodopa
		MAOIs
		Sympathomimetics
		Tricyclic antidepressants

History

- **Acute psychoses/hypomania may be associated with flight of ideas, motor and verbal overdrive, illusions, grandiose plans, and reduced sleep time**.
- The onset is often abrupt, and of relatively short duration (compared with mania) and may be associated with increases in energy out of proportion to the life-limiting illness.
- **Acute psychoses/hypomania needs to be distinguished from delirium (an acute confusional state**; p.29) and from frontal lobe lesions that may cause euphoria or social disinhibition.

Physical examination

Physical examination will often be unremarkable.

Investigations and management

Prognosis measured in hours to days prior to the onset of this problem (symptom control)

In hypomania in the terminal phases of a life-limiting illness, use haloperidol 0.5–2.5 mg orally/SC twice daily. Other choices include olanzapine 2.5–10 mg or risperidone 0.5–2 mg orally in divided doses. These doses will need to be titrated to effect.

Prognosis measured in weeks prior to the onset of this problem (in addition to symptom control)

There are two therapeutic aims of intervention:
- **moderating** mood
- **calming** the person acutely.

The first is best achieved with antipsychotics and the second may require the additional use of benzodiazepines such as diazepam 5–20 mg, depending on the person's body habitus and previous exposure to benzodiazepines, repeated every 2 h until there is a therapeutic effect.

Other medications which may help to moderate mood include sodium valproate or carbamazepine.

Prognosis measured in months to years prior to the onset of this problem (in addition to the above)

If this is an initial episode of acute psychosis/hypomania or part of a pattern of bipolar changes, consider consultation with a psychiatrist if prognosis is measured in months.

Further reading

Saunders KEA, Geddes J (2020). Bipolar disorder (Chapter 26.5.7). In: *Oxford Textbook of Medicine*, 6th ed. Oxford: Oxford University Press. Available at: https://doi.org/10.1093/med/978019 8746690.003.0633

Anxiety ⓘ

- Many people experience anxiety from time to time but this does not meet the criteria of panic or anxiety disorders.
- **Panic attacks** are characterized by a short period with:
  - severe autonomic symptoms (palpitations, sweating or flushes, tremor, light-headedness)
  - somatic symptoms (shortness of breath or choking, chest or abdominal pain)
  - cognitive changes (feeling of dissociation, fear of losing control).
- **Panic disorder** is seen where there are recurring panic attacks with no apparent trigger, leading to ongoing concerns for that person or changed behaviour that persists for >1 month.
- **Acute stress** can occur after any traumatic event. Some reactions may be distant from the event but reflect the impact of that event. Acute stress reactions should rarely be managed with medications. Debriefing after such an event may be of some benefit.
- **Stress management and cognitive behavioural therapy** have important roles when physical causes for the symptoms have been excluded on first presentation.
- In specific circumstances, a short course of a benzodiazepine such as oral diazepam 2 mg twice daily may be justified if there are frequent episodes in a short space of time. **Adjustment disorder with anxious mood** is seen within 3 months of an identified stressor that is not associated with any long-term patterns of behaviour or mental illness. The best treatment is supportive, with counselling, relaxation. stress management, or cognitive behavioural therapy. The aim is to help the person adapt to new circumstances. At times there may be a place for a short (2-week) course of an anxiolytic such as diazepam 2 mg twice daily.
- **Generalized anxiety disorder** is seen in the longer time frame (>6 months). Symptoms include feeling unsettled, fatigue, poor concentration, irritability, muscle tension, and poor sleep patterns. As this is a chronic problem, it is worthwhile ensuring psychiatric input as management may include oral venlafaxine 75 mg in the morning or oral paroxetine 10 mg in the morning titrated to effect. The effects of these antidepressants are seen to work in people who are not clinically depressed. Tremor and palpitations may be treated with a low-dose beta-blocker such as oral propranolol 10 mg twice daily.

Further reading

Sherman KA, Kilby CJ (2021). Fear, anxiety, and adjustment disorder in palliative care (Chapter 13.3). In: *Oxford Textbook of Palliative Medicine*, 6th ed. Oxford: Oxford University Press. Available at: https://doi.org/10.1093/med/9780198821328.003.0073

Watson M et al. (eds) (2019). Psychiatric symptoms in palliative care (Chapter 22). In: *Oxford Handbook of Palliative Care*, 3rd ed. Oxford: Oxford University Press. Available at: https://doi.org/10.1093/med/9780198745655.003.0022

Prolonged grief disorder ⓘ

- There is a wide range of physical, emotional, and social responses that fall within the definition of 'normal' grief.
- Even in the palliative care setting, dying and death may still be perceived to be unexpected by the person with the life-limiting illness, and their family and friends.
- Both the person with the life-limiting illness and their family and friends are likely to experience grief and loss from the time that a life-limiting illness is recognized.
- Grief and bereavement is not a linear process of transition. It is a complex process of adjustment which will see people cycle through a large range of feelings and experiences over quite long periods of time.
- Prolonged grief disorder is where people are unable to move on with their lives and where the symptoms of grief are unchanged over years.
- There should be special concern for someone having difficulty making the transition to life without the person with:
  - high levels of interdependence in the relationship with the person who is dying or has died
  - identifiable and sustained negative aspects of the relationship (e.g. physical or emotional abuse). Expressing the full range of emotions can be difficult except in a trusted therapeutic relationship. Such a person may present to the acute care setting years after the death of the person with little evidence of re-establishing social networks or social reintegration.
- Death of a child, a younger sibling, a spouse, or a partner is a loss that challenges personhood for many people. There are short- and long-term concerns as to how best to support people in this setting. Acutely, support is aimed at allowing expression of grief within the social context of that person.
- Prolonged grief disorder is considered when, over long periods of time (>1 year for adults; >6 months for children) with no tangible improvement, grief continues to be associated with:
  - intense emotions
  - prolonged impairment in social functioning, work, and other roles
  - disturbed sleep.

It is imperative to exclude concomitant psychiatric diagnoses such as generalized anxiety disorder or depression.

Further reading

Kissane D (2021). Bereavement (Chapter 13.5). In: *Oxford Textbook of Palliative Medicine*, 6th ed. Oxford: Oxford University Press. Available at: https://doi.org/10.1093/med/9780198821328.003.0075

Watson M et al. (eds) (2019). Bereavement (Chapter 31). In: *Oxford Handbook of Palliative Care*, 3rd ed. Oxford: Oxford University Press. Available at: https://doi.org/10.1093/med/9780198745655.003.0031

Orthopaedic disorders

Vertebral fracture 274
Threatened or actual fracture of long bones 276
Fat embolism syndrome 278

Vertebral fracture ⊙

- Only one in three vertebral fractures come to medical attention.
- Regardless of the aetiology (Table 12.1), the occurrence of a vertebral fracture increases the likelihood of further fractures within 12 months.
- Vertebral fractures are most likely to occur in the thoracic and lumbar spine.

Table 12.1 Causes of vertebral fractures

	More frequently encountered causes	Less frequently encountered causes
Cancer	Bony metastases	
Intercurrent illness	Primary osteoporosis Osteoporosis secondary to glucocorticoids	Hypogonadism Hypothyroidism Vitamin D deficiency Alcohol

History

- People with vertebral fractures commonly present with **acute onset of back pain, often radiating anteriorly**.
- They may also develop an **acute loss of height** or an **exaggeration of spinal curvature**.
- Rarely, thoracic vertebral fractures may present with acute shortness of breath or neurological symptoms consistent with **spinal cord compression** (p.242) or **cauda equina compression** (p.243).

Physical examination

Physical examination may be unremarkable, even in the presence of early cord compromise. There may be **percussion tenderness** at the level of the fracture.

Investigations and management

Prognosis measured in hours to days prior to the onset of this problem (symptom control)
This is a clinical diagnosis and no further investigations are indicated.

Vertebral fractures may be very painful, especially on movement. Adequate analgesia is imperative. This may require the use of opioids (morphine 2.5–5.0 mg SC every 4 h in someone who is opioid naïve) and paracetamol (1 g orally/IV or 500 mg rectally four times daily). An anti-inflammatory agent, either steroidal (dexamethasone 4–8 mg SC daily) or non-steroidal (ketorolac 10 mg SC four times daily or indomethacin 100 mg rectally daily) may help to reduce movement-related pain.

Prognosis measured in weeks prior to the onset of this problem (in addition to symptom control)

Plain X-rays of the spine are diagnostic. Depending upon the overall condition of the person, further investigations may be indicated. These include inflammatory markers (ESR, CRP), calcium, alkaline phosphatase, and thyroid function.

Additional analgesia may be achieved by the addition of a single infusion of bisphosphonates (pamidronate 60–90 mg IV, zoledronate 4 mg IV).

Prognosis measured in months to years prior to the onset of this problem (in addition to the above)

In people with unexplained fractures, consideration must be given to an underlying malignancy. An **MRI** is indicated in these people, or in people with a known malignancy.

The most important symptom is **pain**. Vertebral fractures are mostly extremely painful and have a major impact on an individual's quality of life. Pain must be addressed promptly to allow people to be as well and as mobile as possible.

Consider **vertebroplasty** in this population but ensure adequate analgesia in the 48 h immediately after the procedure. **Intercostal nerve blocks** may also be considered in people who fail to achieve analgesia by simple means or who are developing adverse effects from prescribed analgesia for thoracic vertebral collapse.

People with vertebral fractures due to malignancy should be considered for a **trial of dexamethasone** (4–8 mg orally/SC daily) and **radiotherapy**.

The **long-term sequelae from vertebral fractures relate to changes in posture**. With progressive kyphosis, changes to gait can occur, making review by a physiotherapist and consideration of walking aids optimal.

The role of calcium and vitamin D supplementation is unclear in vertebral fractures. However, ongoing bisphosphonates have a role in preventing further damage and may assist with pain management.

People with vertebral fractures have an overall increased mortality, with 16% reduction in 5-year survival driven, in part, by the association of vertebral fractures with malignancy.

Further reading

Watson M et al. (eds) (2019). Emergencies in palliative care (Chapter 29). In: *Oxford Handbook of Palliative Care*, 3rd ed. Oxford: Oxford University Press. Available at: https://doi.org/10.1093/med/9780198745655.003.0029

Threatened or actual fracture of long bones :Ö:

- Pathological long-bone fractures most commonly occur in the humerus and femur.
- The most common presenting problem for both actual and threatened fractures is pain.
- The detection of impending fractures allows planned interventions to maintain mobility, improve analgesia, and avoid neurological compromise.
- A relatively small number of aetiologies account for most fractures in people with life-limiting illnesses (Table 12.2).
- Surgical management of impending fractures should be considered in people with a life expectancy of >1 month. Even late in life, adequate surgical immobilization is an excellent way to achieve pain control.

Table 12.2 Causes of actual or impending pathological fractures

	More frequently encountered causes	Less frequently encountered causes
Cancer	Lytic (breast, non-small cell lung cancer) Sclerotic (prostate)	Sarcoma
Intercurrent illness	Paget's disease of bone	Metabolic bone disease
	Osteoporosis	

History

People with **threatened fractures will present with pain**. Initially, this may be pain on movement which settles with rest. Once a fracture has occurred, there will be a **sudden increase in pain** that may become constant. This is often the only clue to the underlying problem. Trauma is a less frequently a way to herald an impending fracture.

Physical examination

There may be very little to find on physical examination of people with impending fractures or there may be localized bone tenderness over the affected region. Once a facture has occurred, there may be **swelling** or **deformity** over the affected bone. **Examination must include an assessment of the neurovascular state of the limb distally**.

Investigations and management

Prognosis measured in hours to days prior to the onset of this problem (symptom control)
This is a clinical diagnosis and investigations are not indicated.

If it appears from the clinical examination that a fracture has occurred, it is good symptom control to immobilize the limb to maximize pain relief, in addition to administration of opioids (morphine 2.5–5.0 mg SC every 4 h in the opioid naïve or titrate to analgesia in people already receiving opioids), paracetamol (1 g orally/IV or 500 mg rectally three times daily), and anti-inflammatory agents (ketorolac 10 mg SC four times daily or indomethacin 100 mg rectally daily).

Despite the very limited prognosis, it may be very good palliation to consider interventional pain relief with an epidural or peripheral nerve block which will allow the person to be comfortably nursed. This includes fractured ribs.

Prognosis measured in weeks prior to the onset of this problem (in addition to symptom control)

The most important investigation is a **plain X-ray**. The X-ray must include the joints above and below the long bone in question and be compared with the contralateral side.

Impending fractures are diagnosed by a combination of X-ray changes where lesions occupy more than two-thirds of the bone's cortex and pain sufficient to interfere with function. Hairline pathological fractures may not be visible on plain X-rays and may be better visualized with a CT scan.

An **orthopaedic consultation** should be sought to establish whether or not surgical stabilization is possible. A **radiotherapy consultation** should also be sought in people with malignancy, even in people who are not well enough for surgery, with the aim of providing a single fraction of radiotherapy in a single visit that includes panning, simulation, and treatment.

Everyone with pain from a threatened or actual fracture needs good analgesia.

A regular bisphosphonate may provide additional pain relief if the fracture is due to a malignancy or osteoporosis.

Once a fracture has occurred, immediate **immobilization of the area will improve analgesia**. If people are not well enough for surgery, consideration of splinting the limb (or traction for fractured necks of femur) should be discussed with the orthopaedic team and physiotherapists.

Prognosis measured in months to years prior to the onset of this problem (in addition to the above)

- These people require **plain X-rays** and an orthopaedic consultation. They may need a **CT scan** to exclude a hairline fracture if their plain X-ray is negative.
- Check **FBC, EUC, LFT, coagulation studies, TFT, and Ca^{2+}**.
- Ensure that these individuals have a **CXR and ECG** in preparation for surgery.
- **Commence DVT prophylaxis**.

The prognosis associated with actual or threatened fracture depends to some extent on the prognosis of the underlying disorder, the site of the problem, and the condition of the surrounding bone. People for whom an operation is not feasible because of advanced disease or comorbidities have a very poor prognosis. People with operable fractures may maintain a prognosis consistent with their disease generally.

Ensure that post-surgery radiotherapy is provided if the fracture is secondary to malignancy.

Further reading

Yakoub M, Healey J (2021). Orthopaedic surgery in the palliation of cancer (Chapter 14.5). In: *Oxford Textbook of Palliative Medicine*, 6th ed. Oxford: Oxford University Press. Available at: https://doi.org/10.1093/med/9780198821328.003.0080

Fat embolism syndrome ☠

- Fat embolism syndrome occurs when people become symptomatic due to fat droplets entering the vasculature (Table 12.3).
- This typically occurs about 12 h after an insult such as a bone fracture.
- There may be a range of presentations from mild hypoxaemia to life-threatening respiratory failure.

Table 12.3 Causes of fat embolism syndrome

	More frequently encountered causes	Less frequently encountered causes
Cancer	Pathological fracture of a long bone	
Intercurrent illness	Traumatic fracture of a long bone	Thrombolysis
	Orthopaedic procedures, surgery	Sickle cell crisis

History

- These people may be very sick.
- They may have **increasing shortness of breath** and may develop respiratory failure. In association with breathlessness, they may have fever.
- Neurological manifestations include **drowsiness, confusion, hemiplegia, seizures, and coma**.

Physical examination

- These people are **breathless and hypoxaemic**. They may be **febrile, tachycardic, and hypotensive**.
- Examine for a **petechial rash**, which typically appears over the oral mucosa and skin of the neck and axilla.
- Neurological examination may disclose a **delirium** (p.29).
- Examine all limbs to ensure that there is no hemiplegia.

Investigations and management

Prognosis measured in hours to days prior to the onset of this problem (symptom control)

- **This is likely to be a terminal event in these people**.
- They require **analgesia, administration of low-flow oxygen if hypoxaemic, treatment of delirium, and control of any bleeding diathesis**.
- Ensure that **crisis medications** (p.53) are available in case there is torrential bleeding.
- If a fracture is present, immediate stabilization may prevent further fat extravasation and improve comfort.

Prognosis measured in weeks prior to the onset of this problem (in addition to symptom control)

- Check FBC, EUC, albumin, and Ca^{2+}.
- FBC may show anaemia and thrombocytopaenia. Other investigations may show hypoalbuminaemia and hypocalcaemia. **Fat globules may be visible in the serum and urine**.
- Check **pulse oximetry** and **arterial blood gases** for hypoxaemia. Organize a **CXR** which may show a patchy infiltrate.
- The management of this problem is supportive.
- These people may be shocked and will require **fluid resuscitation**. Regular pulse oximetry must be instituted and **oxygen** administered to maintain PaO_2 >90 mmHg.
- **Corticosteroids** (methylprednisolone 10 mg/kg/day in divided doses) may improve respiratory function.
- **Attention to symptoms must be considered**. It is likely that these people will be in pain because of the underlying problem. They will be breathless and may have a multifactorial delirium.
- Because of **thrombocytopaenia**, they are at risk of bleeding.

Prognosis measured in months to years prior to the onset of this problem (in addition to the above)

Acute onset of breathlessness, confusion and petechiae are the hallmarks of this syndrome.

These people require **transfer to intensive care for** ventilator support if they have severe respiratory compromise.

If people develop respiratory failure and the adult respiratory distress syndrome, the prognosis is poor. Without respiratory support, >90% of people will suffer respiratory arrest; with support, approximately 60% mortality is expected. There is still a 50% chance that those people who survive will develop progressive pulmonary fibrosis.

Further reading

Bowden G et al. (eds) (2010). Adult trauma (Chapter 9). In: *Oxford Handbook of Orthopaedics and Trauma*, 1st ed. Oxford: Oxford University Press. Available at: https://doi.org/10.1093/med/9780198569589.003.0009

Chapter 13

Genitourological disorders

Upper urinary tract infections 282
Lower urinary tract infections 284
Urinary tract obstruction 286
Urinary retention 288
Acute renal artery occlusion 290
Renal vein thrombosis 292
Genitourinary fistulae 294
Pelvic bleeding 296

Upper urinary tract infections ①

- Upper urinary tract infections include acute pyelonephritis and prostatitis, each with a separate list of potential causes (Box 13.1).
- Upper urinary tract infections are generally parenchymal, while lower tract problems tend to be limited to the mucosa.
- Urinary tract infections may be divided into complicated (instrumentation, indwelling catheters, or structural abnormalities) and uncomplicated.

Box 13.1 Causes of upper urinary tract infections

Pyelonephritis
- Ascending infection.
- Structural abnormalities of the urinary tract.
- Immunodeficiency.
- Complicated lower urinary tract infections.
- Chronic illness.
- Haematogenous spread of infection to the kidneys.

Prostatitis
- Spontaneous.
- Urinary catheters.

History

- People with acute pyelonephritis present with an acute onset of fever, rigors, flank pain, and dysuria.
- Prostatitis presents with fevers, rigors, and dysuria, but is associated with lower back or perineal pain. These people may develop acute urinary retention.

Physical examination

These people may be very unwell.

They may be **febrile or hypothermic, with a thready tachycardia and hypotension**.

People with **pyelonephritis often have tenderness to palpation over the renal angle on the affected side**. Abdominal examination may reveal generalized tenderness with guarding.

Men with **prostatitis will display an extremely tender and soft prostate**. Be careful—examining an inflamed prostate may lead to bacteraemia.

Investigations and management

Prognosis measured in hours to days prior to the onset of this problem (symptom control)

Despite the very limited prognosis of this group, it may be possible to improve comfort by ensuring adequate hydration.

SC or IV infusion fluids and **administration of appropriate antibiotics**. This may be by a single dose of gentamicin 2 mg/kg and ceftriaxone 1 g which may help to control fever and rigor. Other simple interventions to control fever include regular sustained release paracetamol (500 mg rectally three times daily, 1 g orally three times daily) or NSAIDs (ketorolac 10 mg SC every 8 h or indomethacin 100 mg rectally twice daily).

Prognosis measured in weeks prior to the onset of this problem (in addition to symptom control)

The diagnosis of pyelonephritis is based on a combination of history and **the presence of an elevated WCC, raised inflammatory markers** (ESR, CRP), and **positive urine cultures**.

The diagnosis of prostatitis is made on a combination of clinical features including fever, dysuria, and a **tender prostate** and **positive urine cultures**.

People with pyelonephritis may be managed with oral antibiotics (amoxicillin–clavulanic acid every 12 h for 10 days) if they do not have septicaemia or complicated infection (instrumentation, indwelling urinary catheter (IDC)). With nausea and vomiting, hypotension, or a complicated infection, management includes fluid resuscitation and parenteral antibiotics. Cover *Escherichia coli* with ceftriaxone 1 g IV, daily and adjust antibiotics when urine and blood cultures are available.

Acute prostatitis is likely to be due to *E. coli* or *Klebsiella*. Cover with trimethoprim 300 mg daily for 14 days or cefalexin 500 mg every 12 h for 14 days.

Prognosis measured in months to years prior to the onset of this problem (in addition to the above)

Uncomplicated pyelonephritis should resolve. With anatomical abnormalities, long-term use of antibiotics may be necessary in the palliative setting.

Prostatitis carries a reasonably high rate of relapse with the development of resistant organisms. Consider long-term antibiotics or prostatectomy.

Both these disorders may be associated with pain, nausea, and vomiting. Hydrate, provide analgesia, and antiemetic therapy. Significant morbidity may occur in the presence of structural abnormalities.

Further reading

Rothschild JG et al. (2021). Dysuria, frequency, and bladder spasm (Chapter 11.1). In: *Oxford Textbook of Palliative Medicine*, 6th ed. Oxford: Oxford University Press. Available at: https://doi.org/10.1093/med/9780198821328.003.0064

Tomson C, Sheerin N (2020). Urinary tract infection (Chapter 21.13). In: *Oxford Textbook of Medicine*, 6th ed. Oxford: Oxford University Press. Available at: https://doi.org/10.1093/med/9780198746690.003.0503

Lower urinary tract infections ①

Lower urinary tract infections refer to infections of the bladder and urethra. Causes vary depending on the level of infection (Box 13.2).

Box 13.2 Causes of lower urinary tract infections

Urethritis
- Ascending infection.
- Instrumentation of the urinary tract.
- Indwelling catheters.

Additional causes of cystitis
- Prostatitis.
- Fistula formation.

History

Cystitis tends to be more symptomatic in people describing fever, marked dysuria, haematuria, frequency, and the passage of small amounts of urine only. There may be associated suprapubic or lower back pain. A fistula is usually associated with a history of pneumaturia or passage of faecal matter through the urethra (p.294).

In the community, abrupt onset of symptoms is most often due to *Escherichia coli*. *E. coli* or staphylococcal infection are likely when hospital acquired. A more gradual onset of symptoms suggests *Chlamydia* or gonococcal infection in sexually active people. Men may develop urethral discharge.

People with urethritis usually have milder symptoms. Dysuria is reported, and some people may have low-grade fever and urgency of micturition.

Asymptomatic colonization of the urinary tract in someone with an indwelling catheter does not need treatment with antibiotics unless they become systemically unwell.

Physical examination

People may have low-grade fevers and suprapubic tenderness on examination but often nothing else is found.

Investigations and management

Prognosis measured in hours to days prior to the onset of this problem (symptom control)
- Other than a **urinary dipstick, no investigations are indicated**.
- **A single dose of gentamicin (2 mg/kg) IV and ceftriaxone 1 g IV may improve symptoms of pain and fevers**.
- **Ensure adequate hydration**.
- A person may be more comfortable with an **indwelling catheter** to avoid sense of urgency and frequency of micturition.
- Ensure **adequate analgesia** (suprapubic pain) and **regular paracetamol** for any fever.

Prognosis measured in weeks or longer prior to the onset of this problem (in addition to symptom control)

- The diagnosis of these disorders is mostly made on urine examination alone. With urethritis, no abnormalities may be detected on urine collection, but cystitis is almost always associated with microscopic haematuria and a positive urine culture.
- These disorders can usually be managed with oral antibiotics alone.
- Check **WCC** with a differential count of neutrophils and **renal function**.
- **Ensure adequate hydration**.
- **Ensure** that **analgesia** for suprapubic pain and paracetamol for fever is available.

Further reading

Rothschild JG et al. (2021). Dysuria, frequency, and bladder spasm (Chapter 11.1). In: *Oxford Textbook of Palliative Medicine*, 6th ed. Oxford: Oxford University Press. Available at: https://doi. org/10.1093/med/9780198821328.003.0064

Tomson C, Sheerin N (2020). Urinary tract infection (Chapter 21.13). In: *Oxford Textbook of Medicine*, 6th ed. Oxford: Oxford University Press. Available at: https://doi.org/10.1093/med/9780198746690.003.0503

Urinary tract obstruction :✚:

- Urinary tract obstruction is classified as incomplete or complete, unilateral or bilateral. Causes include intraluminal, in the wall of the urinary tract, or due to external compression (Table 13.1).
- As a result of a complete urinary tract obstruction, a person will develop renal failure (p.208).

Table 13.1 Causes of urinary tract obstruction

Within the lumen of the ureters/ urethra	Calculi
	Blood clot
	Papillae sloughing
	Tumour
Within the wall of ureters/urethra	Strictures
	Neurogenic bladder
	Congenital
External pressure on the urinary tract	Tumours
	Retroperitoneal fibrosis
	Granulomatous disease
	Crohn's disease
Other	Surgical trauma

History

- Acute **upper** tract obstruction (kidney and ureters) will present with flank pain that may radiate to the inguinal region or perineum. The pain may increase with fluid intake as a result of pressure from retained urine. There may be deceased or absent urine output.
- An acute **lower** urinary tract obstruction (bladder, urethra) will present with suprapubic pain.
- An incomplete urethral obstruction may be associated with pain, poor stream, or incontinence, and a high risk of infection. Pain may not be present in urinary retention due to a cord lesion (p.242).
- People who are already uraemic may experience drowsiness, nausea, twitching, and itch (p.208).

Physical examination

- **Upper** obstruction may present as loin tenderness or a palpable loin mass only with a significant hydronephrosis.
- **Lower** obstruction may lead to a palpable bladder.
- Check for **fever, hypotension, tachycardia, and dehydration**.
- A **neurological examination** must exclude spinal cord compression (p.242).
- If renal function is deteriorating, uraemia may cause drowsiness, confusion, and myoclonus.

Investigations and management

Prognosis measured in hours to days prior to the onset of this problem (symptom control)

Further investigations are not indicated at this stage.

People who are not passing urine should have an **indwelling urethral catheter (IDC) inserted**. Passing an IDC may relieve lower obstructions. In someone with significant retention, release urine at no more than 500 mL/h to avoid bladder mucosal bleeding. If obstruction is relieved, there may be a large diuresis in which case hydration needs to be carefully monitored. More invasive procedures are not indicated.

People who are anuric will become uraemic and **the symptoms of uraemia must be addressed**. These include nausea (haloperidol 0.5–3.0 mg SC daily), itch (ondansetron wafers 4 mg SL twice daily), and myoclonic jerks (clonazepam 0.5 mg SC/SL twice daily).

An **enlarging renal mass or obstruction may cause pain**. Because of impaired renal function, precautions must be taken when prescribing morphine or hydromorphone. Use lower doses and, if the dose is at its lowest limit, change the dose frequency from 4 h to 6 h or 8 h. Fentanyl is not excreted renally and may be the preferable opioid.

Prognosis measured in weeks prior to the onset of this problem (in addition to symptom control)

- Check **serum electrolytes, renal function, and FBC**.
- Collect **blood cultures if febrile**.
- A **midstream urine sample** should be sent for microscopy and culture.
- Pass an **IDC** to measure residual urine and assess urine output regularly.
- **Plain pelvic X-rays** may display an obstructing calculus. Consider observation, lithotripsy, or removal using a Dormia basket.
- **Upper obstructions require discussions with a urologist and radiologist**.
- Use hyoscine butylbromide 20 mg SC, opioids, and anti-inflammatories until the stone passes.
- A **renal ultrasound** will show the level of obstruction in the upper collecting system.
- **In extrinsic compression, insertion of a ureteric stent may restore renal function**. If this is technically impossible, consider a percutaneous nephrostomy. It is imperative to warn the person that they may have an external drain for the remainder of their lives.
- **Lower obstructions may be relieved by passing an IDC** or **inserting a suprapubic catheter**. (It is unlikely that the catheter will be able to be removed again in this setting.)
- **If febrile, initiate antibiotics after collection of blood and urine cultures**.
- **Ensure IV access for fluid hydration while stabilizing and assessing the person**.

Further reading

Rothschild JG et al. (2021). Dysuria, frequency, and bladder spasm (Chapter 11.1). In: *Oxford Textbook of Palliative Medicine*, 6th ed. Oxford: Oxford University Press. Available at: https://doi.org/10.1093/med/9780198821328.003.0064

Yaqoob MM, McCafferty K (2020). Urinary tract obstruction (Chapter 21.17). In: *Oxford Textbook of Medicine*, 6th ed. Oxford: Oxford University Press. Available at: https://doi.org/10.1093/med/9780198746690.003.0507

Urinary retention ☼

This clinical diagnosis is seen more often in men from a wide range of causes (Box 13.3).

> **Box 13.3 Causes of acute urinary retention**
> - Prostate disease (benign, malignant).
> - Constipation.
> - Infections.
> - Postoperative (abdominal procedures).
> - Neurological dysfunction.
> - Urethral strictures.
> - Medications (especially with anticholinergic effects which are cumulative).

History

People with acute retention of urine may present with suprapubic pain and inability to pass urine. They may have a history of long-standing increasing difficulty of initiating voiding.

For people with chronic urinary retention, pain may be absent but frequency or nocturia is prominent.

Physical examination

These people may be **distressed and are often hypertensive**. The **bladder is distended**, either palpable or percussable, and sometimes tender.

Investigations and management

Prognosis measured in hours to days prior to the onset of this problem (symptom control)

- **Administer analgesia and insert a urinary catheter.** If insertion of a urethral catheter is not possible, a suprapubic catheter may be necessary with specialist urological input.
- A person may have a **post-obstruction diuresis**. **Consider gentle hydration for comfort**.
- Avoid rapid decompression of the bladder to minimize the risk of mucosal haemorrhage. Do not decompress at more than 500 mL/h (and preferably less rapidly).

Prognosis measured in weeks prior to the onset of this problem (in addition to symptom control)

- **This is predominantly a clinical diagnosis**. **Bladder ultrasound** may estimate residual volumes.
- Additional investigations include **renal function tests** and **urine microscopy**.
- **Investigations must not take precedence over relief of retention**. First catheterize.
- Easily reversible causes (infection, constipation) may be addressed.

- More complicated causes of retention (medications that remain essential, neurological causes, clot retention, pelvic tumours) may not be modifiable, leading to a permanent catheter.

Prognosis measured in months to years prior to the onset of this problem (in addition to the above)

- **A urological consult will need to be sought** if a simple cause for retention cannot be found.
- If people need long-term catheterization, it is preferable to consider a suprapubic catheter.

Further reading

Rothschild JG et al. (2021). Dysuria, frequency, and bladder spasm (Chapter 11.1). In: *Oxford Textbook of Palliative Medicine*, 6th ed. Oxford: Oxford University Press. Available at: https://doi.org/10.1093/med/9780198821328.003.0064

Acute renal artery occlusion ☠

- This is a rare problem and may be difficult to diagnose because of the non-specific constellation of symptoms from a range of underlying causes (Box 13.4).
- Although it is not common, it is associated with significant morbidity.

Box 13.4 Causes of renal artery occlusion

- Atrial fibrillation.
- Malignancy.
- Vasculitis.
- Clotting disorders.
- Nephrotic syndrome.

History

Acute onset of flank pain, fever, and haematuria without dysuria is typical.

It is often mistaken for pyelonephritis but, unlike infection, the fever will not respond to antibiotics. Occasionally, people may present with anuria, hypertension, altered mental state, or uraemia.

Physical examination

- People may have **renal angle tenderness on the affected side, fever, tachycardia, and hypertension**.
- An assessment of cognitive state is indicated as confusion can be caused by both malignant hypertension or uraemia.

Investigations and management

Prognosis measured in hours to days prior to the onset of this problem (symptom control)

Pain from an infarcted kidney may be unilateral or bilateral.

The best opioid is fentanyl as it is not excreted through the kidney. Low-dose morphine or hydromorphone may be used with caution. It is advisable to start with low doses every 6–8 h regularly rather than every 4 h.

When bilateral damage has occurred, or there is unilateral damage in a person with previously limited renal reserve, **a person may become anuric and subsequently uraemic**. Control symptoms of uraemia such as itch, nausea, and twitching (p.208).

Prognosis measured in weeks prior to the onset of this problem (in addition to symptom control)

- **Check FBC** (leukocytosis), **renal function** (hyperkalaemia, increased urea, and creatinine), and **coagulation studies** (coagulopathy). These are indicated, although in the early stages after the ischaemic event, they may be within normal limits.
- **A raised LDH** may suggest embolic activity but is very non-specific.
- **Urine microscopy** may show haematuria and leukocytes, but with a negative Gram stain.

- **Doppler ultrasound** allows visualization of the renal blood supply.
- Other investigations (**angiography**) required to diagnose this problem are more invasive and may not contribute to a simple solution for this person.
- The choice of interventions depends upon the chronicity of the obstruction to renal blood flow.
- Unilateral damage to the kidney may not require intervention beyond pain relief and control of other symptoms.
- Bilateral damage may result in precipitous renal failure. An acute disruption to blood flow may respond to thrombolysis or vascular stenting. This decision will depend on other comorbidities.
- A background of chronic narrowing of the renal artery with an acute insult is often a terminal event in this clinical setting. Dialysis is rarely indicated.
- Symptom control includes pain from renal infarcts and headaches from hypertension.

Prognosis measured in months to years prior to the onset of this problem (in addition to the above)

Investigations and management should include the following:

- **ECG** (effects of hyperkalaemia).
- An **IV pyelogram** will display no blood supply but does not differentiate between renal artery spasm, occlusion, avulsion, or an absent kidney.
- **Renal angiography** is the gold standard diagnostic test in people well enough to consider further therapy.

People with chronic renal artery stenosis and renal impairment may require dialysis prior to restoration of blood flow. Immediate restoration of blood flow to the kidney is the most important step in people with no long-term renal damage. Surgical bypass grafting may be considered in people who are functioning well where other therapies are not successful.

In the long term, people require management of hypertension and long-term aspirin. The cause of the obstruction defines other treatment.

People with underlying renal artery stenosis who progress to acute occlusion have a 4-year mortality of 50%.

Further reading

Kalra PA, Vassallo D (2020). Atherosclerotic renovascular disease (Chapter 21.10.10). In: *Oxford Textbook of Medicine*, 6th ed. Oxford: Oxford University Press. Available at: https://doi.org/10.1093/med/9780198746690.003.0500

Renal vein thrombosis ⊙

- This a difficult diagnosis to make, with gradual onset in most people with a limited number of underlying aetiologies (Box 13.5).
- It can occur acutely, leading to renal failure.
- A renal vein thrombosis may propagate, leading to complications such as pulmonary emboli.

> **Box 13.5 Causes of renal vein thrombosis**
> - Nephrotic syndrome.
> - Retroperitoneal fibrosis.
> - Malignancy.
> - Trauma.

History

In the acute situation, people present with **flank pain**, **fevers**, and **haematuria** or a **pulmonary embolus**. In severe cases with bilateral involvement, a person may present with anuria.

Physical examination

There may be **low-grade fever and ipsilateral renal angle tenderness** or a **ballotable kidney**.

Investigations and management

Prognosis measured in hours to days prior to the onset of this problem (symptom control)

The symptomatic management is the same as for people with renal artery occlusion (p.290). Provide analgesia for renal angle tenderness and flank pain, and actively manage headaches.

Prognosis measured in weeks prior to the onset of this problem (in addition to symptom control)

- Check **FBC, serum EUC, LDH, and fibrinogen degradation products**.
- **Urine microscopy** will display haematuria and leukocytosis with no organisms evident.
- **Renal ultrasound and Doppler** are indicated to examine the size of the kidney and blood flow.
- Definite diagnosis is made by **selective venography, CT, or MRI**.

These people should be **commenced on anticoagulation** with therapeutic doses of LMWH. This will need to be life-long. Warfarin is not indicated.

Prognosis measured in months to years prior to the onset of this problem (in addition to the above)

- The initial management will depend upon the degree of venous occlusion.

- In bilateral thrombosis, a person most likely requires dialysis while the definitive therapy is considered.
- Mostly, anticoagulation limits clot propagation. Renal function will return if clot is resorbed.
- In bilateral occlusion, or with pre-existing renal dysfunction, thrombectomy may be indicated.
- Prognosis is largely defined by complications such as pulmonary embolism.

Further reading

Firth JD (2020). Acute kidney injury (Chapter 21.5). In: *Oxford Textbook of Medicine*, 6th ed. Oxford: Oxford University Press. Available at: https://doi.org/10.1093/med/9780198746 690.003.0477

Genitourinary fistulae ①

- A fistula is an abnormal connection between two hollow viscera or a hollow viscus and skin.
- Abnormal communications may occur within the genitourinary tract or between the genitourinary tract and the GIT, blood vessels, the lymphatic system, or the skin. This section focuses on vesicovaginal fistulae and their causes (Box 13.6).

> **Box 13.6 Causes of genitourinary fistulae**
> - Cancer: local invasion.
> - Cancer treatment (surgery, radiotherapy).
> - Local infection.

History

The only history a woman may complain of is **fever and leakage of urine from the vagina**.

Physical examination

- Physical examination may be unremarkable.
- There may be evidence of a frozen pelvis.
- Check for a **fever**.

Investigations and management

Prognosis measured in hours to days prior to the onset of this problem (symptom control)
- **This is a clinical diagnosis and no further investigations are indicated**.
- A person may be more comfortable with an IDC, which can divert the urine flow because of the larger lumen of the urinary catheter.
- **Continence pads** must be used and changed regularly to minimize the risk of skin excoriation.

Prognosis measured in weeks prior to the onset of this problem (in addition to symptom control)
It is unlikely that this group would be considered for surgical repair and therefore further investigations will not be of benefit. An **IDC** may facilitate **spontaneous closure**. Spontaneous closure is less likely in people with a fistula due to cancer.

Prognosis measured in months to years prior to the onset of this problem (in addition to the above)
- **FBC**, **serum EUC**, and **urinalysis** are indicated.
- Cystoscopy and direct visualization of the vaginal vault with the bladder filled with dilute dye.
- In people who are considered for surgical repair, an IV pyelogram should be considered to visualize the patency of the upper urinary tract in the presence of a frozen pelvis.

- Repeat staging if a person develops a urinary fistula during cancer treatment.
- If spontaneous closure with an IDC does not occur, consider surgery for non-cancer causes.
- In cancer, a percutaneous nephrostomy or formation of an ileal conduit may be of benefit.

Further reading

Tilley CP et al. (2021). Palliative wound and ostomy care (Chapter 10.2). In: *Oxford Textbook of Palliative Medicine*, 6th ed. Oxford: Oxford University Press. Available at: https://doi.org/10.1093/med/9780198821328.003.0061

Pelvic bleeding ☼

Bleeding may occur from gynaecological, urological, or GIT viscera of the pelvis (Box 13.7).

> **Box 13.7 Causes of genitourinary bleeding**
> * Gynaecological cancers eroding major vessels.
> * Fungating cancers of the vulva, vaginal vault, cervix, or endometrium.
> * Bleeding from urological structures secondary to tumours, infections, or calculus.
> * Coagulopathy with pelvic pathology.
> * Medications (anticoagulants, NSAIDS).
> * Cytotoxic agents (cyclophosphamide, ifosfamide).

History
* The initial step in the history is to **ascertain the origin of the blood loss**. It is sometimes difficult for people to ascertain whether blood loss is from the GIT or urogenital tract.
* Associated fever and dysuria suggest **infection**, which may be primary or occurring as a complication of obstruction.
* If bleeding is from the genital tract, other symptoms such as pain and offensive discharge are likely.

Physical examination
* **Physical examination may be unremarkable**.
* Check for a **fever**.
* Check for evidence of **petechiae or bruising** suggesting a bleeding disorder.
* Percuss for a **tender or distended bladder**. This may represent clot retention.
* Do a pelvic examination to determine if there is local bleeding that may be amenable to local therapy.

Investigations and manageme nt
Prognosis measured in hours to days prior to the onset of this problem (symptom control)

When erosion of a major vessel has occurred, ensure that **crisis medications** (p.53) are available. These people should be nursed in a single room. Green or red towels help to minimize the visual distress of active bleeding. This is a clinical diagnosis and no further investigations are indicated. Discontinue any medications that may contribute to this problem.
* Genital tract bleeding:
  * These people may be frightened and anxious because if the ongoing blood loss is significant. This may be an indication for sedation.
  * Less torrential bleeding may be well palliated by packing of the vaginal vault with acetone-soaked sponges.
  * Vulval bleeding may be managed with local pressure or epinephrine-soaked sponges.

- Comfort may be improved by insertion of an IDC.
- Urological tract bleeding:
  - Bleeding involving or proximal to the bladder may result in clot retention which should be considered if a person is uncomfortable and unable to pass urine. Even at the end of life, insertion of a three-way catheter with irrigation of the bladder may allow clots to be cleared effectively. Continue regular irrigation to avoid further clots.

Prognosis measured in weeks prior to the onset of this problem (in addition to symptom control)

Collect serum EUC, FBC, and **coagulation studies**. Screen for bleeding complications such as **DIC** (p.196).

- Genital tract bleeding:
  - Investigations to define the site of the bleeding should be undertaken. This may be by direct visualization by inspection of the external genitalia or a speculum examination. Further imaging with a **CT scan** may be necessary.
  - Commence **tranexamic acid** 1 g four times daily orally to help stabilize any clots.
  - If bleeding is from the vaginal vault, consult the gynaecological service for advice about how best to pack the vault and any local options to stem the bleeding.
  - Other options in this prognostic group include embolization of the artery supplying the bleeding site.
- Urinary tract bleeding:
  - Check urine microscopy and culture. Further investigations include **renal ultrasound** or CT scan to define likely bleeding sites.
  - Treat any infection and ensure adequate hydration.
  - In malignancy, a radiotherapy consultation should be considered.

Prognosis measured in months to years prior to the onset of this problem (in addition to the above)

- Transfuse if anaemic. Replace **platelets and FFP** if ongoing torrential bleeding.
- Ensure adequate IV access.
- Maintain blood pressure with adequate hydration.
- **Administer vitamin K 10 mg IV**.
- Consider the best imaging to define the source of bleeding, including selective angiography if the source of bleeding is not obvious.
- Genital tract bleeding:
  - Investigations and initial management should be simultaneously addressed. Seek urgent advice from the gynaecological team.
  - Treat pain, and nausea and vomiting as necessary.
- Urinary tract bleeding:
  - Investigations and management should be simultaneously addressed. Seek urgent advice from urological services.
  - Organize an **urgent renal ultrasound and pelvic CT**.
  - Monitor for clot retention and organize insertion of a three-way catheter if this occurs.

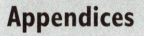

Appendices

1 Australia-modified Karnofsky Performance Scale (AKPS) 301
2 The LANSS pain scale: Leeds Assessment of Neuropathic Symptoms and Signs 302
3 Glasgow Coma Score 304

Australia-modified Karnofsky Performance Scale (AKPS)

Score

100	Normal; no complaints; no evidence of disease
90	Able to carry on normal activity; minor signs or symptoms
80	Normal activity with effort; some signs or symptoms of disease
70	Cares for self; unable to carry on normal activity or to do active work
60	Requires occasional assistance but is able to care for most of own needs
50	Requires considerable assistance
40	In bed more than 50 per cent of the time
30	Almost completely bedfast
20	Totally bedfast and requiring extensive care
10	Comatose or barely rousable
0	Dead

Reproduced from Abernethy, A.P., et al. The Australia-modified Karnofsky Performance Status (AKPS) scale: a revised scale for contemporary palliative care clinical practice [ISRCTN81117481]. *BMC Palliat Care* 4, 7 (2005). https://doi.org/10.1186/1472-684X-4-7 Copyright © 2005, Abernethy et al. This Open Access article is distributed under the terms of the Creative Commons Attribution License (https://creativecommons.org/licenses/by/2.0), which permits unrestricted use, distribution, and reproduction in any medium, provided the original work is properly cited.

The LANSS pain scale: Leeds Assessment of Neuropathic Symptoms and Signs

A PAIN QUESTIONNAIRE

- Think about how your pain has felt over the last week.
- Please say whether any of the descriptions match your pain exactly.

1) **Does your pain feel like a strange, unpleasant sensation on your skin? Words like prickling, tingling, pins and needles might describe these sensations**
   a) NO – My pain doesn't really feel like this .... (0)
   b) YES – I get these sensations quite a lot...................... (5)

2) **Does your pain make the skin in the painful area look different from normal? Words like mottled or looking more red or pink might describe the appearance**
   a) NO – My pain doesn't affect the colour of my skin .... (0)
   b) YES – I've noticed that the pain does make my skin look different from normal .... (5)

3) **Does your pain make the affected skin abnormally sensitive to touch? Getting unpleasant sensations when lightly stroking the skin, or getting pain when wearing tight clothes might describe the abnormal sensation**
   a) NO – My pain doesn't make my skin abnormally sensitive in that area .... (0)
   b) YES – My skin seems abnormally sensitive to touch in that area . (3)

4) **Does your pain come on suddenly and in bursts for no apparent reason when you're still? Words like electric shocks, jumping, and bursting describe these sensations**
   a) NO – I don't really get these sensations .... (0)
   b) YES – I get these sensations quite a lot .... (2)

5) **Does your pain feel as if the skin temperature in the painful area has changed abnormally? Words like hot and burning describe these sensations**
   a) NO – I don't really get these sensations .... (0)
   b) YES – I get these sensations quite a lot .... (1)

B SENSORY TESTING

Skin sensitivity can be examined by comparing the painful area with a contralateral or adjacent non-painful area for the presence of allodynia and an altered pin-prick threshold (PPT).

1) ALLODYNIA

Examine the response to lightly stroking cotton wool across the non-painful area and then the painful area. If normal sensations are experienced in the non-painful site, but pain or unpleasant sensations (tingling, nausea) are experienced in the painful area when stroking, allodynia is present.

a) NO, normal sensations in both areas . . . . (0)

b) YES, allodynia in painful area only   . . . . (5)

2) ALTERED PIN-PRICK THRESHOLD

Determine the pin-prick threshold by comparing the response to a 23 gauge (blue) needle mounted inside a 2 mL syringe barrel placed gently on to the skin in a non-painful and then painful area.

If a sharp pin-prick is felt in the non-painful area, but a different sensation is experienced in the painful area, e.g. none/blunt only (raised PPT) or a very painful sensation (lowered PPT), an altered PPT is present.

If a pin-prick is not felt in either area, mount the syringe on to the needle to increase the weight and repeat.

a) NO, equal sensation in both areas   . . . . (0)

b) YES, altered PPT in painful area . . . . (3)

SCORING

Add values in parentheses for sensory description and examination findings to obtain overall score

TOTAL SCORE (maximum 24)   . . . .

If score <12, neuropathic mechanisms are **unlikely** to be contributing to the patient's pain.

If score ≥12, neuropathic mechanisms are **likely** to be contributing to the patient's pain.

Appendix 3

Glasgow Coma Score

The GCS is scored between 3 and 15, with 3 being the worst, and 15 the best. It is composed of three parameters: best eye response, best verbal response, and best motor response, as given below.

Best eye response (4)
1. No eye opening.
2. Eye opening to pain.
3. Eye opening to verbal command.
4. Eyes open spontaneously.

Best verbal response (5)
1. No verbal response.
2. Incomprehensible sounds.
3. Inappropriate words.
4. Confused.
5. Orientated.

Best motor response (6)
1. No motor response.
2. Extension to pain.
3. Flexion to pain.
4. Withdrawal from pain.
5. Localizing pain.
6. Obeys commands.

Note that the phrase 'GCS of 11' is essentially meaningless, and it is important to break the figure down into its components, such as E3V3M5 = GCS 11. A score of ≥13 correlates with a mild brain injury, 9–12 is a moderate injury, and 8 is a severe brain injury.

Reprinted from The Lancet, 304, 7872, G. Teasdale, and B. Jennett, 'Assessment of coma and impaired consciousness: A practical scale', pp. 81–83, Copyright 1974, with permission from Elsevier.

Index

For the benefit of digital users, indexed terms that span two pages (e.g., 52–53) may, on occasion, appear on only one of those pages.

Note: Tables and boxes are indicated by an italic t and b following the page number.

A

abdomen, acute 156–57, 156t
abdominal aortic aneurysm 112–13, 112t
abdominal cramping 11
abdominal CT 164
abdominal pain 11–13, 150
abscess 41
  cerebral 24, 240t, 259t
  epidural 18, 46–47, 242–43
  intrathecal 242–43
  pelvic 14
acral erythema 95, 95t
ACTH 217t, 233–34
acute
  abdomen 92, 156–57, 156t
  angle glaucoma 21–22
  confusional state 29–31, 35, 51–52, 203, 217, 246–48, 246t, 264t
  generalized exanthematous pustulosis 84–86, 84t
  gout 221–22, 221t
  hepatic failure 12–13, 29–30, 32–33, 41, 177–79, 177t
  hydrocephalus 44
  kidney injury 41, 177–79, 208–11, 208t, 219t, 290–91
  limb ischaemia 116–18, 116t
  myeloid leukaemia 252t
  myocardial infarction 26
  myocardial ischaemia 11
  pancreatitis 11, 26, 174–76, 174t, 196t, 219t
  psychosis 268–69, 268t
  shortness of breath 92, 122
  stress 270
  stroke 240–41, 240t
  tubular necrosis 208t
ACE inhibitors 101–2
acetylcysteine 178
aciclovir 8–9
acid–base balance 208–11
acid suppressants 78t
acquired immune deficiency syndrome (AIDS) 39, 50–52

Addisonian crisis 232–34, 232t
Addison's disease 212t, 220
adhesions 11, 15
adjustment disorders 35
  with anxious mood 270
  with depressed mood 267
adrenal insufficiency 232
  chronic 232
adrenaline 88–89, 115, 192, 199, 296–97
agitation 35–36, 50–51, 52, 235, 268–69
AIDS 39, 50–52
airway obstruction 26–27, 138–39, 138t
akathisia 35
albumin, concentrated 167
alcohol 221t, 249t
  misuse 30, 256t
  withdrawal 175, 247–48
alfentanil 75t
allodynia 303
allopurinol 62t, 73t, 222, 223
alprazolam 66–67, 75t
alveolitis, fibrosing 142
amikacin 60
amiloride 71
aminoglycosides 47, 48–49, 71
amiodarone 60, 62t, 71, 75t, 77t, 79t
amitriptyline 65, 73t, 75t, 77t, 78t
amlodipine 75t
amoxicillin 48–49, 62–63, 71, 73t
amphetamines 64
ampicillin 48–49, 62–63
amyloid deposits 256t
anaemia 26–27, 187–90, 187t
  macrocytic 188–90
  microcytic 188–90
  normocytic 188–90
anaesthetics 70
analgesia, epidural 117
analgesics 62t, 71, 73t, 75t, 77t, 78t, 79t, 80t
anaphylaxis 87t, 88
anastomosis, bronchial 139

aneurysm
  cerebral 256t
  mycotic 108, 109
  rupture, aortic 13, 112–13, 112t
  thoracic aortic 110t, 111
angina, mesenteric 12
angiodysplasia 11, 14
angiography 115, 117–18, 159
  mesenteric 162
  renal 290–91
angio-oedema 90–91, 90t
angiotensin converting enzyme inhibitors 101–2
anterior resection 116t
antiarrhythmics 62t, 75t, 77t, 78t, 79t
antibiotics 62–63, 62t, 63t, 71, 73t, 75t, 78t, 79t
anticholinergic load 29, 68–69, 246t
anticoagulation 72, 73t, 75t, 78t, 79t, 123, 256t
anticonvulsants 9–10
antidepressants 9–10, 62t, 64, 68–69, 73t, 75t, 77t, 78t, 79t, 267
  washout times 65
antiemetics 73t, 77t, 78t
antiepileptics 62t, 63t, 73t, 75t, 77t, 78t, 79t, 80t
antifungals 62t, 63t, 75t, 78t, 79t
antihistamines 68–69
antihypertensives 73t, 75t, 77t, 78t
antineoplastic agents 60, 63t, 73t, 75t, 77t, 78t, 79t
antiphospholipid antibodies 94, 119t, 120–21
antiphospholipid disorders 11
antiplatelet therapy 8–9
antipsychotics 31, 68–69, 73t, 75t, 77t, 78t
antithrombin III 120–21
antivirals 62t, 73t, 75t, 77t, 78t, 79t
anuria 32–33, 287, 292

anxiety 7, 30, 35, 41, 51–52, 247, 270
  generalized, disorder 270
aorta
  aneurysm 13, 112–13, 112t
  dissection 7, 8–9, 110–11, 110t, 112–13
aperients 39
aphasia 35
appendicitis 11, 12–13, 14, 15–16, 46–47
apraxia, constructional 177
arrhythmias, ventricular 249–50
arterial bleed 101–2, 114–15, 114t, 297
  carotid 114t
arterial occlusion
  graft occlusion 116–18
  mesenteric 11
  peripheral artery 116t
  renal 15–16, 290–91
arteriovenous malformations 240t, 256t
arthralgias 46–47
asbestosis 142t
ascites 27, 29–30, 44, 100, 166–68, 166t
  non-malignant causes 167–68
ascitic tap 167
aspiration
  pleural 133t
  pneumonia 126–28, 135
aspirin 74
asterixis 29, 177
ataxia 217
atrial fibrillation 18, 20, 29, 32–33, 116t, 235, 240t, 290–91
atypical pneumonia 127
autoimmune hepatitis 177t
autonomic neuropathy 39
autonomic symptoms (overdrive) 226
azathioprine 73t

B
B symptoms 47
B$_{12}$ deficiency 188–90
back pain 18–19, 242–43, 274
bacterial peritonitis, spontaneous 12–13, 29–30, 46–47, 48–49
barbiturates 75t
basophilia 201
behavioural problems 268–69
benzodiazepines 66–67, 68–69, 71, 73t, 75t, 78t

benztropine 68–69
benzylpenicillin 48–49, 71
biguanides 72
bile salt diarrhoea 39
biliary tract
  sepsis 48–49, 172–73, 172t
  stent 170–71, 172t
bilirubin, indirect 188–90
biopsy, lung 133t
bisphosphonates 9–10, 72, 216
bladder ultrasound 288–89
Blastomyces dermatidis 127
bleeding
  abdominal aortic aneurysm 112–13, 112t
  arterial 101–2, 114–15, 114t, 297
  carotid artery 114t
  genital tract 296–97
  hepatic, subcapsular 11
  intracranial 33, 41, 256–58, 256t
  lower gastrointestinal tract 11, 161–62, 161t
  pelvic 296–97
  respiratory tract 140–41
  retroperitoneal 26
  secondary to coagulopathy 198–99, 198t, 199t
  sentinel 114, 115
  upper gastrointestinal tract 158–60, 158t
  urinary tract 14, 15–16
bleomycin 27
blood loss 187t
blood transfusion 46–47
bone
  fracture 276–77, 276t
  lytic bone metastases 276t
  metastases 9, 14–16, 18, 19, 20, 242–45, 274t
  sclerotic metastases 276t
bone marrow
  examination 185–86
  failure 184–86, 188–90, 194–95, 194t
  infiltration 184–86, 191t
bowel
  blind loop 39
  care, paraplegia 244
  habits, altered 150
  obstruction 44, 163–65, 163t
  obstruction, multilevel 163–65
  perforation 162
breast cancer 144t
breathlessness 26–28, 50–52, 92, 122
bronchiectasis 140t

bronchiolitis obliterans with organising pneumonia (BOOP) 142
bronchitis 26–27
bronchomalacia 139
Brudzinski's sign 253
Budd–Chiari syndrome (hepatic vein) 41, 166t, 166
bullae 92, 133t
buprenorphine 71
bupropion 79t
burr holes 260–61
buspirone 66–67
butyrophenones 72

C
C1 replacement 90–91
C2, 91, 99–123
cachexia 18–19, 27, 28, 30, 31, 33, 44, 50–52, 226t, 226–27
calcium
  channel blocker 8–10
  raised 215–16, 215t, 246t
calculus, renal 15–16
carbamazepine 60, 63t, 66–67, 72, 73t, 75t, 77t, 79t, 250–51
carbimazole 236
carbon dioxide retention 33
carcinoid tumour 39
carcinomatosis, lymphangitis 26–27, 144–45, 144t
cardiac decompensation, acute 26–27, 100–3, 100t, 106, 108–9, 129–30, 219t
cardiac tamponade 26–27, 104–5, 104t
cardiomyopathy 27
carotenaemia 169t
carotid artery 114t
  disease 240t
carotid dissection 21–22
catastrophic terminal events 53
catheter
  central venous 46–47, 133t
  Tenckhoff 167–68
  urinary 243–44, 284–85, 287, 288
  urinary suprapubic 287, 288
  urinary three-way 15–16, 296–97
cation exchange resins 212
cauda equina damage 15–16, 18, 242–43
ceftazidime 47, 48–49, 71
ceftriaxone 48–49, 282–83

cellulitis 46–47, 48–49
central cyanosis 126, 129, 142
central nervous system
  infections 48–49
  tumours 32
central venous catheter 46–47, 133t
cephalosporins 62–63
cerebellar metastases 41, 44
cerebral abscess 24, 240t, 259t
cerebral aneurysm 256t
cerebral bleeds 256t, 256–57, 259t
cerebral ischaemic injury 259t
cerebral metastases 29–31, 35, 41, 44, 246t, 249t
cerebral oedema 42, 44, 177, 217, 219–20, 240–41
cerebral tumours 259t
cerebrospinal fluid 254
  blood-stained 257–58
  evaluation 254–55
cerebrovascular accident 266t
cervical disc prolapse 242t
Charcot's triad 172
chemotherapy
  acral erythema 95, 95t
  mucositis 12–13
  neutropenia 46–47
  pneumonitis 142–43, 142t
chest drain 130, 133
chest infection 8–9, 26, 47, 126–28
chest X-ray 101–2, 127, 134
Cheyne–Stokes respiration 259
chlorpromazine 73t, 75t, 77t
cholangitis 11, 172–73
cholecystectomy 173
cholecystitis 11, 12–13, 46–47
cholestasis 172–73
cholestyramine 39–40, 63t
chronic liver disease, stigmata 166
chronic obstructive pulmonary disease 26–27
ciclosporin 60, 73t, 75t, 77t
cimetidine 47, 62t, 75t, 77t, 78t, 79t
ciprofloxacin 62t, 78t
cirrhosis, liver 167–68, 219t
cisapride 75t
citalopram 65, 77t, 79t
clarithromycin 62t, 75t, 78t, 79t

clavulanate 47, 48–49
clavulanic acid 71, 73t
clindamycin 62–63, 73t
clomipramine 64, 65, 73t, 77t, 78t
clonazepam 66–67, 73t, 75t, 250
clopidogrel 79t
Clostridium difficile 39, 151, 153
clot retention 14
clotrimazole 75t
clozapine 78t
clubbing 142
coagulation, laser 141
coagulation studies 188–90, 192–93
coagulopathy 18, 20, 21–22, 32, 114t, 115, 177–79, 290–91
  bleeding secondary to 198–99, 198t, 199t
Coccidiodes immitis 127
codeine 71, 73t, 77t
colic, ureteric 14
colitis 11, 12–13, 153–55, 153t
  ischaemic 15–16, 153, 156–57
  pseudomembranous 39
  radiation 153t
colonic polyp 11
colonoscopy 162
community-acquired pneumonia 26, 27, 46–47, 126–28
comorbid illnesses 4–5, 6, 81
complement levels 91
concentrated albumin 167
conduit, ileal 294–95
confusional state, acute 29–31, 35, 51–52, 203, 217, 246–48, 246t, 264t
consciousness, decreased level 32–34, 217, 304
constipation 11, 35, 37–38, 37t
  faecal overflow 39
  hypercalcaemia 215
constructional apraxia 177
contrast, radiological 47, 235t
cord, spinal
  compression, compromise 7, 8–9, 14, 18, 19, 20, 242–45, 242t
  multilevel 243
coronary syndrome, acute 8–9, 100, 266t

corticosteroids 29, 63t, 75t, 79t, 217t, 233, 244
cortisol 75t
cortisol levels, serum 233–34
costochondritis 7
co-trimoxazole 62t
counselling 267
Courvoisier's sign 172
Creutzfeldt–Jakob disease 55
crisis
  medications 53
  sickle cell 205–6
cryoprecipitate 197
cryptococcal meningitis 252t
CT scan, abdominal 164
CTPA 120–21
Cullen's sign 175
cultures
  blood 46–47
  stool 151
Cushing's syndrome 217t
cutaneous vasculitis 92–93
cyanosis, central 126, 129, 142
cyclophosphamide 63t, 73t, 75t, 79t
cyst, ruptured ovarian 14, 15–16
cystectomy 116t
cystitis 284–85
cystoscopy 294–95
cytarabine 73t
cytochrome P450 75–80, 75t
Cytomegalovirus 39
cytotoxic chemotherapy 60, 63t, 73t, 75t, 77t, 78t, 79t

D

D dimer 192–93
D vitamin 215–16, 215t
dantrolene 66–67, 70
deaminates 64
deconditioning 19
decreased fluid intake 217t, 246t
deep vein thrombosis
  prophylaxis 277
deficiency
  B₁₂ 188–90
  folate 188–90
  thiamine 24, 188–90
dehydration 29–30, 32–33, 246t
delirium 29–31, 35, 51–52, 246–48, 246t
delusions 264t

demeclocycline 220
dementia 30, 31, 33
deoxygenated
    haemoglobin 205–6
deprescribing 81
depressed mood, adjustment
    disorder 267
depression 30, 35, 264t,
    266–67, 266t
    agitated 35
    major 267
desipramine 77t, 78t
desquamation 85
dexamethasone 8–9, 28,
    68–69, 75t, 79t, 233,
    244, 260
dextromethorphan 64, 66–
    67, 75t, 77t
dextropropoxyphene
    62t, 71
diabetes mellitus 228–31,
    240t, 266t
    type 1 228–31
    type 2 228–31
diabetic ketoacidosis 32,
    214t, 228–31
diabetic nephropathy 208t
dialysis, haemo 223, 290–
    91, 292–93
diaphragmatic
    innervation 244–45
diarrhoea 39–40
    bile salt 39
    hypokalaemia 214
diazepam 71, 73t, 74, 75t,
    78t, 79t, 250
DIC 192–93, 196–97, 196t
dicloxacillin 48–49, 62–
    63, 63t
diflunisal 71
dignity, loss of 249–51
digoxin 60, 68–69, 71,
    75t, 101–2
diltiazem 68–69, 75t
disc prolapse, cervical 242t
disease-modifying therapy 6
disease progression 4–5
disopyramide 60, 75t
disorientation 31
dissection
    aortic 7, 8–9, 110–11,
        110t, 112–13
    thoracic aneurysm 26
disseminated intravascular
    coagulation 192–93,
    196–97, 196t
diuresis, post-
    obstruction 288
diuretics 167–68, 217t, 219t
    thiazide 220t

diverticulitis 11, 12–13, 14,
    15–16, 46–47
dopamine 64
Doppler ultrasound 290–
    91, 292
dothiepin 65
doxepin 65, 77t
doxorubicin 73t
doxycycline 73t
DRESS syndrome 84–86,
    84t, 96t, 97
dressings, sterile
    paraffin 85–86
drowsiness 229
drug reaction with
    eosinophilia and
    systemic symptoms
    84–86, 84t
drug reactions 84–86, 84t,
    87–89, 87t, 96–97, 96t
drug withdrawal 249t
drug withdrawal (illicit) 24
dyspnoea 26–28, 50–52,
    92, 122
dysuria 14, 15–16

E
ecchymoses 192
ECG
    electrical alternans 105
    hyperkalaemia 210
    saddle-shaped ST
        elevation 106–7
echocardiography 102–
    3, 105
effusion
    pericardial 8–9, 27, 104t
    pleural 27, 28, 129–30,
        130t, 131
electrolytes 208–11
embolectomy 117, 120–21
embolization, selective
    arterial 115
embolus
    arterial 116t
    fat 26, 278–79, 278t
    pulmonary 8–9, 129
    saddle 9
    septic 11, 108–9
emphysema,
    subcutaneous 136
empyema 26, 48–
    49, 131–32
enalapril 75t
encephalitis 21–22
    of unknown cause 55
encephalopathy 11, 32–
    33, 177–79

hepatic 249t
    uraemic 211
    Wernicke's 24, 227
end stage organ
    failure 50–52
endocarditis, infective 24,
    41, 48–49, 108–9, 108t
endometriosis 14–15
endoscopy, upper
    GIT 159–60
energy levels, improved 268
enteritis 11
enterocolonic fistula 39
eosinophilia 201
ephedrine 64
epididymitis 14, 15–16
epidural abscess 18, 46–
    47, 242–43
epidural catheter 18
epilepsy 29–30, 32, 33, 217,
    249–51, 249t, 256t
epinephrine 88–89
epinephrine-soaked gauze/
    sponge 115, 192,
    199, 296–97
ERCP 170, 175
erythematous skin changes
    84t, 85, 88, 94, 95,
    95t, 180
erythromycin 62t, 75t,
    78t, 79t
escitalopram 65
ethanol 61, 79t
etoposide 75t
expected deterioration
    4–5, 32
extrinsic compression, large
    airways 159t
exudate 129–30, 130t

F
facial oedema 122
factor V Leiden 94,
    119t, 120–21
factor Xa inhibitors 198t
faecal overflow 39
failure
    cardiac 100, 129–30
    hepatic 12–13, 29–30,
        32–33, 41, 177–79,
        177t, 246t
    renal 26–27, 41, 177–79,
        208–11, 208t,
        219t, 246t
fallopian tube, torsion 14
famciclovir 8–9
famotidine 68–69
fasciitis, necrotizing
    14, 15–16

fasciotomy 117
fat embolus 26, 278–79,
    278t
fear 35, 41, 51–52
febrile neutropenia 48–49
feculent vomiting 163
felodipine 75t
fentanyl 71, 287
ferritin 188–90
fever 26–27, 29–30, 32, 35,
    46–49, 126–27
FFP 197, 199, 199t
fibrillation, atrial 18, 20,
    29, 32–33, 116t,
    235, 290–91
fibrinogen degradation
    products 141, 292
fibrosing alveolitis 142
fistula 180–82, 180t
  bronchial 139
  gastrointestinal tract 39,
      180–82, 180t
  genitourinary 180,
      294–95
  tracheo-oesophageal 135
fitting 217
  see also seizures
flecainide 79t
flight of ideas 268
flucloxacillin 48–49
fluconazole 62t, 75t, 79t
fludrocortisone 233
fluid
  balance 208–11
  intake decreased
      217t, 246t
  peritoneal 166–68
  restriction 220
fluoxetine 65, 75t, 77t, 79t
fluranes 70
flutamide 75t, 78t
fluticasone 68–69
fluvastatin 79t
fluvoxamine 65, 75t, 77t,
    78t, 79t
folate deficiency 188–90
fracture
  immobilization 276–77
  long bone 116t, 276–77,
      276t, 278t
  rib 7
  vertebral 274–75, 274t
free gas, sub-
    diaphragmatic 162
fresh frozen plasma 197,
    199, 199t
frusemide 68–69
frustration 35
functional status 6, 301
fungating cancers 296–97

G

gabapentin 72
gait disorders 203
gallstones 7, 169t, 180
gastric compression 41
gastric outlet obstruction 41
gastric secretions 44
gastric splash 163–64
gastritis 41
gastroenteritis 11, 39–40
Gastrografin® swallow 135,
    164, 181
gastrointestinal tract
  bleeding, lower 11, 161–
      62, 161t
  bleeding, upper 158–60,
      158t
  ischaemia 11
  mucositis 150–52, 150t
  obstruction 11
gastroparesis 41, 42–43
gastroscopy 159–60
G-CSF 185
generalized anxiety
    disorder 270
generalized bullous fixed
    drug eruptions 84–86
genital ulcers 85
gentamicin 48–49,
    60, 282–83
Giardia lamblia 39
Gilbert syndrome 169t
Glasgow Coma Score 304
glaucoma, acute
    angle 21–22
glibenclamide 62t, 73t, 79t
gliclazide 72
glipizide 72
gliquidone 72
glomerular filtration
    rate 208–11
glomerular nephritis 208t
glucagon 178–79
glucocorticoid use 18, 63t,
    75t, 79t, 217t, 244
  acute confusional
      state 29–30
  sudden withdrawal 232t
glucose, 50% 210
glucose, blood
  high 228–31, 228t
  low 226–27, 226t
glycaemic control 29–30,
    226–27, 228–31
glycopyrrolate 68–69
GM-CSF 185
gout
  acute 221–22, 221t
  chronic 221

grading
  ascites 166
  encephalopathy 177
  gastrointestinal tract
      mucositis 151t
  oral mucositis 148–49, 151t
graft, arterial 116–18
graft-versus-host
    disease 196t
grandiose thinking 268
Grey–Turner's sign 175
grief, prolonged 271
griseofulvin 63t
growth factors 185
Guillain–Barré syndrome
    20, 242t
guilt 264t

H

haematemesis 158
haematoma, subdural 33
haematuria 14, 15–16, 284
haemodialysis 223, 290–
    91, 292–93
haemoglobin
  low 187–90
  S 205–6
haemolysis 26–27, 187t, 188–90
haemolytic uraemic
    syndrome 191t, 192–93
haemophilia 198t, 198
haemopoiesis,
    ineffective 187t
haemoptysis 92, 140–41, 140t
haemorrhage
  intracerebral 256t, 256–57
  subarachnoid 33,
      256t, 256–57
  subdural 256t, 256–57
  terminal phase 53
haemorrhagic stroke 21–
    22, 241
haemorrhoids 161t
haloperidol 75t, 77t, 78t,
    220t, 268
halothane 70
hand–foot syndrome 95, 95t
haptoglobins 188–
    90, 192–93
headache 21–23, 21t, 122,
    203, 259, 260
heart failure 100, 129–30
heart valve, prosthetic 29
height loss 274
heparin 72, 73t
  induced thrombocytopenia
      192–93
  low molecular weight 94,
      120–21

hepatic bleed, subcapsular 11
hepatic failure
  acute 12–13, 29–30, 32–33, 41, 177–79, 177t, 246t
  fulminant 177–79
  medication dosing 73, 73t
  tumours 226t, 226–27
hepatic vein thrombosis 41
hepatitis
  acute viral 177t
  autoimmune 177t
  B virus 55
hepatomegaly 41, 44
hernia, strangulated 11, 14, 164–65
herpes simplex virus 39
herpes zoster, acute 7, 8–9, 22–23
Histoplasma capsulatum 127
HIV 55
HIV/AIDS medications 75t, 77t, 78t
hormone agents 62t, 75t, 77t, 78t, 79t
Horner's syndrome 138
hospital-acquired pneumonia 126–28, 178–79
HUS 191t, 192–93
hydrocephalus 33, 41, 44
hydrocodone 77t
hydrocortisone 233
hyoscine butylbromide 28, 287
hyperactive delirium 246–48
hypercalcaemia 29–30, 32–33, 215–16, 215t, 246t
hypercholesterolaemia 240t
hyperglycaemia 32, 33, 228–31, 228t, 229t
hyperkalaemia 212–13, 212t
hyperleukocytosis 192–202
hypernatraemia 217–18
hyperosmolar hyperglycaemia 228–31
hyperparathyroidism 215t
hyperphosphataemia 223
hyper-reflexia 217
hypersensitivity reactions 87–89, 87t
hypertension 8–9, 21–22, 240t
  portal 158t, 169–70
hypertensive nephropathy 208t
hyperthermia, malignant 70
hyperthyroidism 29–30, 39, 47, 235–36, 235t
hyperuricaemia 221–22

hyperviscosity 203–4, 203t
hypoactive delirium 246–48
hypoadrenal crisis 232–34, 232t
hypoalbuminaemia 27
hypoaldosteronism 212t
hypoglycaemia 29–30, 32, 33, 35, 178–79, 226–27, 226t
hypoglycaemic agents 62t, 72, 73t, 226–27
hypokalaemia 214, 214t
hypomania 35, 246t, 268–69, 268t
hyponatraemia 29–31, 33, 35, 219–20, 219t, 260–61
hypoperfusion, renal 208t
hyposplenism 206
hypotension 11, 26–27, 35, 158–59, 232
hypothermia 35, 237
hypothyroidism 188–90, 220t, 237–38, 237t
hypovolaemia 212
hypoxaemia 28, 29–31, 32, 35

I

ICD 54
icterus 169–70
idiopathic thrombocytopenic purpura 191–93, 191t
IgE 87t
ileal conduit 294–95
ileal resection 39–40
ileus 153
  gallstone 11, 180
illusions 268
imatinib 75t
imipramine 65, 75t, 77t, 78t
immunocompromise 32, 41
immunosuppressants 73t, 75t, 77t
immunotherapy, skin reactions 96–97, 96t
impaired mobility 18
implantable defibrillator 54
inappropriate antidiuretic hormone secretion 29–30, 220, 220t
incarcerated hernia 14
incontinence 242–43
indinavir 73t, 75t, 77t
indirect bilirubin 188–90
indomethacin 71
infarction
  mesenteric 13
  micro 196–97

myocardial 26, 27
pulmonary 140t
renal 11, 15–16
splenic 11
infection 29, 46–49
  biliary tract 7, 48–49, 172–73, 172t
  cerebral abscess 24, 48–49
  endocarditis 24, 41, 48–49, 108–9, 108t
  inadequate treatment 47
  lower respiratory tract 48, 126–28
  mediastinum 8–9, 135, 136–37, 136t
  meninges 252–53
  organ donation 55
  osteomyelitis 24
  peritonitis, spontaneous bacterial 14, 29–30, 46–47, 48–49
  pleural space 131–32
  prostate 15
  pyelonephritis 15–16
  respiratory tract 8–9, 48–49
  urinary tract – lower 46–47, 48–49, 284–85
  urinary tract – upper 15–16, 46–47, 48–49, 282–83
inflammation
  mediastinitis 136–37, 136t
  pneumonitis 143
inflammatory bowel disease 15–16, 39–40, 153, 157, 180t
insulin 60, 64, 226–27, 229
  sliding scale 229t
insulin–glucose infusion 213
intercurrent illnesses 4–5, 6
intracranial bleeding 33, 41, 256–58, 256t
intracranial pressure, raised 44, 177–79, 259–61, 259t
intrathecal abscess 242–43
intrathecal catheter 18
iodine load 235t
ipratropium bromide 28
iron deficiency 188–90
irritable bowel syndrome 15
ischaemic colitis 15–16, 153, 156–57
ischaemic gastrointestinal tract 11
ischaemic heart disease 26–27, 100, 266t
ischaemic limb 116–18, 116t
ischaemic priapism 14, 15–16

ischaemic skin 196
ischaemic stroke 21–22
isocarboxazid 64
isoniazid 62t
itch, cholestatic 172–73
ITP 191–93, 191t
itraconazole 75t

J

jaundice 169–71, 169t

K

Karnofsky performance
    status 301
Kernig's sign 184, 253
ketoacidosis, diabetic 32
ketoconazole 62t, 75t, 78t, 79t
kidney injury, acute 41,
    177–79, 208–11, 208t,
    219t, 290–91
kidneys, polycystic 208t
Kussmaul breathing 228–29
Kussmaul's sign 104–5

L

labetalol 77t
lansoprazole 79t
LANSS 302–3
large airway obstruction
    138–39, 138t
large bowel obstruction
    163–65
laryngeal oedema 122
laser coagulation 141
laxatives 38
left-sided cardiac failure 100
leptomeningeal disease 41,
    44, 246t
leukaemia 11, 223
leukocytosis 200–2, 200t
level of consciousness 32–
    34, 217, 304
levothyroxine 60
lidocaine 60, 75t, 77t, 78t
life-limiting illness 4–5, 6
limb ischaemia 116–18, 116t
lithium 60, 66–67, 72
liver
    cirrhosis 167–68
    disease 166, 198t
loperamide 68–69
lopinavir 73t
loratidine 75t, 77t
L-tryptophan 66–67
lumbar puncture 254
    cytology 254
lung
    biopsy 133t

collapse – pneumothorax
    133–34, 133t
    malignancy 140t
    small cell cancer 220t, 223
lymphangitis carcinomatosis
    26–27, 144–45, 144t
lymphocytosis 201
lymphoedema, infected 46–47
lymphoma 11, 223, 252t
lytic bone metastases 276t

M

major depression 267
malaria 55
malignancy 129–30, 196–97,
    292–93
    breast 144t
    lung 144t
malignant hyperthermia 70
marrow
    examination 185–86
    failure 184–86, 188–90,
        194–95, 194t
    infiltration 184–86, 191t
mediastinal infection 135
mediastinitis 7, 8–9, 26, 135,
    136–37, 136t
    descending necrotic 9
mediastinoscopy, video-
    assisted 137
medications
    acute confusional state 29
    adverse reaction 46–47
    anticholinergic load 68–69
    antidepressants 65
    antihypertensives 29–30
    deprescribing 81
    dosing 71–73
    glucocorticoid withdrawal
        232t
    metabolism 75–80, 75t
    monoamine oxidase
        inhibitors 64
    non-compliance (thyroid)
        237t
    overuse headache 22–23
    protein binding 74
    reaction 84–86, 84t, 87–
        89, 87t, 96–97, 96t
    review 29–30, 33
    serotonin syndrome 66–67
    therapeutic index 60
    toxicity 41
    warfarin interactions 62–
        63, 62t, 63t
    withdrawal 29–30, 35
medroxyprogesterone 73t
megacolon, toxic 153
melaena 158
meningism 184, 243, 254

meningitis 18, 21–22, 46–
    47, 252–55, 252t
    bacterial 252t
    carcinomatous 252t
    cryptococcal 252t
    intercurrent sepsis 252t
    toxoplasmosis 252t
    viral 252t
meningococcal meningitis
    252t, 253
mentation, slowed/altered
    215, 237
mesalazine 39–40
mesenteric vessels,
    ischaemia 11, 13
metastases
    bone 9, 14–16, 18, 19, 20,
        242–45, 274t
    cerebellar 41, 44
    cerebral 29–31, 35, 41, 44,
        246t, 249t
    vertebral body 242t
metformin 72, 73t
methadone 75t, 77t, 78t, 80t
methotrexate 73t
methylphenidate 62t, 64
metoclopramide 73t
metoprolol 77t
metronidazole 48–49, 62t,
    73t, 75t, 79t
mexiletine 77t
mianserin 65
micro-infarcts 196–97
microthrombi 196–97
midazolam 52, 71, 75t, 250
migraine, chronic 22–23
mirtazapine 65, 75t, 78t
mitral stenosis 140t
mobility, impaired 18
moclobemide 64, 65,
    77t, 79t
modafinil 64, 75t, 77t, 79t
monoamine oxidase
    inhibitors 64
monocytosis 201
mononeuritis multiplex 20
morphine 9–10, 28, 40, 52,
    53, 64, 71, 73t, 77t, 287
mouth care 51–52, 149
moxifloxacin 48–49
MRI 244
mucositis
    chemotherapy induced
        12–13, 39
    gastrointestinal tract 11,
        12–13, 15–16, 150–
        52, 150t
    oral 148–49, 148t, 151t
    radiation induced 12–13,
        39

multiple myeloma 203t, 252t
multiple sclerosis 22–23,
    242t, 266t
Murphy's sign 172
myalgias 46–47
Mycobacterium tuberculosis
    127
*Mycoplasma avium–
    intracellulare* 39
Mycoplasma spp. 126–27
mycotic aneurysm 108, 109
myelitis, transverse 242t
myelodysplasia 188–90
myelosuppression, late
    46–47
myocardial infarction,
    acute 26
myocardial ischaemia
    11, 100
myxoedema 237–38

N

naloxone 38
naproxen 47
nausea 35, 41–43
necrosis, papillary 15–16
necrotic mediastinitis 9
necrotizing fasciitis 14,
    15–16
nephritis
    glomerular 208t
    interstitial 208t
nephropathy
    diabetic 208t
    hypertensive 208t
nephrostomy, percutaneous
    287
nephrotic syndrome 219t,
    290–91, 292–93
nerve, intercostal nerve
    damage 7
neuralgia, post-herpetic 8–9
neurodegenerative diseases
    50–52
neuroendocrine tumour
    39–40
neuroglycopenic symptoms
    226
neuropathic pain, diagnosis
    302–3
neuropathy, autonomic 39
neutropenia 18, 184–86
neutropenic sepsis 46–47,
    48–49, 184–86
neutrophilia 201
neutrophils
    destruction 184–86
    impaired production
        184–86
    sequestration 184–86

nevirapine 75t
nifedipine 68–69, 73t, 75t
nitrates 8–10
nitrazepam 71
Nocardia 127
noisy respirations 28, 51–52
non-steroidal anti-
    inflammatory
    medications 8–10
norepinephrine 64
norfloxacin 48–49, 75t,
    78t, 79t
norproxyphene 71
nortriptyline 65, 77t

O

obstipation 11, 37
obstruction
    airway 26–27, 138–39,
        138t
    bowel 41, 44
    large bowel 163–65
    multilevel bowel 163–65
    small bowel 163–65
    superior vena cava 32–33,
        122–23, 122t
    ureteric 41, 208t
    urinary tract 32–33, 208t,
        286–87, 286t
occlusion, renal artery 15–
    16, 290–91
occupational lung disease
    142t
octreotide 39–40, 181
odynophagia 148–49
oedema
    cerebral 42, 44, 177, 217,
        219–20, 240–41
    facial 122
    laryngeal 122
    pulmonary 210, 211
oesophageal pain 7, 8–9
oesophageal perforation
    135, 136t
oesophageal reflux 7
oesophageal spasm 7, 8–9
oesophageal stenting 7
oesophageal varices 160,
    166
oesophagitis, pain 7, 8–9
oestrogen 75t
olanzapine 75t, 77t, 78t, 268
oliguria 211
omeprazole 62t, 75t,
    78t, 79t
ondansetron 40, 77t, 78t
opioids
    constipation 38
    dyspnoea 28
oral contraceptives 75t

oral hypoglycaemic agents
    62t, 64, 72, 73t, 226–27
oral intake, reduced 226t
oral mucositis 148–49,
    148t, 151t
organ donation request 55
organ failure, end-stage
    50–52
osteomyelitis 24
osteoporosis 18, 274t, 276t
outlet obstruction, gastric 41
ovarian cyst
    bleed 14
    rupture 14, 15–16
ovarian torsion 14, 15–16
oxybutynin 68–69
oxycodone 77t
oxygen, dyspnoea 28

P

P450, cytochrome 75–80,
    75t
paclitaxel 75t, 77t, 79t
Paget's disease of the bone
    276t
pain 35
    abdominal 11–13, 150
    back 18–19, 242–43, 274
    bone 14–15
    chest 7–10
    epigastric 11
    flank 14
    incident 276
    ischaemic chest 7
    left lower quadrant 11
    neuropathic 20
    oesophageal 7
    pelvic 14–17
    penile 14
    perineal 14–15
    post-thoracotomy 8–9
    previous substance misuse
        24–25
    prostatic 15–16
    radicular 18
    right upper quadrant 11
    scrotal 14, 15–16
    spinal 20
    suprapubic 14
    symmetrical peripheral
        (glove and stocking)
        20
    visceral 14–16
palmar–plantar
    erythrodysaesthesia
        95, 95t
palsy
    phrenic nerve 138
    recurrent laryngeal nerve
        138

pamidronate 72
pancreatic cancer 220t
pancreatic enzyme
    replacement 39–40
pancreatic pseudocyst
    12–13
pancreatitis 7, 11, 216
    acute 11, 12–13, 26, 174–
        76, 174t, 196t, 219t
    chronic 12
    haemorrhagic 11
    severity 174–76
panic attack 270
panic disorder 270
papillary necrosis 15–16,
    286t
papilloedema 259
papules 92
paracetamol 47, 48, 62t, 71,
    73t, 73, 75t, 78t
    overdose/toxicity 12–13,
        41, 177t, 178–79
paraneoplastic disease
    92–93
paraplegia, bowel care 244
para-pneumonic pleural
    effusion 131
paroxetine 65, 75t, 77t,
    78t, 79t
patent foramen ovale 240t
patient assessment,
    palliative care 6
pelvic abscess 14
pelvic bleeding 296–97
pelvic inflammatory disease
    14
Pemberton's sign 122
penicillin 48–49, 62–63
peptic ulcer disease 12–13,
    41, 158t
percutaneous nephrostomy
    287
perforated bowel 162,
    163–65
performance status 6, 301
perhexiline 60, 77t
pericardial drainage 105
pericardial effusion 8–9,
    27, 104t
pericardial pain 7, 8–9
pericardial rub 104–5, 106
pericardial window 105
pericarditis 8–9, 26, 104t,
    106–7, 106t
peripheral vascular disease
    32–33
peristaltic agents 44
peritoneal disease 41
peritoneal fluid 166–68
peritoneal–venous shunt
    167–68

peritonitis 11, 12–13, 14,
    46–47, 48–49, 219t
petechiae 108–9, 192
pethidine 64, 66–67, 77t
pharmacokinetics
    linear (first order) 61
    non-linear (zero order) 61
phenacetin 78t
phenelzine 64, 65
phenobarbital 60, 63t, 73t,
    75t, 77t, 78t, 79t, 80t,
    178, 250–51
phenothiazines 72
phenytoin 60, 61, 62t, 63t,
    72, 73t, 74, 75t, 77t,
    78t, 79t, 178, 250–51
phimosis 14, 15–16
phrenic nerve palsy 138
physiotherapist 9
PICC line 46–47
pigmentation 232
pin-prick sensation 243,
    302–3
piperacillin 47, 62–63, 71
piroxicam 62t
plasmapheresis 195, 203–4
platelets
    function 191–93, 191t
    low 191–93, 191t
pleural aspiration 133t
pleural effusion 27, 28, 129–
    30, 130t, 131
pleural fluid 130, 131–32
pleurisy 7
pleuritic pain 7
pleurodesis 130
pneumaturia 284
pneumomediastinum 136
pneumonia
    aspiration 126–28, 135
    atypical 26–27, 127
    community-acquired 26,
        27, 46–47
    hospital-acquired 126–28,
        178–79
    lobar 11, 48–49
    pleural effusion 129, 131
    SIADH 220t
    ventilator-associated
        126–28
pneumonitis 142–43, 142t
    chemotherapy induced
        142–43, 142t
    radiotherapy induced 142–
        43, 142t
pneumothorax 7, 8–9, 26,
    133–34, 133t
    tension 133
polycystic kidney disease
    208t
polycythaemia 14, 203t

polyethylene glycol 38
polyp, colonic 11, 14
portal hypertension 158t,
    169–70
positioning, terminal care
    51–52
post-herpetic neuralgia 8–9
post-obstruction diuresis
    288
postural drop 161
potassium, serum
    lowered 214, 214t
    raised 212–13
potassium-sparing diuretics
    212t
prednisolone 68–69, 75t
pressure, intracranial 44,
    177–79, 259–61, 259t
pressure area care 18
priapism, ischaemic 14,
    15–16
primidone 60
procainamide 60
procarbazine 78t
prochlorperazine 68–69
progesterone 75t, 79t
prognosis-modifying
    therapy 6
prolapse, cervical disc 242t
prolonged grief disorder
    271
promethazine 68–69, 73t
propantheline 68–69
propoxyphene 75t
propranolol 62t, 73t, 74,
    77t, 79t
propylthiouracil 63t
prostatitis 14–15, 282–83
prosthetic heart valve 29,
    188–90
protein C deficiency 94,
    120–21
protein S deficiency 94,
    120–21
prothrombin complex
    concentrate 199, 199t
proton pump inhibitors
    79t, 160
pseudomembranous
    colitis 39
Pseudomonas aeruginosa 128
psychosis, acute 268–69,
    268t
psychotherapy 267
pulmonary embolus 7,
    8–9, 129
    saddle embolus 9
pulmonary oedema 210, 211
pulmonary
    thromboembolism,
    acute 26

pulsus paradoxus 104–5
purpura 92–93
pyelonephritis 14, 15–16, 208t, 282–83

Q

quetiapine 75t
quinidine 60, 62t, 75t, 77t

R

radiation colitis 153t
radiation mucositis 12–13, 39
radiculopathy 7
radiological contrast 47, 235t
radiotherapy
    induced pneumonitis 142–43, 142t
    upper abdominal 41
    vertebral column 244
raised intracranial pressure 44, 177–79, 259–61, 259t
ranitidine 63t, 68–69, 73t, 164
Raynaud's phenomenon 116
rectum, tumour 39
recurrent laryngeal nerve palsy 138
reflux oesophagitis 7
refractory nausea 42
renal angiography 290–91
renal angle tenderness 282, 292
renal artery
    occlusion 15–16, 290–91
    stenosis 291
renal calculus 15–16
renal failure
    acute 41, 177–79, 208–11, 208t, 219t, 246t, 290–91
    decompensated chronic 208t
    end-stage 26–27
    intrinsic 208–11, 208t
    medication dosing 71–72
    medications 208t, 209
    post-renal 208–11, 208t
    pre-renal 208–11, 208t
renal hypoperfusion 208t
renal tubular dysfunction 214t
renal ultrasound 287
renal vein thrombosis 292–93
resonium 210, 212

respiratory secretions 28, 51–52
respiratory tract, infection 8–9, 48–49
response (consciousness)
    eye 304
    motor 304
    verbal 304
restless legs 36
retention, urinary 14, 15–16, 35, 288–89, 296–97
reticulocyte count 188–90, 206
retroperitoneal fibrosis 292–93
rhabdomyolysis 70, 212t, 214
rheumatoid arthritis 106t
    pneumonitis 142t
rib, fracture 7
right-sided cardiac failure 100
risperidone 75t, 77t, 268
ritonavir 62t, 73t, 75t, 77t, 78t, 79t
roxithromycin 48–49
RTOG mucositis grading 151t

S

SAAG 167–68
sacral pressure areas 18
saddle sensation 18, 243
salbutamol, dyspnoea 28
salicylates 61
salmeterol 68–69
salpingitis 14
saquinavir 73t, 75t, 77t
sarcoidosis 215t
SCARs 84–86, 84t
schizophrenia 35
sclerotic bone metastases 276t
scrotal pain 15–16
seizures 29–30, 32, 33, 217, 249–51, 249t, 256t
    focal 249–51
    generalized 249–51
    partial 249–50
    status epilepticus 249–51
selective serotonin reuptake inhibitors 36, 62t, 64, 65, 66–67
selective venography 292
selegiline 64
sensation
    light touch 243, 302–3
    pin-prick 243, 302–3
    saddle 18, 243

sepsis 19, 29–30, 33, 41, 46–49, 196–97, 196t, 237t, 246t
    meningococcal 116t
    neutropenic 46–47, 48–49, 184–86
    pneumococcal 116t
    see also infection
sequestration, splenic 184–86
serotonin 64
serotonin syndrome 66–67
sertraline 65, 75t, 77t, 79t
serum
    ascites albumin gradient 167–68
    cortisol levels 233–34
    urate 223
severe cutaneous adverse reactions 84–86, 84t
shock 11, 158–59, 169t, 232
short bowel syndrome 39
shunt, peritoneal–venous 167–68
sickle cell disease 11, 14, 205–6
sigmoidoscopy 162
skin
    biopsy 93
    erythema 84t, 85, 88, 94, 95, 95t, 180
    necrosis 87–88, 94
    target lesion 85
sleeplessness 268
sliding-scale insulin 229t
small bowel obstruction 163–65
small cell lung cancer 220t, 223
SNRI 66–67
sodium, serum
    lowered 219–20, 219t
    raised 217–18, 217t
sodium valproate 60, 72, 79t, 250–51
spinal cord compression, compromise 7, 8–9, 14, 18, 19, 20, 242–45, 242t
spironolactone 71
splash, gastric 163–64
spleen
    infarction 11
    torsion 11
splenomegaly 108–9, 184–86
spondyloarthropathy 18–19
spontaneous bacterial peritonitis 12–13, 29–30, 46–47, 48–49

sputum
  cytology 144
  purulent 126
SSRIs 36, 62t, 64, 65, 66–67
Staphylococcus aureus 127, 128
statins 62t, 63t, 70, 75t
steatorrhoea 39
stenosis, mitral 140t
stent
  biliary 46–47
  gastrointestinal tract 164
  ureteric 46–47
sterile paraffin dressings 85–86
steroids 29, 63t, 75t, 79t, 217t, 233, 244
Stevens–Johnson syndrome 84–86, 84t, 96t, 97
stigmata, chronic liver disease 166
Stokes–Adams attack 249–50
strangulated hernia 11, 14, 164–65
Streptococcus pneumoniae 126–27
streptokinase 117
stress, acute 270
stricture, ureteral 286t
stridor 138
stroke 20, 21–22, 240–41, 240t, 266t
subacute thyroiditis 235t
subarachnoid haemorrhage 21–22, 33
subcapsular hepatic bleed 11
subcutaneous emphysema 136
subdural haematoma 33
substance misuse 24–25
succinylcholine 70
sucralfate 63t
suicide risk assessment 35–36, 264–65, 264t, 266
sulindac 71
sulphonylureas 72
sumatriptan 66–67
superior vena cava obstruction 32–33
suprapubic urinary catheter 287, 288
supraventricular tachycardia 235
swallow, Gastrografin® 135, 164, 181
syncope, vasovagal 249–50
syndrome
  acquired immune deficiency 39, 50–52

Budd–Chiari 41, 166t, 166
carcinoid 39
cauda equina 15–16
DRESS 84–86, 84t, 96t, 97
fat embolus 26, 278–79, 278t
Guillain–Barré 20, 242t
Horner's 138
hyperviscosity 203–4, 203t
inappropriate antidiuretic hormone secretion 29–30, 220, 220t
Stevens–Johnson 84–86, 84t, 96t, 97
tumour lysis 223
Zollinger–Ellison 40
syphilis 55
systemic lupus erythematosus 106t
systemic vasculitis 47

T

tachycardia 235–36
tacrolimus 60, 75t, 77t
tamoxifen 62t, 75t, 77t, 78t, 79t
tamponade, cardiac 26–27, 104–5, 104t
  low-pressure 105
tap, ascitic 167
target lesions, skin 85
targeted therapy, skin reactions 96–97, 96t
tazobactam 47, 62–63, 71
temazepam 71
temporal arteritis 21–22
tenderness, renal angle 282, 292
tension headache, chronic 22–23
tension pneumothorax 133
terfenadine 75t
terminal phase
  care in the 30–31, 50–52
  catastrophic events 53
testis 14
testosterone 75t, 77t, 79t
tetracycline 62–63, 62t
tetrahydrocannabinol 79t
thalassaemia 188–90, 205–6
theophylline 60, 61, 73t, 78t
therapeutic index 60
thiamine 24, 188–90, 227, 247–48, 250–51
thiazide diuretics 220t
thioridazine 66–67, 77t
thoracic aneurysm, dissecting 26
thoracic surgery 104t

thoracoscopy, video-assisted 130
thoracotomy, pain 8–9
threatened fracture 276–77
thrombectomy 292–93
thrombocytopenia 18, 20, 191–93, 191t
thromboembolic disease, venous 27
thrombolysis 8–9, 117
thrombosis
  deep vein, prophylaxis 277
  hepatic vein 41
  renal vein 292–93
  superior vena cava 122–23
  venous 116t, 116–17
thrombotic stroke 240–41
thrombotic thrombocytopenic purpura 191t, 192–93
thyroid
  hyper- 47, 235–36, 235t
  hypo- 188–90, 220t, 237–38, 237t
  storm 235–36, 235t
thyroid function tests 236, 237–38
thyroiditis 235t
thyroxine 62t
TIA 240
ticarcillin 47, 48–49, 62–63
tissue plasminogen activator 117
tobramycin 60
Todd's paresis 250
torsion
  ovary 14
  testis 14, 15–16
toxic epidermal necrolysis 84–86, 84t, 96t, 97
toxic erythema of the palms and soles 95, 95t
toxic megacolon 153
tracheal obstruction 26–27, 138
tracheal shift 133
tracheo-oesophageal fistula 135
tramadol 64, 66–67, 77t
transfusion
  blood 46–47
  reaction 188–90
transient ischaemic attack 240
transudate 129–30, 130t
transverse myelitis 242t
tranylcypromine 64, 65
triamterene 71
triazolam 75t
tricyclic antidepressants 220t

trifluperidol 77t
trigeminal neuralgia 22–23
trimethoprim 48–49, 71
trimipramine 65
L-tryptophan 66–67
TTP 191t, 192–93
tuberculosis 55, 127
tubular necrosis, acute renal 208t
tumour
carcinoid 39
colonic 39
neuroendocrine 39–40
rectal 39
tumour lysis syndrome 223
tyramine 64

U

ulcer disease, peptic 12–13, 41, 158t
ulcers, genital 85
ultrasound
bladder 288–89
Doppler 290–91, 292
renal 287
unexpected changes 4–5
uraemia 35, 287
uraemic encephalopathy 211
urate, serum 223
ureteral stricture 286t
ureteric obstruction 41, 208t
urethritis 284–85
urinary calculi 286t
urinary catheter 243–44, 284–85, 287, 288
suprapubic 287, 288
three-way 15–16, 296–97
urinary catheterization 243–44, 284–85, 287, 288
urinary clot 286t
urinary fistula 180, 294–95
urinary output, decreased 32–33, 208–11
urinary retention 14, 15–16, 35, 288–89, 296–97
urinary three-way catheter 15–16, 296–97
urinary tract infection
lower 46–47, 48–49, 284–85
upper 15–16, 46–47, 48–49, 282–83

urinary tract obstruction 32–33, 208t, 286–87, 286t
urticaria 92

V

valproate, sodium 60, 72, 79t, 250–51
valve, prosthetic heart valve 29
valvular heart disease 46–47
vancomycin 39–40, 48–49, 60, 71
varices, oesophageal 160, 166
vascular disease, peripheral 32–33
vascular stent, aortic 113
vasculitis 14, 20, 47, 92–93, 290–91
cutaneous 92–93
vena cava, obstruction 32–33, 122–23, 122t
venlafaxine 62t, 64, 65, 75t, 77t
venography, selective 292
venous catheter, central 46–47, 133t
venous Doppler 120
venous thromboembolic disease 27, 119–21, 119t
venous thrombosis
hepatic 41
renal 292–93
ventilator-associated pneumonia 126–28
ventricular arrhythmias 249–50
verapamil 73t, 75t, 78t
vertebral fracture 274–75, 274t
vertebroplasty 275
vestibular apparatus 41, 44
video-assisted mediastinoscopy 137
video-assisted thoracoscopy 130
vigabatrin 72
vinblastine 73t, 75t, 77t
vincristine 73t
viral gastroenteritis 39–40
viral hepatitis 177t

virus
Cytomegalovirus 39
Epstein–Barr 177t
herpes simplex 39
vitamin B_{12} deficiency 188–90
vitamin D metabolism 215–16
vitamin K 62–63, 63t
vitiligo 232
volvulus, colonic 11, 164–65
vomiting
feculent 163
hypokalaemia 214
nausea and 41–43, 163
unheralded 44–45, 260
von Willebrand disease 198t

W

warfarin 60, 68–69, 94
medication interactions 62–63, 62t, 63t, 72, 73t, 73, 74, 75t, 78t, 79t, 198t
Wernicke's encephalopathy 24, 227
West Nile virus 55
white cell count
high 200–2
low 184–86
WHO grading, mucositis 148–49
'WHY' framework 4–5
withdrawal
alcohol 175, 247–48
glucocorticoids 232t
illicit drugs 24
medications 29–30

X

xanthochromia 257–58
X-ray, chest 101–2, 127, 134

Z

zidovudine 73t
ziprasidone 75t
Zollinger–Ellison syndrome 40
zopiclone 75t
zoster, herpes 7, 8–9, 22–23